Contributors

Connie J. Beehler, MD
Research Fellow
University of Colorado Health
  Sciences Center
Denver, Colorado

Elaine M. Berger, BS
Instructor, University of
  Colorado Health Sciences
  Center
Denver, Colorado

Kenneth L. Brigham, MD
Professor of Medicine and
  Director Pulmonary
  Circulation Center
Vanderbilt University School of
  Medicine
Nashville, Tennessee

Peter R.B. Caldwell, MD
Associate Professor of Medicine
College of Physicians and
  Surgeons
Columbia University
New York, New York

Jeffrey A. Cooper, MD
Department of Physiology
Albany Medical College of
  Union University
Albany, New York

Edward D. Crandall, PhD, MD
Professor of Medicine
Director, Will Rogers Institute
  Pulmonary Research
  Laboratory
University of California
Los Angeles, California

Richard M. Effros, MD
Professor of Medicine
Division of Respiratory
  Physiology and Medicine
Harbor–UCLA Medical Center
Torrance, California

Joseph G. Garcia, MD
Department of Physiology
Albany Medical College of
  Union University
Albany, New York

Barbara E. Goodman, PhD
Will Rogers Institute
  Pulmonary Research
  Laboratory
Department of Medicine
University of California
Los Angeles, California

Jon M. Grazer, MPH
Research Assistant
Department of Pharmacology
Tulane University School of
  Medicine
New Orleans, Louisiana

Gail Gurtner, MD
Associate Professor of Medicine
Johns Hopkins University
  School of Medicine
Baltimore, Maryland

Charles A. Hales, MD
Associate Professor of Medicine
Harvard Medical School
Associate Physician
Massachusetts General Hospital
Boston, Massachusetts

Albert L. Hyman, MD
Professor of Surgery, Medicine
and Pharmacology
Tulane University School of
Medicine
New Orleans, Louisiana

Louis J. Ignarro, PhD
Professor of Pharmacology
Tulane University School of
Medicine
New Orleans, Louisiana

Arnold Johnson, PhD
Department of Physiology
Albany Medical College of
Union University
Albany, New York

Kent J. Johnson, MD
Associate Professor of Pathology
The University of Michigan
Medical School
Ann Arbor, Michigan

Rosemary C. Jones, PhD
Research Associate
Children's Hospital
Assistant Professor of Pathology
Harvard Medical School
Boston, Massachusetts

Philip J. Kadowitz, PhD
Professor of Pharmacology
Tulane University School of
Medicine
New Orleans, Louisiana

Homayoun Kazemi, MD
Chief, Pulmonary Unit
Massachusetts General Hospital
Professor of Medicine
Harvard Medical School
Boston, Massachusetts

Kwang-Jin Kim, PhD
Will Rogers Institute Pulmonary
Research Laboratory
Department of Medicine
University of California
Los Angeles, California

H.L. Lippton, MD
Tulane University School of
Medicine
New Orleans, Louisiana

Siu K. Lo
Department of Physiology
Albany Medical College of
Union University
Albany, New York

Asrar B. Malik, PhD
Professor of Physiology
Albany Medical College of
Union University
Albany, New York

Denis Martin
Faculty of Medicine
C.H.U. de Grenoble
Grenoble, FRANCE

Gregory R. Mason, MD
Assistant Professor
Division of Respiratory
Physiology and Medicine
Department of Medicine
Harbor-University of California
Los Angeles Medical Center
Los Angeles, California

Dennis B. McNamara, PhD
Professor of Pharmacology
Tulane University School of
Medicine
New Orleans, Louisiana

Irving Mizus, MD
Clinical Instructor
University of California School
    of Medicine
Los Angeles, California

Myron B. Peterson, MD, PhD
Director, Critical Care Medicine
Floating Hospital for Infants
    and Children
Associate Professor of Pediatrics
Tufts University School of
    Medicine
Boston, Massachusetts

Marc B. Perlman, MD
Department of Physiology
Albany Medical College of
    Union University
Albany, New York

Lynne M. Reid, MD
Simeon Burt Wolbach Professor
    of Pathology
Harvard Medical School
Pathologist-in-Chief
Children's Hospital
Boston, Massachusetts

John E. Repine, MD
Professor of Medicine and
    Pediatrics
University of Colorado Health
    Sciences Center
Denver, Colorado

Sami I. Said, MD
Professor of Medicine
University of Oklahoma Health
    Sciences Center
Veterans Administration
    Medical Center
Oklahoma City, Oklahoma

Michael T. Snider, MD, PhD
Associate Professor of
    Anesthesia
Hershey Medical Center
Hershey, Pennsylvania

Norman C. Staub, MD
Professor of Physiology
Cardiovascular Research
    Institute and Department of
    Physiology
University of California
San Francisco, California

Warren Summer, MD
Professor of Medicine
Chief, Pulmonary/Critical Care
    Medicine
Louisiana State University
    Medical Center
New Orleans, Louisiana

Aubrey E. Taylor, PhD
Professor and Chairman
Department of Physiology
College of Medicine
University of South Alabama
Mobile, Alabama

Gerd O. Till, MD
Associate Professor of Pathology
The University of Michigan
    Medical School
Ann Arbor, Michigan

Karen M. Toth, BS
Medical Student II
University of Colorado Health
    Sciences Center
Denver, Colorado

Peter A. Ward, MD
Professor and Chairman
Department of Pathology
The University of Michigan
  Medical School
Ann Arbor, Michigan

W. David Watkins, MD, PhD
Professor and Chairman
Department of Anesthesiology
Professor of Pharmacology
Duke University Medical Center
Durham, North Carolina

Carl W. White, MD
Assistant Professor of Pediatrics
University of Colorado Health
  Sciences Center
Denver, Colorado

K.S. Wood, BS
Tulane University School of
  Medicine
New Orleans, Louisiana

Warren M. Zapol, MD
Associate Professor of
  Anesthesiology
Harvard Medical School
Anesthetist
Massachusetts General Hospital
Boston, Massachusetts

Contents

viii

Introduction

Adult Respiratory Distress Syndrome (ARDS) is a multifactorial disorder of diverse etiology with a high mortality rate. The syndrome is associated with diffuse injury of pulmonary vascular endothelium and the alveolar epithelium. Proteolytic enzymes released by neutrophils, activation of the coagulation cascade, prostanoids and other vasoactive peptides all have been incriminated in the pathophysiology of this disorder.

This symposium on Acute Lung Injury and its relationship to ARDS focuses on new knowledge in areas of pulmonary physiology, pathology, biochemistry and pharmacology and their role in lung injury. The contributors have all been intensely involved in studies of pathophysiology of ARDS.

The symposium was organized under the auspices of the Cardiopulmonary Council of the American Heart Association and was held in Dallas, Texas, in September 1984. The organizers of the symposium gratefully acknowledge grants from the AHA, the Division of Lung Diseases, National Heart, Lung and Blood Institute, NIH, and the Upjohn Company.

We are also indebted to the staff of the AHA, in particular Mr. Leonard P. Cooke and Ms. Stephanie Stansfield, for their invaluable assistance in organizing the symposium.

Lastly, PSG Publishing Company and its president, Dr. Frank Paparello, have been particularly helpful in putting the proceedings of the symposium together and expediting their publication, and we express our special appreciation to them.

Albert J. Hyman
Philip J. Kadowitz
Homayoun Kazemi, Chairman
Program Committee for the Symposium
Cardiopulmonary Council of the
American Heart Association

1 The Pulmonary Vascular Bed in Acute Lung Injury— An Overview

Homayoun Kazemi

This symposium addresses the pathophysiology and therapeutic approaches to acute lung injury. The concept of acute lung injury causing severe respiratory insufficiency, failure, and in many instances death, is relatively recent and has been identified as a clinical syndrome for less than 20 years.

Adult respiratory distress syndrome (ARDS) is one of varied etiology and is characterized by a constellation of clinical features and physiologic aberrations in the respiratory system. The cardinal features of ARDS are its relatively acute onset, presence of dyspnea and a rapid respiratory rate, arterial hypoxemia and decreased lung compliance, diffuse infiltrates on x-ray films of the chest and, physiologically, a leaky alveolar-capillary membrane.

The role of the pulmonary vascular bed is becoming more and more important in the pathogenesis of ARDS. In addition to the leaky alveolar-capillary membrane, there are other special features in the pulmonary vascular bed that are of particular interest and relevance to our understanding of this syndrome: There is significant loss of capillary units, there is invariably pulmonary arterial hypertension, there is clotting in large and small vessels, and on pathologic examination there is structural remodeling of precapillary pulmonary vessels. This intriguing and complex syndrome is believed to occur in about 150,000 persons per year in the United States and has a mortality rate of around 50% — in some series it may be as high as 90%[1] — and therapeutic modalities have not been particularly effective in saving patients with this syndrome in the past.

In their classic monograph on adult respiratory failure in 1972, Pontoppidan et al[2] devote a large part of their writing to the mechanical abnormalities of the lung and gas exchange derangements in ARDS and an equal amount to its management. However, little was said then about the vascular bed since at that time little was known about the role of the pulmonary vascular bed and particularly about the vascular endothelial cells and interaction between formed elements in the blood and the vessels in the lung. In the recent past it has become apparent that the role of the vascular bed is a significant and possibly crucial part of the syndrome.

The pulmonary circulation and vascular bed, however, have been the subject of interest to physicians and physiologists going back to the thirteenth century. The first description of the vascular bed was given by Ibn-El-Nafis, a native of Damascus working in Cairo, who said that "the blood of the right ventricle passes through the vena arteriosa to the lung, spreads through its substance, mixes with air and becomes completely purified; then it passes through the arteria venosa to reach the left chamber of the heart." In Europe, Michael Servetus, the Spanish monk, working in Paris in the sixteenth century, wrote of "the vital spirit. It is generated in the lungs from a mixture of inspired air with elaborated subtle blood which the right ventricle of the heart communicates to the left . . . blood becomes reddish-yellow and is poured from the pulmonary artery into the pulmonary vein."[3] His book *Christianismi restitutio* was considered heretical by both Catholics and Protestants and he was burned at the stake by the Calvinists in Geneva in 1553.

In ARDS the area of particular interest in the pulmonary circulation is the alveolar-capillary (A-C) membrane. Looking at the ultrastructure of the A-C membrane, one can wonder about the behavior of the cell lining of both the epithelial and the endothelial surfaces of the membrane and their interaction with formed elements in blood in causing the disease. In terms of pathogenesis of ARDS, one point of view is that there is first injury and damage to the A-C membrane leading to development of the leaky membrane. Edema formation then creates the physiologic abnormalities in the lung, but at the same time there are alterations in the metabolic behavior of both epithelial and endothelial cells and in their interaction with leukocytes in the blood — all culminating in the development of the classic pictures of ARDS. Later chapters in this book will address the questions of how injury to the A-C membrane might occur and what role specific cells play. In considering the pulmonary vascular bed physiologically, two aspects of it need to be emphasized: (1) reactivity of the vessels and (2) permeability characteristics of the A-C membrane.

As far as reactivity is concerned, the pulmonary vessels may be more reactive than any other vascular bed in the body in reacting to changes in their environment. Specifically, the mechanical forces within the thorax, the interstitial pressure of the lung and the state of alveolar distention affect vessel caliber and blood flow. Furthermore, the pulmonary vessels are particularly sensitive to changes in oxygen tension in the alveolar air and to a lesser extent to oxygen saturation in blood. The response of the vessels to a fall in alveolar oxygen tension, as demonstrated by the shift of perfusion away from areas of alveolar hypoxia, is the major mechanism for adjustment of distribution of regional perfusion to ventilation. This remarkable vasoreactivity to alveolar hypoxia is demonstrated in Figure 1-1, and was reported from our laboratory earlier.[4] In this example, the anesthetized dog is mechanically ventilated through a double-lumen endotracheal tube to separate ventilation of one lung from the other. Distribution of perfusion to the lungs is quantitated by intravenous (IV) injection of a bolus of nitrogen 13 (^{13}N) in solution and positron scintigraphy of the chest. When both lungs are ventilated on room air, blood flow is relatively equal to both lungs. As soon as the inspired gas mixture to one lung is switched to a low O_2 mixture, despite continued mechanical ventilation, blood flow to the hypoxic lung is markedly reduced.

The question in ARDS is whether this normally present hypoxic pulmonary vasoconstriction contributes to development of pulmonary hypertension and vascular remodeling. The evidence at hand would say yes. Mechanisms of vasoconstriction are probably several and among others include the sympathetic system[5] and a number of chemical mediators which are either elaborated in the lung or modified in their passage through the pulmonary vascular bed. Of these, histamine and prostanoids seem particularly relevant at the moment.

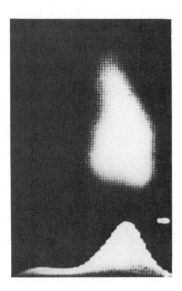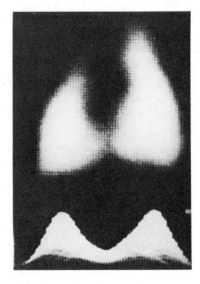

Figure 1-1 Positron scintigraphy of distribution of pulmonary perfusion with nitrogen 13 in the anesthetized supine dog. The upper half of the picture is the perfusion image and the lower half the summation of all counts from each lung. Left panel is control perfusion when both lungs are ventilated on room air and the right panel the pattern of perfusion after the right lung was ventilated with 100% nitrogen. Perfusion to the alveolar hypoxic lung is reduced by 54%. (Reproduced with permission from Hales et al.[4])

Despite the reduction in pulmonary capillary bed, the marked pulmonary hypertension, and the high pulmonary vascular resistance in ARDS, it is possible to increase flow through these vessels by increasing cardiac output.[6] This finding implies that there may be recruitment of new vessels with a possible critical opening pressure or further distention of already patent vessels or both.

The A-C membrane leaks in ARDS. Assessing permeability of the membrane and quantitating regional lung water has been one of the challenges to our understanding of ARDS. To quantitate regional lung water in an isolated lung model that spontaneously developed pulmonary edema, we have used the short-lived positron-emitting isotopes oxygen 15 (^{15}O) with a half-life of two minutes to measure total lung water with $H_2^{15}O$, the intravascular volume with carbon monoxide-labeled hemoglobin (Hgb-$C^{15}O$), and the difference between the two to calculate the extravascular lung water volume. With positron camera scintigraphy one can regionalize the extravascular lung water.[7] Using such a technique, we found that extravascular lung water increased in all regions of the lung from apex to base (Figure 1-2) as the wet/dry ratio increased from 3.6 to 6.0 and the increase in extravascular water matched the intravascular volume closely, suggesting that leakiness of the membrane is fairly uniform from apex to base of the lung, but that *fluid accumulation* after fluid leaving the vascular bed is greater at the lung base due to gravitational forces.

In summary, then, it is apparent that the pulmonary vascular bed has a major and significant role in the development of ARDS. There are structural as well as reactive changes in the vessels. Endothelial cell injury and biochemical events following the injury are significant factors in ARDS, and finally mechanisms of permeability changes in the A-C membrane should be the focus of further study.

REFERENCES

1. Rinaldo JE, Rogers RM: Adult respiratory distress syndrome. *N Engl J Med* 1982;306:900–909.
2. Pontoppidan H, Geffin B, Lowenstein E: Acute respiratory failure in the adult. *N Engl J Med* 1972;287:690–697,743–752,799–806.
3. Perkins JF: Historical development of respiratory physiology, in Fenn WO, Rahn H (eds): *Handbook of Physiology. Respiration.* Washington, American Physiological Society, 1964, vol 1 pp 1–62.

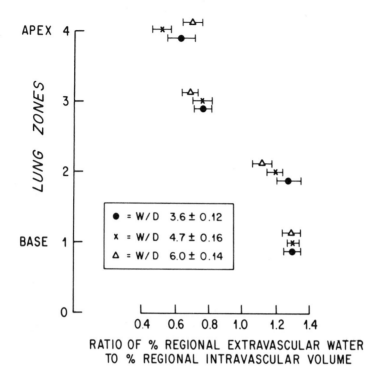

Figure 1-2 Distribution of regional extravascular lung water compared to regional intravascular volume in 17 isolated, perfused lungs which developed spontaneous pulmonary edema. There is no change in distribution of lung water with increasing edema, but there is a gravity-dependent increase from apex to base of the same magnitude at all levels of pulmonary edema. (Reproduced with permission from Hales et al.[7])

4. Hales CA, Ahluwalia B, Kazemi H: Strength of pulmonary vascular response to regional alveolar hypoxia. *J Appl Physiol* 1975;38:1083–1087.
5. Dauber IM, Weil JV: Lung injury edema in dogs. Influence of sympathetic ablation. *J Clin Invest* 1983;72:1977–1986.
6. Zapol WM, Snider MT: Pulmonary hypertension in severe acute respiratory failure. *N Engl J Med* 1977;296:476–480.
7. Hales CA, Kanarek DJ, Ahluwalia B, et al: Regional edema formation in isolated perfused dog lungs. *Circ Res* 1981;48:121–127.

2 Pathology of Pulmonary Vascular Bed in Adult Respiratory Distress Syndrome (ARDS)

Lynne M. Reid
Rosemary C. Jones

There is a time "to lump" and a time "to split." In the clinical setting, we can be "lumpers" since treatment of patients with the acute respiratory distress syndrome (ARDS) is essentially similar, regardless of cause. Furthermore, as the care of ARDS patients has improved we less frequently see the acute stages of the injury, and in the subacute and chronic stages structural changes in the lung correlate with the duration of the disease rather than with the cause.

In considering the experimental studies of ARDS we can be "splitters" in the attempt to identify the particular pathogenetic pathways by which a given cause produces lung disease. It is necessary to analyze separately the mechanisms responsible for the early acute injury from those that lead to its amplification and fatal outcome. One set of questions concerns the way nonthoracic injury damages the pulmonary microvasculature to cause the increased permeability and hemorrhage that give us the symptoms and signs of acute respiratory failure. Another set of questions is concerned with the evolution of the acute changes, with or without artificial ventilation using high partial pressure of oxygen. Resolution, healing with varying degrees of scar, or fatal outcome are possibilities at this stage.[1-9]

The presence of edema and hemorrhage as hallmarks of the acute stage of ARDS and the early presence and steady progression of pulmonary hypertension point to injury of the pulmonary circulation at all stages. The most puzzling form of ARDS is the severe lung damage that follows a primary injury at some distance from the lung such as peripheral trauma or abdominal sepsis. In such cases its vascular channels are likely also to be the route by which attack on the lung is delivered.

The human disease is first described here after consideration of the normal microcirculation of the lung, then selected animal models are considered for their relevance either to the cause of ARDS or its treatment.

7

8

NORMAL STRUCTURE
OF PULMONARY VASCULAR BED

The lung has a double arterial supply (pulmonary and bronchial) and a double venous drainage (pulmonary and true bronchial), but the regional distributions of the two systems do not correspond. The alveolar capillary region receives the whole of the cardiac output of mixed venous blood via the pulmonary artery and its many branches. The capillary bed in the wall of conducting airways, as far as the terminal bronchiolus, is supplied from the left side of the heart via the bronchial arteries. Intrapulmonary blood whether from alveoli or bronchi, drains to the pulmonary veins and the left atrium. It is only a small region near the hilum that drains to the so-called true bronchial veins which drain to the superior vena cava and the right side of the heart via the azygos system. In the normal subject the bronchial artery blood that drains to the left atrium supplies several percent venous admixture. Elevation of left atrial pressure causes raised pulmonary venous pressure with its sequela of edema in airway walls as well as in alveoli.

In the normal lung precapillary anastomoses are present between pulmonary and bronchial arteries, but these are normally closed. In disease such vessels often open. For example, block of a central pulmonary artery leads to increase in bronchial flow with filling of the distal pulmonary artery through bronchopulmonary arterial anastomoses. Infection, as in bronchiectasis or lung abscess, also opens up these channels. Such bronchial flow has a protective role in infection; its effect in ARDS is not known.

Microcirculation

The alveolar wall vessels are especially affected in human ARDS and in experimental studies of lung injury. The structure of the normal pre- and postcapillary unit is described here. In the adult human, resistance arteries are present in the alveolar wall. Along any pulmonary arterial pathway a level is reached where the fully *muscular* coat gives way to a segment where muscle is incomplete and is arranged as a spiral—a *partially muscular* artery—before disappearing—a *nonmuscular* artery—still in vessels larger than capillaries. The largest partially muscular artery is about 150 μm. The above are the features apparent by light and electron microscopy. By electron microscopy cells can be identified in the nonmuscular wall, namely the pericyte and intermediate cell which in response to injury and in disease give rise to mature smooth muscle cells causing "extension" of a medial muscle coat into more peripheral arteries than is normal. On the venous side of the capillary a postcapillary unit is present which has a similar structure.

The pulmonary and bronchial arteries run with the airway, at the center of any respiratory unit, be it segment or acinus, forming a bronchoarterial bundle. The veins run separately at the periphery of any unit.

The lung is well supplied with lymphatics but none are found in the alveolar wall. Lymphatics lie in the connective tissue of the pleura, in the perivascular connective tissue sheaths, and in interlobular septa where these are present.

VASCULAR CHANGES IN HUMAN ARDS

Quantitative Analysis
of Pulmonary Vascular Bed

We have analyzed quantitatively, using light and electron microscopy, vascular changes in the lungs of 22 patients who, between 1977 and 1983, died from ARDS in the respiratory intensive care unit at Massachusetts General Hospital, Boston.[10,11]

We recognize early, intermediate, and late stages, which correspond to key pathologic events (Figure 2-1). In the *early* group the interval between intubation and death is less than nine days (three days is the shortest interval) and the mean pulmonary artery pressure (PAP) measured near to death is 36 ± 7.3 mmHg (five patients): patients in the *intermediate* group (ten to 19 days) have a mean PAP of 42 ± 9.4 mmHg (eight patients): patients in the *late* stage (20 days and more) have a mean PAP of 42 ± 3.8 mmHg (nine patients).

The lungs in the *early* stage of edema and hemorrhage are heavy, airless, and dark red-blue. Microscopically, interstitial edema, micro-

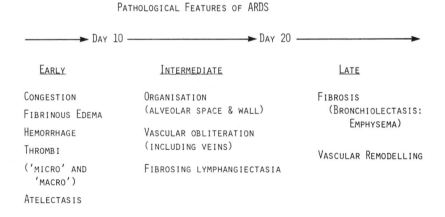

Figure 2-1 Pathologic changes at various stages of ARDS.

thrombi (Figure 2-2), intra-alveolar hemorrhage, hyaline membranes, and fibrin in alveoli and bronchioli are seen (Figure 2-2). In the *intermediate* stage organization is beginning. The lungs are more fleshy in texture with lung architecture less obvious: the consolidated peripheral regions show a patchy mixture of red-brown and yellow-gray areas. Microscopically, proliferation of alveolar epithelial cells is apparent and exuberant granulation tissue is especially prominent in alveolar ducts, sometimes even obliterating the air space. In the *late* stage dense interstitial and intra-alveolar fibrosis is present, with distortion and obliteration of alveolar and bronchiolar spaces.

The origin of thromboemboli is controversial. In burn and trauma patients thrombi in the lung are thought to originate as systemic venous thrombi, such microemboli being a "mechanism" of lung injury.[12,13] On the other hand, the severe and widespread pulmonary endothelial cell injury seen in ARDS could well cause localized intravascular coagulation, with local propagation of clot.[14-17]

Pulmonary macrothrombi in arteries that have a lumen of 1 mm diameter are present in all three stages of ARDS, although less common

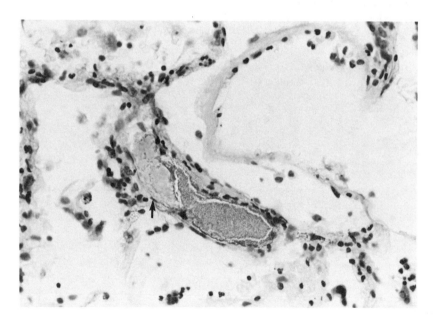

Figure 2-2 Platelet-fibrin thrombus (arrow) obstructing the flow of contrast medium in an alveolar wall artery in ARDS (six days after aspiration of gastric contents). A hyaline membrane is below and extravasated red blood cells to the right of the thrombosed vessel (H & E × 250). (Reproduced with permission from Tomashefski et al.[11])

in the late stage. Microthrombi also are found at all stages and are numerous in the early stage of illness. The number of *macrothrombi* is highest in patients with pulmonary artery filling defects. Filling defects seen by balloon occlusion arteriography (BOPA) are also associated with microthrombi.[16] Some patients had pulmonary artery thromboemboli at autopsy, although the diagnosis of diffuse intravascular coagulation was not made clinically. If the most sensitive coagulation tests are used, most patients with ARDS have evidence of intravascular clotting.

Even if such pulmonary arterial occlusions are numerous, the lung often shows little necrosis, and no infarction. Although an infarct is defined as a lung hemorrhage, this has a special distribution related to the zone of pulmonary artery supply or to the drainage by pulmonary vein. Perhaps because of the lung's double arterial supply, in the normal lung an infarct is not caused just by blocking a pulmonary artery or a bronchial artery. It is necessary to have concomitant elevation of pulmonary venous pressure or capillary damage.

Pulmonary Arteriography

Arteriograms show uneven filling (Figures 2-3–2-6). Filled vessels are not seen even microscopically in hemorrhagic or fibrotic zones. Reduced background haze is most striking in the intermediate and late stage: in filled regions the pattern is often abnormal. The degree of filling varies within a lung and within a single lobe. By contrast, in the lungs of some patients with ARDS resulting from infection, a widespread *increase* in microvascular filling is apparent. Pleural "arcade" arteries filling from pulmonary artery to pulmonary artery are sometimes numerous. When the veins are injected, irregular filling and reduction in background haze is also apparent, often with subpleural regions of nonfilling.

Pulmonary thromboemboli In pulmonary arteriograms thromboemboli cause intravascular filling defects or nonfilling of distal vessels. We assessed semiquantitatively the number of pulmonary thromboemboli — macroscopically in 1-cm-thick slices of fixed lung, and microscopically in tissue sections — and correlated the findings with those of BOPA.[16]

The lumen of veins is obliterated by hyaline material, onionskin in appearance (Figure 2-7). Obstruction to pulmonary lymphatics, interlobular and subpleural, is caused by similar tissue. Coagulation of proteinaceous edema also obstructs lymphatics doubtless impeding removal of interstitial fluid (Figure 2-8). Endolymphatic obstruction involves relatively large interlobular channels, implying widespread obstruction to the smaller ones.[11]

Chronic vascular remodeling In the intermediate and late stages of ARDS structural changes affect both preacinar and intra-acinar arteries: small artery filling is much less than in the normal lung or during the first

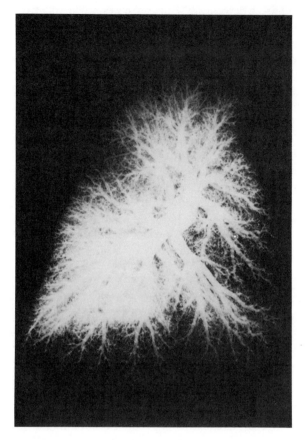

Figure 2-3 Normal human adult pulmonary arteriogram (× 0.5). (Reproduced with permission from Reid L: The angiogram and pulmonary artery structure and branching in the normal and with reference to disease). *Proc R Soc Lond* 1965;58:681–684.

days of acute injury.[11] In the late stage of ARDS preacinar and intra-acinar arteries appear tortuous in the arteriogram; such arteries are in regions of dense fibrosis (Figure 2-6). Through nests of dilated capillaries the injection medium sometimes crosses to pulmonary veins. Obliteration of small precapillary arteries also occurs. The thickness of the medial muscle coat of partially muscular and muscular arteries increases with duration of illness. The mean external diameter of partially muscular and muscular arteries decreases. Muscle develops in normally nonmuscular arteries. All these changes contribute to reduction of cross-sectional area of the vascular bed. The hemodynamic behavior will be a balance between the dilating and obliterative lesions.

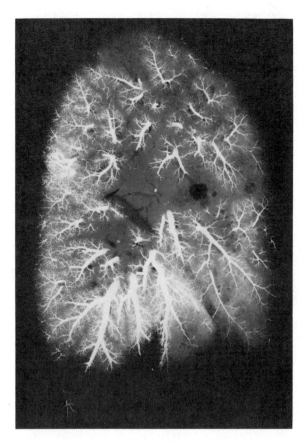

Figure 2-4 A Arteriogram of 1-cm-thick lung slice ($\times$ 0.5) in ARDS. **B** Macroscopic view of lung slice (x 0.5) from same patient shown in (**A**) 15 days after drug overdose and aspiration of gastric contents. The arteries are injected with barium-gelatin sulfate and appear white; filled vessels are irregularly distributed throughout the lung and large areas, centrally placed within the slice (in upper part of lower lobe, and in middle lobe), contain few filled vessels. **C** Macroscopic view of another lung slice from same patient as in (**A**) showing areas of congestion-hemorrhage, liquefaction, and fibrosis (single arrow) ($\times$ 2.2). Regions of congestion-hemorrhage and fibrosis are demarcated by interlobular septa (double arrow). (Reproduced with permission from Jones et al.[9])

ANIMAL MODELS RELEVANT TO CAUSE AND TREATMENT OF ARDS

Clinical studies such as those of Carvalho et al[17] have given leads to differences in the various types of ARDS that correspond with the original cause of injury. Detailed studies of pathogenesis can only be made satisfac-

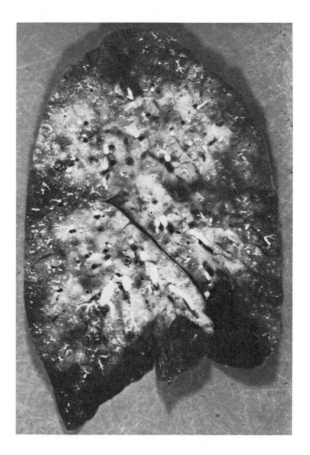

Figure 2-4B

torily in the experimental animal. Sepsis, endotoxemia, and pulmonary contusion simulate common causes of ARDS seen clinically. The subacute or chronic injury of hyperoxia needs also to be identified, since high fractions of inspired oxygen (FiO_2) may be necessary for the patient's survival. The experimental models chosen for brief mention here represent recent or current studies from our laboratory.

Oxygen Toxicity

The acute injury of high oxygen is well recognized and the effect of longer exposure on the capillary bed also has been described.[18-20] It is the subacute injury to the other segments of the lung's vasculature that we describe here.[21-23] It is striking how quickly the necrotic debris produced in the first few days of oxygen injury is cleared. The remaining tissue adapts by hypertrophy and hyperplasia with striking vascular remodeling at all

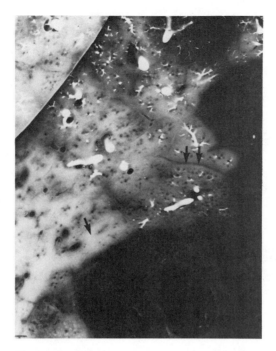

Figure 2-4C

levels, and major occlusive vascular injury particularly to the microcirculation. The obliterative nature of many of the lesions means they are irreversible.

Whereas exposure to 95% to 100% O_2 (normobaric) is fatal to adult rats within a few days, the lower concentrations of 80% to 90% allow the animals to survive the early period of acute pulmonary edema and respiratory failure. The rats recover and continue in a satisfactory clinical condition for several weeks.[21-23] This tolerance parallels an increase in antioxidant enzyme activity: after breathing 85% O_2, adult rats increase superoxide dismutase activity by half.[19] On return to air, superoxide dismutase levels fall and tolerance is lost.[19]

Seven days in an atmosphere of 87% O_2 causes obliteration of many small arteries.[23] There is striking arterial remodeling (Figure 2-9), that histologically is seen to include narrowing of preacinar arteries, increased thickness of the muscular arterial coat, and the appearance of muscle in normally nonmuscular arteries and intimal proliferation in the microcirculation. These changes are accentuated by longer exposure.[22] Cross-filling of the bronchial arteries with injection medium indicates that hyperoxia opens precapillary anastomoses between pulmonary and bronchial arteries. Right ventricular hypertrophy parallels the severity of these

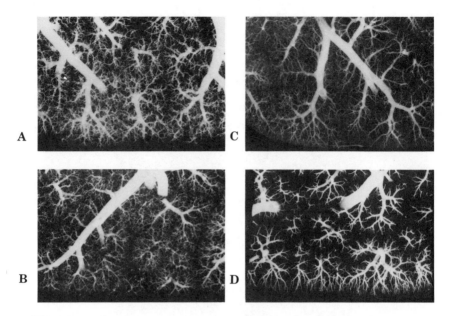

Figure 2-5 Pulmonary arteriograms – pleural surface at lower edge ($\times$ 2.4). **A** Normal adult lung. **B** Early ARDS (six days after aspiration of gastric contents) showing reduced preacinar filling of small arteries and prominent, edematous interlobular septa. **C** Intermediate stage ARDS (after 16 days, viral pneumonia) showing marked reduction of filled small vessels and prominent interlobular septa. **D** Intermediate stage ARDS (16 days after toxic inhalation) showing more extensive reduction of filled small arteries due to intimal obliteration. Stretching of subpleural branches of the pulmonary artery about large air spaces gives a "picket-fence" appearance. (Reproduced with permission from Tomashefski et al.[11])

changes: the PAP after 28 days is rather more than doubled (control PAP 17.8 ± 1.75 mmHg, hyperoxia PAP 39.0 ± 8.09 mmHg).

Return to air is fatal to these animals; weaning through gradually lowered oxygen tensions is necessary. During the seven days we have used for weaning right ventricular hypertrophy increases, pointing to an increase in PAP.[22] Paradoxically, while some arterial structural changes start to regress, others progress; there is a "weaning injury." During subsequent recovery in air the right ventricular hypertrophy regresses but muscle continues to appear in more of the peripheral arteries that are normally nonmuscular. Even recovery causes injury. We have demonstrated a pulmonary constrictor response when rats are returned rapidly to air.[23] After adaptation to high oxygen, air is an abnormal environment and calls for further adaptation.

Sepsis

Various species (rat, dog, baboon, rabbit) have been used to develop models of intra-abdominal sepsis[24-26] using various methods (eg, cecal ligation and perforation, intraperitoneal inoculation of infected material). A subacute model of intraperitoneal sepsis has recently been produced by Kirton et al[27,28] using a modification of the method of Onderdonk.[26] The bacterial flora and dose are defined and a reproducible bacteremia with a chronic course develops.

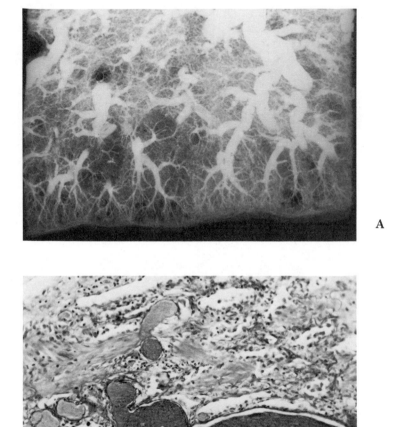

A

B

Figure 2-6 **A** pulmonary arteriogram — pleural surface at lower edge ($\times$ 2.4); late stage ARDS (after 28 days, bacterial pneumonia and sepsis), showing marked arterial tortuosity. **B** Pulmonary arteriogram — pleural surface at lower edge ($\times$ 2.4); late stage ARDS (26 days after aspiration) showing marked arterial tortuosity, increased filling of small arteries, and stretching of arteries about honeycomb "cystic" spaces. (Reproduced with permission from Tomashefski et al.[11])

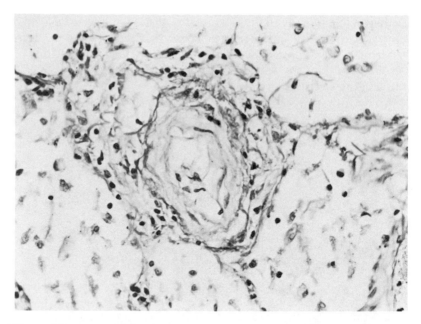

Figure 2-7 Lumen of an intralobular vein narrowed by loose connective tissue; intermediate stage ARDS (20 days after trauma) (elastic van Gieson stain, × 365). (Reproduced with permission from Tomashefski et al.[11]).

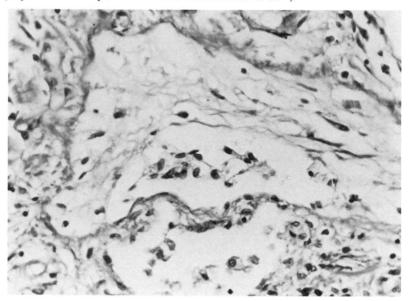

Figure 2-8 Intermediate stage ARDS (20 days after trauma); lymphatic duct lumen narrowed by loosely organized sparsely cellular connective tissue. The surrounding interlobular septum is fibrotic (elastic van Gieson stain, × 365). (Reproduced with permission from Tomashefski et al.[11])

Single implants at weekly intervals over four or eight weeks (*intermittent bacteremia*) causes more severe restructuring of pulmonary arteries than *continuous* bacteremia of shorter duration (produced by a total of four implants given on alternate days). The results of intermittent bacteremia are described here.

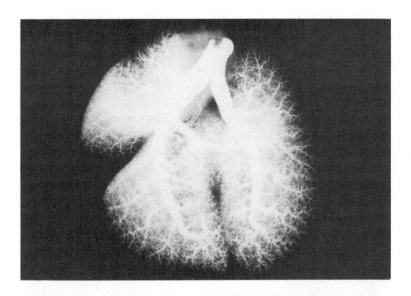

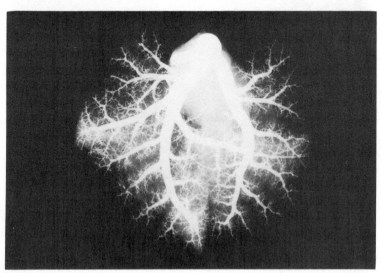

Figure 2-9 Rat pulmonary arteriograms ($\times$ 2), normal above, after hyperoxia below, showing reduced background haze, due to reduced density of small filled arteries. (Reproduced with permission from Jones et al.[9])

After four or eight implants abdominal abscesses are found, the white cell count is significantly increased while the platelet count is normal. There is no change in pulmonary hemodynamic findings, and arterial blood gas tensions and pH are normal. Plasma levels of the prostaglandin 6-keto-$PGF_{1\alpha}$ are increased after four, but not after eight implants. Thromboxane B_2 (TxB_2) levels are unaffected at any time studied.

There is progressive injury to the lung (Figure 2-10): inflammatory cell infiltration of the alveolar wall and space increases due mainly to neutrophils and nonspecific mononuclear cells. The arteriogram reveals a diffuse dilatation of small vessels including capillaries, so that the injection medium passes to the veins. The endothelial cells and precursor cells of the preacinar arteries are hypertrophied but the capillary walls are very thin.

Endotoxemia

By infusion of purified *Escherichia coli* endotoxin lipopolysaccharide (LPS B4-0111, Difco Distributors, Detroit, Mich, 300 μg daily) through indwelling catheters placed in the jugular vein, we have also developed models of intermittent and continuous endotoxemia.[28,29]

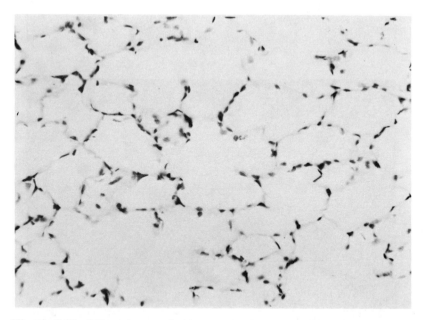

Figure 2-10 Photomicrograph of rat lung after intra-abdominal inplants of *Bacteroides fragilis* and *Escherichia coli* (H & E, × 488). **A** Normal lung. **B** After four implants. **C** After eight implants. (Reproduced with permission from Kirton et al.[27])

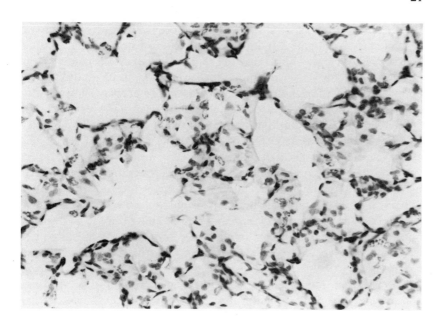

B

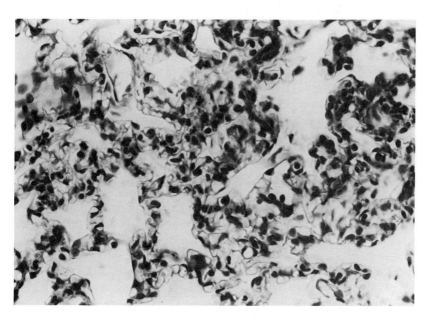

C

Given *continuously* for seven days, endotoxemia causes an increase in white blood cell count and in the proportion of neutrophils. Thrombocytopenia is present until day 3 but thereafter the platelet count is near normal. Pulmonary arteriography shows some regions of nonfilling and others of increased background haze. Quantitative analysis shows dilatation of nonmuscular and partially muscular arteries in the alveolar wall, an increase in the medial thickness of muscular and partially muscular arteries, and an increase in the relative number of muscularized vessels at the expense of nonmuscular ones.[28,29]

The continuous endotoxin infusion causes a significant rise of PAP by 24 hours (9 mmHg in awake rats); subsequently the pressure fluctuates but is still elevated at day 6. At no time is pulmonary vascular resistance (PVR) significantly changed. Fifteen minutes and 24 hours of infusion both produce elevated plasma levels of 6-keto-PGF$_{1\alpha}$ while TxB$_2$ is unchanged; the PAP and PVR have returned to normal 24 hours after the last infusion.

Intermittent endotoxemia causes a striking increase in white cell count and a relative increase in neutrophils. Light microscopy shows alveolar walls thickened by inflammatory cells, monocytes, and polymorphs which have also accumulated in the alveolar space. The walls of some small arteries undergo lysis and occasional arteries show plaques, produced by intimal cell proliferation; necrosis is a feature. Electron microscopy shows that endothelial cells and precursor smooth muscle cells within the pulmonary microcirculation are hypertrophied.

These findings demonstrate that the pulmonary vascular injury caused by sepsis has different features from that of endotoxin, indicating that endotoxemia alone is not the cause of ARDS in sepsis. It is striking that intermittent challenge causes more severe injury than continuous challenge. Continuous exposure seems to allow a protective adaptation while intermittent periods of recovery seem to restore sensitivity to injury or enhance it.

Pulmonary Contusion

In a sheep model of pulmonary contusion, arteriograms have been performed on the lungs. Within four hours intravascular filling defects and regional nonfilling is apparent.[30] Some defects and nonfilling are caused by intravascular thrombi. These are present both in the regions of direct contusion or contrecoup, as well as in more distant regions where local formation of a clot would seem to be responsible. Despite the use of a hypertensive perfusion pressure some narrowing and nonfilling on the arteriogram correlate histologically with patent arteries but with intramural edema.

ACKNOWLEDGMENT

This work was supported by the National Heart, Lung, and Blood Institute (NHLBI), Specialized Center of Research (SCOR), grant 23591.

REFERENCES

1. Moon VH: The pathology of secondary shock. *Am J Pathol* 1948;24: 235–273.
2. Ashbaugh DG, Bigelow DB, Petty TL, et al: Acute respiratory distress in adults. *Lancet* 1967;2:319–323.
3. Blaisdell FW, Lewis FR: *Respiratory Distress*. Philadelphia, W.B. Saunders, 1977.
4. Hill JD, Ratliff JL, Parrott JCW, et al: Pulmonary pathology in acute respiratory insufficiency: Lung biopsy as a diagnostic tool. *J Thorac Cardivasc Surg* 1976;71:64–69.
5. Fallat RJ, Lami M, Koeniger E, et al: Use of physiologic and pathologic correlations in evaluating adult respiratory distress syndrome, in Zapol WM, Qvist J (eds): *Artificial Lungs for Acute Respiratory Failure. Theory and Practice.* New York, Academic Press, 1976, pp 391–404.
6. Pratt PC, Vollmer RT, Shelburne JD, et al: Pulmonary morphology in a multihospital collaborative extracorporeal membrane oxygenation project. I. Light microscopy. *Am J Pathol* 1979;95:191–214.
7. Murray JF: Conference report — Mechanisms of acute respiratory failure. *Am Rev Respir Dis* 1977;115:1071–1078.
8. Jones R, Reid L: Pulmonary vascular changes in adult respiratory distress syndrome, in Artigas A, Lemaire F, Suter P, et al (eds): *Adult Respiratory Distress Syndrome.* London, Churchill Livingstone, in press.
9. Jones R, Tomashefski JF, Kobayashi K, et al: Pulmonary microvascular pathology: Human and experimental studies, in Zapol WM, Falke KJ (eds): *Acute Respiratory Failure*, vol 24: in Lenfant C (exec ed): *Lung Biology in Health and Disease.* New York, Basel, Marcel Dekker, Inc, 1985, pp 23–160.
10. Snow RL, Davies P, Pontoppidan H, et al: Pulmonary vascular remodelling in adult respiratory distress syndrome. *Am Rev Respir Dis* 1982;126:887–892.
11. Tomashefski JF Jr, Davies P, Boggis C, et al: The pulmonary vascular lesions of the adult respiratory distress syndrome. *Am J Pathol* 1983;112: 112–126.
12. Eeles GH, Sevitt S: Microthrombis in injured and burned patients. *J Pathol Bacteriol* 1976;93:275–293.
13. Saldeen T: The microembolism syndrome: a review, in Saldeen T: *The Microembolism Syndrome.* Stockholm, Almquistad Wiksell, 1979, pp 7–44.
14. Bone RC, Francis PB, Pierce AK: Intravascular coagulation associated with the adult respiratory distress syndrome. *Am J Med* 1976;61:585–589.
15. Schneider RC, Zapol WM, Carvalho AC: Platelet consumption and sequestration in severe acute respiratory failure. *Am Rev Respir Dis* 1980;122:455–451.
16. Greene R, Zapol WM, Snider MT, et al: Early bedside detection of pulmonary vascular occlusion during acute respiratory failure. *Am Rev Respir Dis* 1981;124:593–601.
17. Carvalho ACA, Bellman SM, Saullo VJ, et al: Altered factor VIII in acute respiratory failure. *N Engl J Med* 1982;307:1113–1119.

18. Crapo JD, Peters-Golden M, Marsh-Salin J, et al: Pathologic changes in the lungs of oxygen-adapted rats. A morphometric analysis. *Lab Invest* 1978;39: 640–653.
19. Crapo JD, Tierney DF: Superoxide dismutase and pulmonary oxygen toxicity. *Am J Physiol* 1974;226:1401–1407.
20. Kapanci Y, Weibel ER, Kaplan HP, et al: Pathogenesis and reversibility of the pulmonary lesions of oxygen toxicity in monkeys II. Ultrastructural and morphometric studies. *Lab Invest* 1969;20:101–116.
21. Jones R, Zapol WM, Reid LM: Pulmonary artery remodeling and pulmonary hypertension after exposure to hyperoxia for 7 days. *Am J Pathol* 1984;117:273–284.
22. Jones R, Zapol WM, Reid L: Progressive and regressive structural changes in rat pulmonary arteries during recovery from prolonged hyperoxia. *Am Rev Respir Dis* 1982;125:227.
23. Jones R, Zapol WM, Reid L: Pulmonary artery remodelling and pulmonary hypertension after exposure to hyperoxia for 7 days: A morphometric and hemodynamic study. *Am J Pathol* 1984;117:273–285.
24. Clowes GHA, Zuchneid W, Slobodan D, et al: The nonspecific pulmonary inflammatory reactions leading to respiratory failure after shock, gangrene and sepsis. *J Trauma* 1968a;8:899–914.
25. Bartlett JC, Onderdonk AB, Louie T, et al: Lessons from an animal model of intra-abdominal sepsis. *Arch Surg* 1978;113:853–857.
26. Onderdonk AB, Weinstein WM, Sullivan NM, et al: Experimental intraabdominal abscesses in rats: quantitative bacteriology of infected animals. *Infect Immun* 1974;10:1256–1259.
27. Kirton OC, Jones R, Zapol WM, et al: Structural and hemodynamic changes in rat lung after intra-abdominal infection: a model of subacute lung injury. *Surgery* 1984;96:384–394.
28. Kirton O: *Pulmonary structural and hemodynamic alterations induced by intraabdominal sepsis and endotoxemia: new models of subacute lung injury*, thesis (honors in special field), Harvard Medical School, Boston, 1983.
29. Jones R, Kirton OC, Zapol WM, et al: Pulmonary microvascular injury produced by intermittent infusions of *Escherichia coli* endotoxin over 21 days. Submitted for publication.
30. Upton MP, Jones R, Zapol WM, et al: Narrowing and reduced perfusion of pulmonary arteries in sheep after blunt chest trauma: morphologic and angiographic correlates. *Fed Proc* 1984;43:884.

3 Pulmonary Hemodynamics in Adult Respiratory Distress Syndrome (ARDS)

Warren M. Zapol
Michael T. Snider

PULMONARY HYPERTENSION IN ARDS

We have reported a major increase of the pulmonary vascular resistance during ARDS.[1] In the absence of systemic hypoxemia, patients with mild acute respiratory failure (ARF) have a moderately elevated (22 to 27 mmHg) mean pulmonary artery pressure (PAP). Moderate or severe ARDS patients have a higher PAP (27 to 35 + mmHg). Thus the severity of lung injury during ARDS is related to the level of elevation of the pulmonary artery pressure. This increase of pulmonary vascular resistance can occur within a few hours after the onset of acute respiratory failure. The presence of mild pulmonary hypertension is so common in ARDS of all causes that one must doubt ARDS is the correct diagnosis in any patient with mean PAP less than 20 mmHg at a cardiac index (CI) greater than 2.5 L/min·m^2. Clinical hemodynamic studies in ARDS patients after septicemia and trauma[2-4] confirm our findings that pulmonary artery hypertension results from an elevated pulmonary vascular resistance (PVR).

All patients with moderate and severe ARDS develop pulmonary artery hypertension (PAH) (Figure 3-1) because the pulmonary vascular resistance (PVR has risen to two to three times the normal value (Figure 3-2).[1] Pulmonary vascular resistance is calculated as the difference between the mean pulmonary artery (PAP) and capillary wedge pressure (PCWP) divided by the cardiac output (CO). The normal value in adults is approximately 56 ± 24 dyne/s/cm^5.[5] The normal PVR is often erroneously reported to be higher. For each patient there is an inverse relationship between the pulmonary vascular resistance and the CI (Figure 3-3). The values in Figure 3-3 were obtained using venoarterial cardiopulmonary bypass to vary the CI during severe posttraumatic ARDS while stabilizing the mixed venous and arterial gas tensions.[6] In any pa-

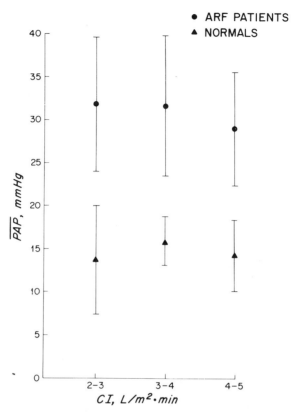

Figure 3-1 Mean pulmonary artery pressure (PAP) as a function of cardiac index (CI) for 30 patients with acute respiratory failure (ARF) and for 33 normal controls.

tient sequential measurements of PVR must be referred to a specific CI and a PVR-CI curve should be constructed before changes of the PVR are interpreted as alterations in the status of the pulmonary vessels.

It is unclear precisely what determines the shape of the PVR-CI curve. In early ARDS, endothelial and interstitial cells swell and as microvascular permeability increases, the matrix fills with plasma exudate and thrombus (fibrin). The lungs increase in weight up to 2 or 3 kg (Figure 3-4). It is our belief that during ARDS a markedly increased lung interstitial pressure raises the "opening pressure" of the pulmonary vessels from 5 to 10 to 20 to 30 mmHg and thus increases the mean pulmonary artery pressure (Figure 3-5), but the evidence for such a hypothesis of reversible vascular compression is inferential. In sheep, despite severe acute inflammatory pulmonary edema and a threefold increase of lung weight after pure oxygen breathing for three days, there was no increase of either the

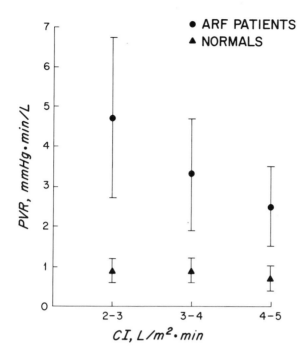

Figure 3-2 Pulmonary vascular resistance (PVR) as a function of cardiac index (CI) for 30 patients with acute respiratory failure (ARF) and for 33 normal controls.

PVR or the PAP.[7] Prior studies with hydrostatic pulmonary edema showed this did not cause vascular compression.[8] Nevertheless, it is unlikely that animal acute lung injury models approach the degree of pulmonary inflammatory engorgement and vascular pathology that occurs during clinical ARDS. Species differences may also be vital in this regard. Indeed, serial hemodynamic studies in humans suggest reversible vascular compression may contribute to vascular obstruction. Figure 3-6 illustrates serial measurements of PAP and CI during control and periods of isoproterenol infusion in a patient recovering from posttraumatic ARDS. With intensive care therapy, lung function improved and the patient progressed from moderate ARDS to mild ARF, his radiographic infiltrates cleared and the pulmonary vascular "opening pressure" may have decreased.

LUNG VASCULAR RECRUITMENT OR DISTENTION IN ARDS

During early hemodynamic studies we infused isoproterenol to increase the heart rate and cardiac output of patients with ARDS. This

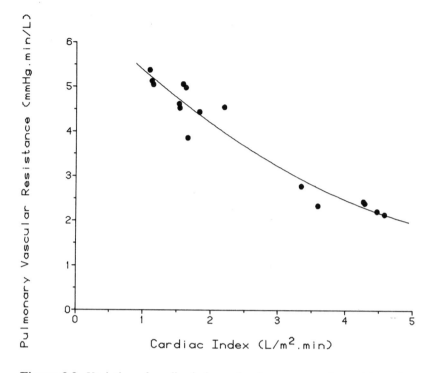

Figure 3-3 Variation of cardiac index and pulmonary vascular resistance by a change in bypass blood flow rate during severe posttraumatic acute respiratory failure (closed circles). Isoproterenol 1 μg/min was infused during 13 of the 16 measurements over 34 hours.

technique is illustrated in Figure 3-7, which charts the course of a patient with early posttraumatic ARDS. An isoproterenol infusion doubled his CO from 3.5 to 7 L/min but increased the PAP only 3 mmHg (from 44 to 47 mmHg). Three days later his respiratory failure had become more severe and the PAP had increased to 55 mmHg. At that time, despite the infusion of large quantities of inotropic drugs, we were unable to increase the CO above 4.2 L/min. The patient appeared unable to increase his cardiac output due to the elevated PVR and PAP, probably due to right ventricular dysfunction.

These early hemodynamic studies posed questions about the nature of lung vascular pathophysiology during ARDS. Was the elevated PVR due to obstructed or destroyed lung vessels? Did moderate and severe ARDS patients have lung vessels remaining to be recruited (or dilated) by increasing the CO (and thereby slightly increasing the PAP)? To answer these questions, we prospectively studied (after obtaining informed consent from relatives) pulmonary hemodynamics in patients with mild lung

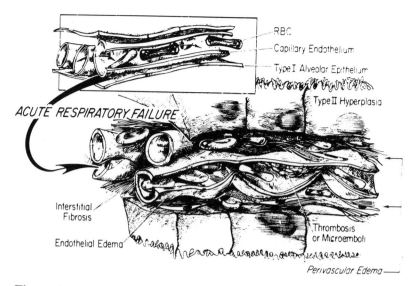

Figure 3-4 A comparison of pathologic alterations of lung structure in severe ARF with the normal structure. Vascular occlusion by endothelial and interstitial edema, thrombosis, and microembolism is shown. Type II cell hyperplasia is prominent and increases the diffusion distance for respiratory gas exchange.

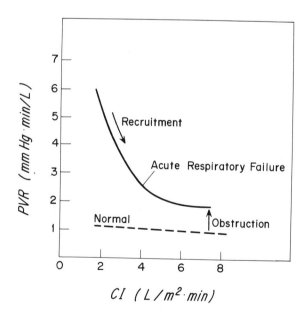

Figure 3-5 Schema of possible physiologic events that may influence the relationship of pulmonary vascular resistance (PVR) with the cardiac index (CI).

30

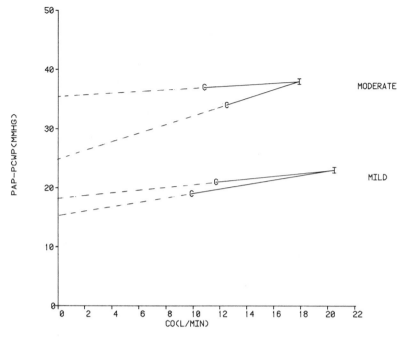

Figure 3-6 Pulmonary artery pressure (PAP) minus pulmonary capillary wedge pressure (PCWP) during posttraumatic ARF. C = control, I = isoproterenol infusion. Linear intercepts to zero cardiac output (CO) may provide an indication of interstitial lung pressure. The intercept pressure rises in moderate and severe ARDS.

injury as well as moderate and severe ARDS patients after pharmacologically increasing their cardiac output. Our hypothesis was that if the majority of the pulmonary vasculature was destroyed, a major increase of cardiac output (eg, by a factor of two) would require a marked increase (eg, doubling) of the mean PAP.

Fifteen mild ARF and moderate ARDS patients were studied soon after admission to the respiratory intensive care unit. Their hemodynamic and gas exchange data are summarized in Tables 3-1 and 3-2. After control measurements were obtained, isoproterenol was infused intravenously (IV) and the dosage slowly increased for 15 minutes until the heart rate approached 120 beats/min (see Table 3-1). There was no change of the mean systemic arterial pressure (SAP) or the PCWP. A mean of 3.3 ± 2.3 μg/min of isoproterenol was infused (all data mean $\pm$ SD). The CO increased from 6.6 ± 2.0 to 10.8 ± 4.9 L/min and the heart rate increased from 94.5 ± 19.6 to 124.5 ± 16.4 beats/min (Figure 3-8). The mean CO increased by over 60%; however, the mean PAP (see Figure 3-9) increased only 2.5 mmHg (from 30.4 to 32.9 mmHg). After the measurements were obtained the isoproterenol infusion was stopped. These hemodynamic

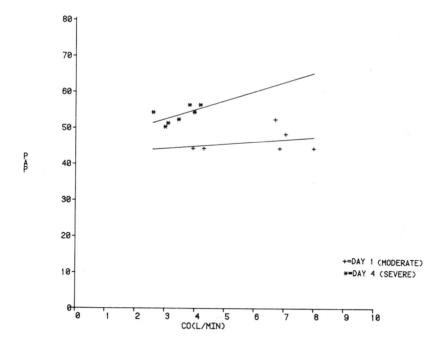

Figure 3-7 Mean pulmonary artery pressure (PAP) (mmHg) for one patient plotted against cardiac output during moderate (+) and severe (*) respiratory failure.

data provide evidence that in the majority of early ARDS patients the pulmonary vasculature is available for dilation and/or recruitment. In most instances pulmonary blood flow can be increased by opening or dilating vessels without markedly increasing the PAP.

During isoproterenol infusion we found that a reduced arterial oxygen tension (PaO_2) accompanied an increase in the CO and that the right-to-left shunt ($\dot{Q}_S/\dot{Q}_T$) increased from 20.8 to 28.8% (Figure 3-10). It is possible that the additional pulmonary blood flow increased the PAP, thereby recruiting lung vessels in poorly or nonventilated regions of the lung, and increased the $\dot{Q}_S/\dot{Q}_T$. Another possibility is that as the CO and mean mixed venous oxygen tension (PvO_2) increased (from 36 to 42 mmHg), the degree of hypoxic vasoconstriction of injured lung regions declined, and $\dot{Q}_S/\dot{Q}_T$ increased.

DIFFUSE VASOCONSTRICTION IN ARDS

Vasodilators infused during the late stages of severe ARDS did not reduce the PVR. Figure 3-11 illustrates serial hemodynamic measurements of a previously healthy patient who developed severe ARDS within a few

Table 3-1
Isoproterenol Infusion during ARF (Mean ± SD)

	n	Base Line	Isoproterenol	Mean	t	p
PAP	15	30.4 ± 9.8	32.9 ± 9.6	+ 2.5	− 2.75	< .02
PAS	13	43.2 ± 13.2	48.7 ± 15.8	+ 5.5	− 2.82	< .02
PAD	13	20.8 ± 5.3	21.5 ± 6.1	± .7	− 0.56	< .6
PCWP	15	14.5 ± 5.1	13.4 ± 5.6	− 1.1	1.32	< .3
RVEDV	13	216.2 ± 87.7	248.3 ± 108.1	+ 32.1	− 2.92	< .02
CO	15	6.6 ± 2.0	10.8 ± 3.9	+ 4.2	− 5.80	< .01
PVR	15	2.5 ± 1.2	1.9 ± .08	− .6	3.92	< .01
HR	13	94.5 ± 19.6	124.5 ± 16.4	+ 30	− 8.39	< .01
MAP	13	89.2 ± 18.8	90.9 ± 19.8	+ .3	− 0.57	< .6
SAP	13	132.1 ± 15.9	148.7 ± 26.0	+ 16.6	− 1.88	< .2
DAP	12	65.5 ± 18.1	63.2 ± 20.9	− 2.3	0.76	< .5
$\dot{Q}_S/\dot{Q}_T$	15	20.8 ± 10.1	28.8 ± 12.3	+ 8	− 5.13	< .01
PaO_2	15	113.7 ± 41.3	95.1 ± 21.8	− 17.9	2.23	< .05
$PaCO_2$	15	42.9 ± 9.6	45.5 ± 10.0	+ 2.6	− 4.60	< .01
pHa	15	7.4 ± 0.06	7.4 ± .06	0	−	−
PvO_2	15	35.5 ± 5.4	41.7 ± 6.2	+ 6.2	− 4.4	< .01
$PvCO_2$	15	46.7 ± 10.1	49.3 ± 11.2	+ 2.6	− 3.22	< .01
pHv	15	7.42 ± 0.06	7.39 ± 0.06	− .03	4.35	< .01
Temp	15	98.3 ± 3.0	98.5 ± 3.0	− .2	− 0.97	< .4
SVR	15	12.0 ± 6.1	7.9 ± 5.0	± 4.1	4.83	< .01
PEEP	15	11.4 ± 4.8	11.4 ± 4.8			
Dose (μg/min)	15	0	3.3 ± 2.3			
FiO_2	15	.58 ± .2	.58 ± .2			

Abbreviations and units for Tables 3-1 and 3-2: PAP = mean pulmonary artery pressure (mmHg), PAS = systolic pulmonary artery pressure (mmHg), PAD = diastolic pulmonary artery pressure (mmHg), PCWP = pulmonary capillary wedge pressure (mmHg), RVEDP = right ventricular end-diastolic pressure (mmHg), RVEDV = right ventricular end-diastolic volume (ml), CO = cardiac output (L/min), PVR = pulmonary vascular resistance (mmHg·min/L), HR = heart rate (beats/min), MAP = mean arterial pressure (mmHg), SAP = systolic arterial pressure (mmHg), DAP = diastolic arterial pressure (mmHg), $\dot{Q}_S/\dot{Q}_T$ = right-to-left shunt (%), PaO_2 = arterial O_2 tension (mmHg), $PaCO_2$ = arterial CO_2 tension (mmHg), pHa = arterial pH, PvO_2 = mixed venous O_2 tension (mmHg), $PvCO_2$ = mixed venous CO_2 tension (mmHg), pHv = mixed venous pH, Temp = body temperature (°F), SVR = systemic vascular resistance (mmHg·min/L), PEEP = positive end-expiratory pressure (cm H_2O), FiO_2 = fraction of inspired O_2.

hours after ingesting an overdose of drugs and aspirating gastric contents.[6] Twelve hours after aspiration the patient had a markedly elevated PVR of 5.5 mmHg·min/L. Large doses of several vasodilators were infused IV without producing any pulmonary hemodynamic effect; after five days of intensive care and despite concomitant infusion of three vasodilators, isoproterenol (8 μg/min), phentolamine (250 μg/min), and nitroprusside (80 μg/min), the PAP and PVR were not reduced.

Although in late stages of severe ARDS these pulmonary vasodilators proved ineffective, a major question for study remained. Could PVR be reduced by IV vasodilator infusions early in the hospital course of mild

Table 3-2
Nitroprusside Infusion during ARF (Mean ± SD)

	n	Base Line	Nitroprusside	Mean	t	p
PAP	15	29.6 ± 10.6	24.2 ± 9.3	− 5.4	8.12	<.01
PAS	12	40 ± 14.3	34.8 ± 14.3	− 5.2	7.43	<.01
PAD	12	19.7 ± 7.1	16.5 ± 7.2	− 3.2	3.73	<.01
PCWP	15	13.5 ± 6.0	10.4 ± 6.1	− 3.1	6.11	<.01
RVEDP	13	14 ± 5.4	10.7 ± 5.5	− 3.3	5.13	<.01
CO	15	6.9 ± 1.9	8.75 ± 3.1	+ 1.85	3.69	<.01
PVR	15	2.2 ± 1.0	1.5 ± 0.6	− .7	4.4	<.01
HR	13	98.5 ± 19.9	108.3 ± 12.0	+ 9.8	− 3.16	<.01
MAP	12	89.6 ± 19.7	70.5 ± 17.6	− 19.1	4.86	<.01
SAP	12	134.6 ± 15.2	114.7 ± 23.9	− 19.9	2.70	<.02
DAP	12	67.7 ± 19.9	53.4 ± 16.8	− 14.3	3.94	<.01
$\dot{Q}_S/\dot{Q}_T$	15	23.0 ± 9.4	31.6 ± 14.4	+ 7.6	− 4.09	<.01
PaO_2	15	105.3 ± 45.5	74.7 ± 23.1	− 30.6	3.40	<.01
$PaCO_2$	15	43.3 ± 8.4	45.4 ± 10.1	+ 2.1	− 2.29	<.05
pHa	15	7.4 ± 0.05	7.4 ± 0.07	0	−	−
PvO_2	15	36.9 ± 6.4	35.1 ± 4.4	− 1.8	2.0	<.1
$PvCO_2$	15	48.5 + 9.2	48.9 + 9.3	+ .4	− 0.57	<.6
pHv	15	7.4 ± 0.05	7.4 ± 0.06	0	−	−
Temp	15	98.3 ± 3.3	98.2 ± 3.2	− .1	0.73	<.5
SVR	12	10.4 ± 5.5	6.2 ± 2.8	− 4.2	3.82	<.01
PEEP	15	11.5 ± 4.8	11.5 ± 4.8			
Dose (μg/min)	15	0	150.7 ± 112.5			
FiO_2	15	.58 ± .2	.58 ± .2			

For abbreviations and units, see footnote to Table 3-1.

ARF or moderate ARDS patients? If infusing a vasodilator agent reduced both the PAP and PCWP while increasing the CO, then diffuse pulmonary vasoconstriction would be evidenced. After obtaining informed consent from relatives control hemodynamic measurements were obtained in 15 mild ARF and moderate ARDS patients. We then slowly infused increasing IV doses of sodium nitroprusside until the mean SAP was reduced to 70 mmHg. We continued this infusion for 15 minutes until the CO and other hemodynamic measurements were stable. The measurements we obtained are reported in Table 3-2. Cardiac output increased by 28% from 6.9 to 8.8 L/min, while the PAP was reduced from 29.6 to 24.2 mmHg (Figure 3-12) and the PCWP decreased from 13.5 to 10.4 mmHg (Figure 3-13). Thus, despite the 28% increase in CO, nitroprusside reduced both the PAP and PCWP. Nitroprusside infusion produced widespread pulmonary vasodilation. These data support the hypothesis that diffuse pulmonary vasoconstriction occurs in early ARDS.

During nitroprusside infusion the venous admixture increased from 23% to 31.6% (Figure 3-14) and the PaO_2 decreased from 105 to 75 mmHg, while both the PVR and the PvO_2 were significantly decreased.

34

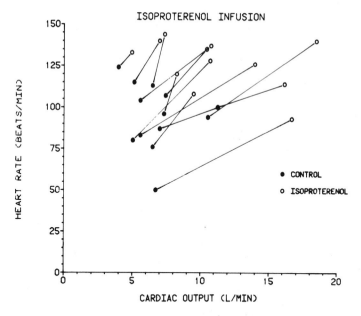

Figure 3-8 Heart rate in the control period (closed circles) and after isoproterenol infusion (open circles) during acute respiratory failure plotted against the cardiac output (see Table 3-1).

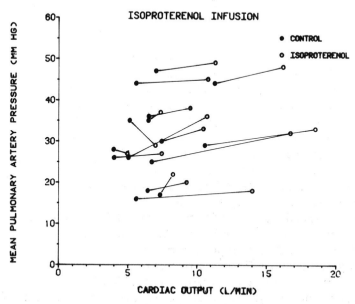

Figure 3-9 Mean pulmonary artery pressure in the control period (closed circles) and after isoproterenol infusion (open circles) during acute respiratory failure plotted against the cardiac output (see Table 3-1).

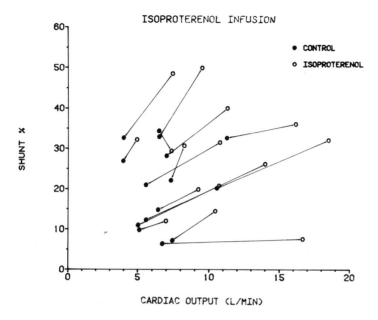

Figure 3-10 Mean right-to-left venous admixture (shunt %) in the control period (closed circles) and after isoproterenol infusion (open circles) during acute respiratory failure graphed against the cardiac output (see Table 3-1).

After measurements were obtained during nitroprusside infusion (about 30 minutes) the nitroprusside infusion was stopped.

THE PCWP IN ARDS

The PAP may be elevated during ARDS in part due to an increase of the PCWP. In many cases of moderate and severe ARDS the PCWP may not be elevated. We have reported that 16 patients with moderate ARDS of diverse etiology had a similar mean PCWP compared with the normal value (Figure 3-15). The PCWP should be measured in each ARDS patient, as an elevated PCWP can contribute to the elevated PAP and increase the microvascular leak.

AIRWAY PRESSURE IN ARDS

Increasing airway pressure in ARDS minimally alters the PAP or CO.[1] There are several mechanisms for this insulation. Firstly, the increase of intrapleural pressure with the application of positive end-expiratory pressure (PEEP) is proportional to the product of the chest

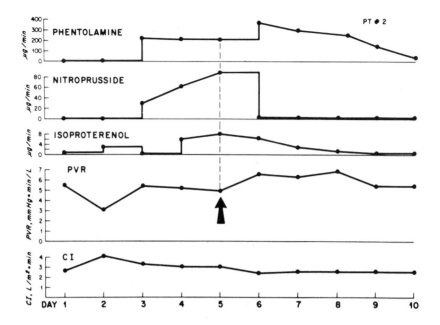

Figure 3-11 In a patient with severe ARDS several days after gastric acid aspiration, vasodilator infusion was unsuccessful in lowering the pulmonary vascular resistance (PVR) from markedly elevated levels. Note that the cardiac index (CI) remains fixed despite large doses of isoproterenol, nitroprusside, and phentolamine (concomitantly).

wall compliance (which is usually unchanged in ARDS) with the increase of lung volume. The low lung compliance of severe ARDS permits the lung to increase its volume by only a small amount due to an increasing alveolar pressure. Thus, there is only a small directly transmitted increase of intrapleural pressure. This can be readily documented by observing the PAP while disconnecting the endotracheal tube from the ventilator during intensive therapy of a patient with severe ARDS (Figure 3-16). In a group of ten patients with severe ARDS, we measured the PAP before and five seconds after disconnecting 20.5 ± 4.8 cm H_2O PEEP. The mean PAP was reduced by only -3.00 ± 3.21 mmHg (mean $\pm$ SD), and the mean PCWP by -2.33 ± 2.29 mmHg.[1]

In addition to the minimal increase of intrathoracic pressure with PEEP during ARDS, there is little evidence for airway pressure compressing or occluding the lung's microvasculature during severe ARDS. In the normal lung a positive pressure ventilation would be expected to raise the PAP by compressing or distorting lung (alveolar) vessels and thereby raising the PVR (Figure 3-17). In the normal lung we expect a low interstitial

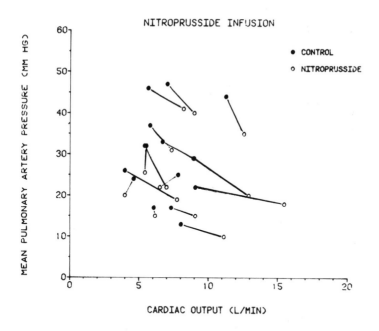

Figure 3-12 Mean pulmonary artery pressure in the control period (closed circles) and after nitroprusside infusion (open circles) during acute respiratory failure plotted against the cardiac output (see Table 3-2).

pressure and little shunt (venous admixture). In contrast, during severe ARDS the lung's interstitium is filled with edema, thrombi, and cells and the interstitial pressure rises (although a precise measurement has not been reported). If we hypothesize that the large interstitial pressure compresses the lung's vessels then a vascular "waterfall" of 10 to 20 mmHg has been created (Figure 3-18). In that circumstance increasing the alveolar pressure to 10 or 20 cm H_2O would not elevate the PAP, as the alveolar pressure would remain beneath the interstitial pressure. To visualize this barrier, we obtained balloon occlusion wedge angiograms during severe ARDS that provided evidence of stringlike vessels with diffuse narrowing.[9] As an additional mechanism to reduce the PAP the presence of a large nonventilated intrapulmonary shunt could provide a passage for pulmonary artery blood to run off should alveolar compression have increased the PAP. The above-described mechanisms are unproven and hypothetical. It remains for future clinical research to demonstrate which if any of the mechanisms are important during ARDS to isolate the pulmonary circulation from alveolar pressure.

38

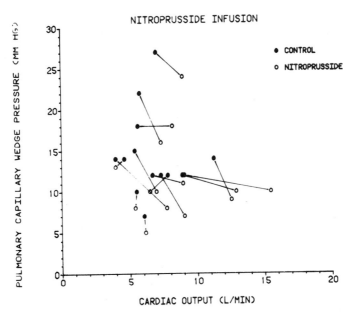

Figure 3-13 Pulmonary capillary wedge pressure in the control period (closed circles) and after nitroprusside infusion (open circles) during acute respiratory failure plotted against the cardiac output (see Table 3-2).

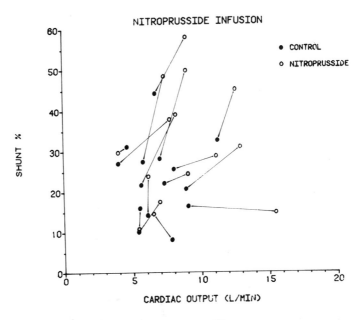

Figure 3-14 Right-to-left shunt (shunt %) in the control period (closed circles) and after nitroprusside infusion (open circles) during acute respiratory failure plotted against the cardiac output (see Table 3-2).

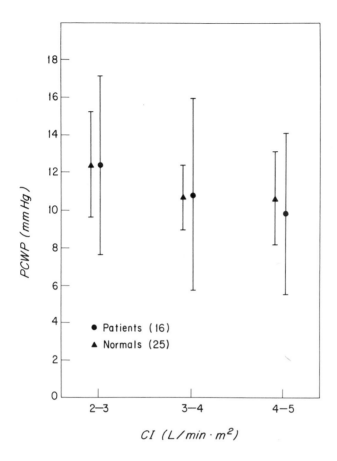

Figure 3-15 The pulmonary capillary wedge pressure (PCWP) of 16 patients with moderate and severe ARDS and 25 normals plotted against the cardiac index (CI). There is no statistically significant difference.

In summary, during ARDS evidence has been reported here and elsewhere[10] that:

1. Mild pulmonary hypertension (mean PAP 30 mmHg) is a universal hallmark of moderate to severe ARDS regardless of etiology.[1]
2. Pulmonary hypertension is due to an elevated PVR.
3. The calculated PVR appears to be an inverse function of the CO.
4. The $\dot{Q}_S/\dot{Q}_T$ increases as CO increases.[11]
5. Both increasing PEEP and decreasing the pulmonary blood flow favor reduction of $\dot{Q}_S/\dot{Q}_T$ but appear to act by separate physiologic mechanisms.[12]

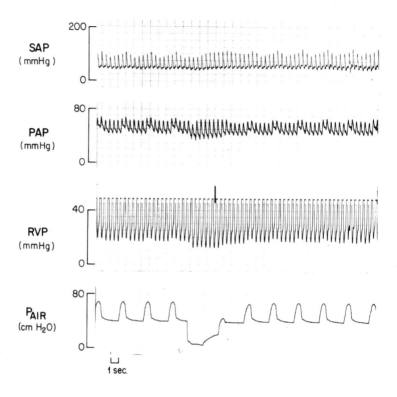

Figure 3-16 Minimal decrease of the pulmonary artery pressure and right ventricular pressure (RVP) removing 40 cm H_2O airway pressure (PEEP) during severe ARDS.

6. By infusing nitroprusside into 15 patients with moderate and severe ARDS, we were able to lower both the mean PAP (from 30 to 24 mmHg) and the PCWP, despite increasing the CO by 28%.[10] This supports the hypothesis that diffuse pulmonary vasoconstriction contributes to the early increase of PVR.

7. By infusing isoproterenol into 15 patients with moderate and severe ARDS, we increased the mean CO by 64%. However, the mean PAP increased by only 2.5 mmHg.[10] Thus, in the majority of patients during ARDS, lung vessels can be recruited with only a small increase of the mean PAP.

8. An elevated pulmonary vascular resistance (≥ 2.5 mmHg$\cdot$min/L) correlated with the presence of thromboembolic pulmonary macrovascular occlusions ascertained by balloon occlusion pulmonary angiography in 19 of 40 patients.[9,13]

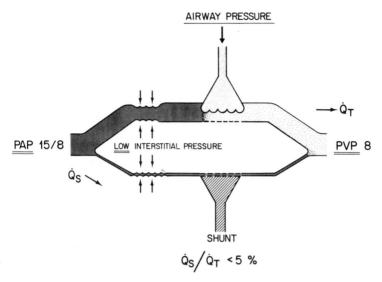

Figure 3-17 Schema of hydrostatic events surrounding the normal intrathoracic pulmonary circulation. Applied airway pressure (PEEP) raises the pulmonary vascular resistance (PVR) and pulmonary artery pressure (PAP) in the presence of a small shunt (less than 5%) and a low lung interstitial pressure.

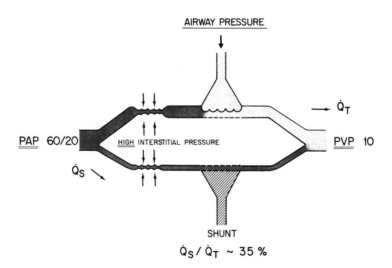

Figure 3-18 Schema of hydrostatic events surrounding the intrathoracic pulmonary circulation during severe ARDS. Applied airway pressure (PEEP) causes little increase of pulmonary vascular resistance (PVR) as the pulmonary artery pressure (PAP) remains above the level of the interstitial pressure (waterfall effect). Airway pressure (PEEP) is less than interstitial pressure. The large shunt via nonventilated but perfused lung acts as a runoff if the PVR in the ventilated zones should be increased by alveolar pressure.

42

9. Pulmonary artery occlusion, medial hypertrophy of pulmonary arteries, and extension of medial musculature into distal alveolar arteries occur during ARDS and each may contribute to coagulative necrosis of the distal lung.[14,15]

10. The precise cause of the elevated PVR remains unclear but a number of diverse and complex phenomena probably contribute to it. The causes of the early increase of PVR (eg, vasoconstriction, transient leukocyte obstruction, alveolar collapse) may differ from the later causes of an increased PVR (eg, medial hypertrophy, thrombosis, interstitial fibrosis). The latter events appear more irreversible, and lead to microvascular and lung tissue destruction.

11. Positive airway pressure has little effect on the PVR in severe ARDS.[10] It is uncertain why the vasculature is shielded from the increased airway pressure. Shielding may result from widespread shunting of pulmonary artery blood, from altered mechanical properties of the interstitium, or from an increased pressure on the vessels of the lung (waterfall effect).

Clinical and laboratory research into the causes of the elevated PVR of ARDS will eventually unravel the precise causes of the pulmonary artery hypertension. Pulmonary artery hypertension during ARDS with an elevated microvascular permeability can exacerbate pulmonary edema. Careful examination of each factor contributing to the increased pulmonary vascular resistance may allow us to reverse some of its causes and partly salvage the lung's microvasculature, allowing injured pulmonary tissue to heal and the severely ill ARDS patient to survive.

ACKNOWLEDGMENTS

The authors thank Ms Janice Lauer for assistance with the hemodynamic studies, and Dr M.B. Laver, and Dr S. Permutt for helpful discussions of the hemodynamic effects of lung injury.

Figures 3-1 and 3-2 are reproduced with permission from Zapol and Snider[1]; Figures 3-3, 3-8, 3-9, 3-10, 3-12, 3-13, 3-14, and 3-15 from Zapol et al[10]; Figures 3-4, 3-5, 3-6, and 3-7 from Zapol et al[16]; and Figure 3-11 from Zapol et al.[6] Tables 3-1 and 3-2 are from Zapol et al.[10]

REFERENCES

1. Zapol WM, Snider MT: Pulmonary hypertension in severe acute respiratory failure. *N Engl J Med* 1977;296:476–480.
2. Clowes Jr GHA, Hirsch E, Williams L, et al: Septic lung and shock lung in man. *Ann Surg* 1975;181:681–692.

3. Weigelt JA, Gewertz BL, Aurbakken CM, et al: Pharmacologic alterations in pulmonary artery pressure in ARDS. *J Surg Res* 1982;32:243-248.
4. Sibbald WJ, Anderson RR, Reid B, et al: Alveolocapillary permeability in human septic ARDS. *Chest* 1981;79:133-142.
5. Barratt-Boyes BG, Wood EH: Cardiac output and related measurements and pressure values in the right heart and associated vessels, together with an analysis of the hemodynamic response to the inhalation of high oxygen mixtures in healthy subjects. *J Lab Clin Med* 1958;51:72-90.
6. Zapol WM, Snider MT, Schneider RC, et al: Pulmonary hypertension in severe acute respiratory failure, in Zapol WM, Qvist J (eds): *Artificial Lungs for Acute Respiratory Failure: Theory and Practice.* New York, Academic Press, 1976, pp 435-454.
7. Liland AE, Zapol WM, Qvist J, et al: Positive airway pressure in lambs spontaneously breathing air and oxygen. *J Surg Res* 1976;20:85-92.
8. Ritchie BC, Schanberger G, Staub N: Inadequacy of perivascular edema hypothesis to account for distribution of pulmonary blood flow in lung edema. *Circ Res* 1969;24:807-814.
9. Greene R, Zapol WM, Snider MT, et al: Early bedside detection of pulmonary vascular occlusion during acute respiratory failure. *Am Rev Respir Dis* 1981;124:593-601.
10. Zapol WM, Snider MT, Rie M: Pulmonary circulation during ARDS, in Zapol WM, Falke K (eds): *Acute Respiratory Failure*, in Lenfant C (exec ed): *Lung Biology in Health and Disease.* New York, Marcel Dekker, 1985, vol 24, pp 241-274.
11. Lemaire F, Jardin F, Regnier B, et al: Pulmonary gas exchange during venoarterial bypass with a membrane lung for acute respiratory failure. *J Thorac Cardiovasc Surg* 1978;75:839-846.
12. Snider MT, Zapol WM: Assessment of pulmonary oxygenation during venoarterial bypass with aortic root return, in Zapol WM, Qvist J (eds): *Artificial Lungs for Acute Respiratory Failure: Theory and Practice.* New York, Academic Press, 1976, pp 257-273.
13. Greene R, Boggis CRM, Jantsch H-S, et al: Radiography and angiography of the pulmonary circulation in ARDS, in Zapol WM, Falke K (eds): *Acute Respiratory Failure*, in Lenfant C (exec ed): *Lung Biology in Health and Disease.* New York, Marcel Dekker, 1985, vol 24, pp 275-302.
14. Snow RL, Davies P, Pontoppidan H, et al: Pulmonary vascular remodelling in adult respiratory distress syndrome. *Am Rev Respir Dis* 1982;126:887-892.
15. Tomashefski JF, Davies P, Boggis C, et al: The pulmonary vascular lesions of the adult respiratory distress syndrome. *Am J Pathol* 1983;112:112-126.
16. Zapol WM, Trelstad RL, Snider MT, et al: Pathophysiologic pathways of the adult respiratory distress syndrome, in Tinker J, Rapin M (eds): *Care of the Critically Ill Patient.* Heidelberg, Springer-Verlag, 1983, pp 341-358.

4 Active Transport and Permeability Properties of the Alveolar Epithelium in the Lung

Edward D. Crandall
Kwang-Jin Kim
Barbara E. Goodman

The characteristics of net fluid flow across adult mammalian lung alveolar epithelium are not well understood. Although we have reasonable estimates of the osmotic and hydrostatic pressures of interstitial fluid, little is known of these quantities on the air side of the alveolar epithelial barrier. Nevertheless, insight into fluid balance across alveolar epithelium relevant to alveolar pulmonary edema will require greater knowledge not only of these driving forces but also of the barrier properties of the alveolar epithelium itself. At least two major transport characteristics are likely to be involved in alveolar fluid balance: (1) active transport of solutes; and, (2) resistance to the passive transport of solutes and water.

ACTIVE TRANSPORT BY ALVEOLAR EPITHELIUM

One of the distinguishing characteristics of epithelia both in vivo and in vitro is the presence of transepithelial solute transport mechanisms, especially active transport processes. These active transport properties of epithelia have been well characterized in intestine, skin, gallbladder, and kidney epithelia, but relatively neglected in lung epithelia. A good deal of work on isolated upper airway epithelia has been performed in recent years, dating back to 1975,[1] focused primarily on the active ion transport properties of this barrier. Studies have been conducted on mammalian upper airway epithelia, usually mounted in Ussing chambers in vitro.[2] Tracheal epithelium exhibits active chloride transport into the lumen, and generates a spontaneous potential difference of about 30 mV[1] and a tissue resistance of about 400 ohm-cm[2].[1,3] Substitution for sodium and exposure to ouabain decrease net chloride secretion.[4] Active chloride secretion and active sodium reabsorption are both found in canine large airway epithelia, with the former process predominating in the trachea and the latter in the segmental bronchi.[1,5]

Fetal lungs which are normally fluid-filled have also been shown to actively transport chloride from blood to lumen.[6] Olver et al[7] found evidence for sodium reabsorption across fetal lamb pulmonary epithelium which increased with gestational age and after exposure to epinephrine. Fetal lung liquid is very low in bicarbonate, suggesting that acid secretion takes place.[8] A potential difference of 4.3 mV between airway fluid and blood has been measured across the fetal lung.[9] Bullfrog lung generates a spontaneous potential difference of 18 mV[11] and has a tissue resistance of 2000 ohm-cm[2].[10,11] The bullfrog alveolar epithelium actively transports chloride into the alveolar space,[10] similar to tracheal epithelium and fetal lung epithelium.

Experiments performed on whole lungs either in vitro or in vivo have been useful for elucidating the transport properties of the pulmonary epithelial barrier. Unfortunately, due to the complex anatomical structure of mammalian lungs (parallel pathways for transport of airways v alveolar epithelium and series pathways of epithelium, interstitium, and endothelium), it has not been possible to determine precisely the characteristics and mechanisms of transport across the mammalian alveolar epithelium alone. Recently, primary cultured monolayers of isolated rat alveolar epithelial cells have been used as a model for intact mammalian alveolar epithelium.[12,13] Using techniques frequently employed by renal and other epitheliologists, we have been able to provide evidence for the presence of a regulable active solute transepithelial transport mechanism in the pulmonary alveolar epithelium of mammalian lungs.

In order to study mammalian alveolar epithelium in isolation, we have harvested rat lung cells by enzymatic digestion with elastase.[12] The lung cell mix has been further purified by a discontinuous metrizamide density gradient followed by a differential adherence technique.[12,14] Confluent monolayers of harvested, purified type II cells on nonporous surfaces form domes within four days in culture[12] (Figure 4-1). Domes are thought to result from active transport of solute from medium to substratum, with water following passively.[15,16]

When dome-forming confluent monolayers of type II alveolar epithelial cells (five to seven days after plating) were exposed to the metabolic inhibitors 2,4-dinitrophenol (DNP), potassium cyanide (KCN), and 4°C, domes disappeared rapidly. This implies that the solute transport mechanism resulting in dome formation is energy-dependent; ie, an active process. Sodium transport inhibitors (ouabain, amiloride, and or-

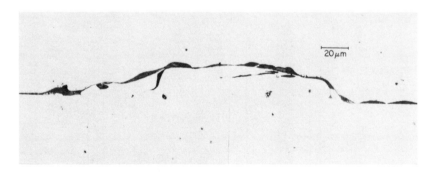

Figure 4-1 Light photomicrograph of a cross section of a typical dome from a five-day plate. Note that dome is a fluid-filled structure consisting of a monolayer of cells raised above the plastic surface. (Reproduced with permission from *J Appl Physiol.*[18])

thovanadate) added to the medium above the cell monolayers also caused rapid disappearance of domes. When monolayers were exposed to the chloride transport inhibitors (furosemide, 4,4′-diisothiocyano-2,2′-disulfonic stilbene [DIDS], and indacrinone), dome density did not change significantly compared to control. Substitution for sodium (Figure 4-2) in the medium (with choline, tris(hydroxymethyl)methylamine (Tris), K^+, or tetraethylammonium) always led to dome disappearance, while domes remained present following chloride substitution (nitrate or gluconate). These observations provide strong evidence that an active sodium transport process results in dome formation by cultured monolayers of alveolar epithelial cells and is probably also present in intact mammalian alveolar epithelium.[17]

In subsequent studies using dome-forming monolayers, we have investigated the effects of substances expected to increase intracellular cAMP (or analog) concentrations on active transport across alveolar epithelial cells.[18] Cyclic adenosine monophosphate (cAMP) is known to increase active ion secretion in many secretory epithelia, including stomach, salivary gland, and pancreas, and to increase active ion absorption in absorptive epithelia, including toad urinary bladder, frog skin, and renal collecting tubule.[19] Beta-adrenergic activity has been shown to increase intracellular cAMP in many systems, including dog kidney.[20] Therefore, we investigated the effects of cAMP analogs, phosphodiesterase inhibitors, and β-agonists on active transport (as evidenced by dome formation) in primary cultured monolayers of alveolar epithelial cells. Monolayers exposed to cAMP analogs, phosphodiesterase inhibitors, and β-agonists exhibited large increases in dome density compared to monolayers maintained in control medium alone (Figure 4-3). The presence of the β-blocker pro-

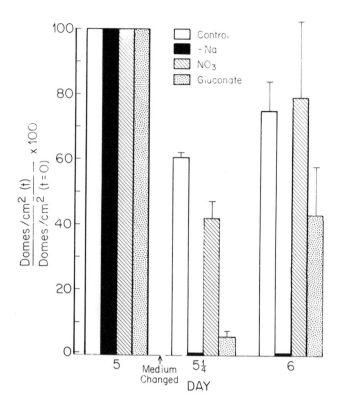

Figure 4-2 Effects of substitution for NA$^+$ and Cl$^-$ on dome formation in primary cultured monolayers of type II alveolar epithelial cells. Day 0 is day of initial cell plating. Bars indicate SE (control, n = 6; − Na, n = 6; NO$_3$, n = 3; gluconate, n = 3). (Reproduced with permission from *Am J Physiol.* [17])

pranolol had no effect on dome density by itself and eliminated the terbutaline-induced increase in dome formation (Figure 4-3).

In a recent publication,[21] Sugahara et al have utilized a vibrating microelectrode to detect small currents flowing in the medium above dome-forming monolayers of type II alveolar epithelial cells. They found that electrical current flowed out of the domes, was inhibitable by amiloride and ouabain, and was dependent on the presence of sodium in the medium. Their data seem to suggest that sodium may be transported across the entire monolayer and leak back mainly through the domes. Whether domes are sites of increased transport or sites of solute leak, either mechanism is consistent with the premise that domes result from active sodium transport across the monolayer.

Quantitating domes as an indicator of active transepithelial transport has proved to be useful for screening molecules which may affect the

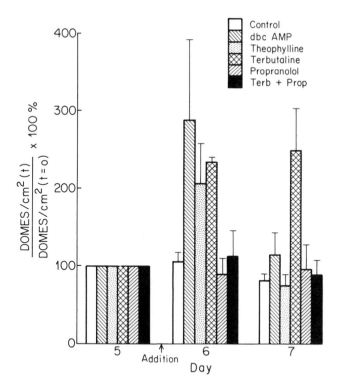

Figure 4-3 Effects of representative substances expected to increase intracellular cAMP (or analog) concentrations on dome formation in primary cultured monolayers of type II alveolar epithelial cells. Abscissa represents number of days after initial cell plating. At 24 hours, dbcAMP, theophylline, and terbutaline are significantly different from control ($P < .05$). (control, n = 9; dbcAMP, n = 4; theophylline, n = 3; terbutaline, n = 4; propranolol, n = 4; terb + prop, n = 4) (Reproduced with permission from *J Appl Physiol*. [18])

transport processes of the pulmonary alveolar epithelium. Nevertheless, more direct evidence of active transport of ions across cultured monolayers can be obtained from dome micropuncture or study of cells grown on porous filters. These techniques permit access to both the apical and basolateral surfaces of the alveolar epithelium for manipulations and measurements.

Using type II cell monolayers grown on porous filters (rat-tail collagen-coated millipore and nucleopore filters) and studied in water-jacketed 37°C Ussing chambers, we have been able to verify that the cultured monolayer is a tight barrier to the movement of small molecules. Primary cultured monolayers grown on porous filters generate a spontaneous potential difference of up to 4 mV, with a resistance of as much as 600 ohm-cm^2, and are relatively impermeable to sodium-22 (^{22}Na) and carbon-14 (^{14}C)-hydroxymethylinulin.[22] Using type II cell monolayers grown on collagen-coated millipore filters, Mason et al[13] obtained transepithelial potential differences measured in two laboratories of 0.7 ($\pm$0.1) mV to 1.3 ($\pm$0.1) mV (mean $\pm$ SEM), apical side negative, with resistances of 217 ($\pm$11) ohm-cm^2 and 233 ($\pm$12) ohm-cm^2. Terbutaline produced a transient decrease and then a sustained increase in potential difference. Amiloride (10^{-4} mol/L) abolished the potential difference when added apically and ouabain (10^{-3} mol/L) inhibited potential difference more effectively from the basal side. In a preliminary report on sheep with lung lymph fistulas,[23] amiloride (10^{-3} mol/L) caused a significantly decreased liquid volume removal rate, perhaps due to inhibition of sodium transport (alveolar to interstitial) across the pulmonary epithelium. In preliminary experiments in our laboratory, the permeability of the bare filter to ^{22}Na was 2 × 10^{-4} cm/s, while ^{22}Na flux across a collagen-coated filter covered by a monolayer was 1 × 10^{-5} cm/s. ^{14}C-inulin permeability across tight monolayers[22] was 3 × 10^{-7} cm/s (compared to 1.2 × 10^{-7} cm/s for dog lung[24] and 0.3 × 10^{-7} cm/s for bullfrog alveolar epithelium.[25]) We have also found that exposure to amiloride (10^{-3} mol/L) from the apical (alveolar) surface but not the basolateral (serosal) surface causes a rapid decrease in spontaneous potential difference. Ouabain (10^{-3} mol/L) causes a slower decrease in spontaneous potential difference only when added to the basolateral reservoir.

Using standard micropuncture techniques (similar to those used by renal physiologists to study nephron function), we have been able to sample the fluid within individual domes. In preliminary results, dome [Na$^+$] had a mean value greater than medium [Na$^+$] and dome [Cl$^-$]. These data are consistent with active transport of sodium from medium to substratum across the dome. The mean concentration of sulfur compounds was also elevated within the dome, which may indicate an active transport process for sulfate, amino acids, or other sulfur-containing substances. In a few experiments, we were able to measure the spontaneous potential difference across individual domes with microelectrodes filled with KCl by backfilling. Preliminary results indicate that the potential difference across the dome was 0.6 mV, apical side negative. This value is also consistent with active Na$^+$ transport from medium to substratum.

Measurements in preliminary experiments on intact perfused lungs isolated from rats are consistent with active transepithelial sodium transport across the pulmonary epithelium. In these experiments, ^{22}Na is instilled into the airways of degassed isolated perfused lungs.[26,27] Appearance of radioisotope in the recirculating perfusate is used as a measure of flux from alveolar to vascular space. The flux of sodium appears to increase after the addition of terbutaline to the perfusate, consistent with the findings on dome formation by monolayers of type II cells. These observations suggest the presence of an active sodium transport mechanism in the alveolar epithelium of intact mammalian lungs.

PERMEABILITY PROPERTIES
OF THE ALVEOLAR EPITHELIAL BARRIER

To date, almost all the information available on passive transport properties of the alveolar epithelial barrier has been obtained using the fluid-filled mammalian lung model. Several investigators have shown, by physiologic and morphologic studies, that the epithelia lining the air spaces of the lung offer the greatest resistance to the movement of fluid and solutes across the air-blood barrier. Studies using fluid-filled mammalian lungs indicate that the pulmonary epithelial barrier can be characterized by a majority of small pores with radii 0.55 to 1.0 nm occupying most of the available pore area,[28,29] and a few large pores whose radii may be greater than 8 nm.[24] The epithelial barrier offers significant resistance to the diffusion of electrolytes and other small hydrophilic solutes.[30-32] Hemoglobin, cytochrome C, and horseradish peroxidase have all been shown to easily traverse the endothelial but not the epithelial junctions of the lung barrier.[33-35] Fetal lung liquid contains essentially no protein, indicating that prenatal lung epithelia are impermeable to proteins.[8] On the other hand, several biochemical analyses have demonstrated albumin, immunoglobulin G, and α_1-globulin in alveolar fluid, although the distinction between normal components of surfactant and contaminants from the blood during lung lavage or homogenation of the lung was a confounding problem.[36-43] Autologous serum albumin and immunoglobulin G were visualized on the alveolar epithelial surface of the adult rat lung,[44] suggesting an important role for these proteins in lung fluid balance.

Although these findings are important and useful, there are several problems involved in interpreting data from the mammalian whole lung model (as noted briefly above). There are barriers in series and/or in parallel when solutes and water are instilled into the airways (airway v alveolar epithelial barrier; epithelium, interstitium, and endothelium and/or lymphatics), surface area and distribution volumes of solutes cannot be precisely defined, and presumably very large unstirred layers exist next to each barrier. To circumvent all or part of these inherent problems, hollow amphibian lungs have been used extensively to study alveolar epithelial transport properties in isolation. The bullfrog lung has proven to be a viable and reliable tissue suitable for studying a number of transport properties of the alveolar epithelial barrier.

Passive Nonelectrolyte Fluxes
of Bullfrog Lung[11,45]

Diffusional fluxes of water and small hydrophilic solutes across the bullfrog alveolar epithelium have been measured using radiotracer techniques. Unidirectional fluxes of solutes and water obtained were used to estimate the apparent permeability coefficients of each substance. Table 4-1 summarizes the normal bullfrog lung permeabilities of water and some hydrophilic solutes. All the permeability values were corrected for unstirred layer effects.[46,47] The last two columns of Table 4-1 contain the normalized permeabilities (P) and free diffusion coefficients (D) in reference to 2-deoxyglucose. These data suggest that the alveolar epithelial barrier offers significant resistance to the passive permeation of solutes and water. This, in turn, favors a very restricted passage of solutes and water leaking from the lung interstitial and vascular spaces into the alveolar air space. It can be noted that the permeability properties of the bullfrog alveolar epithelium are very similar to those of other tight epithelia such as toad urinary bladder and frog stomach.[48,49]

Equivalent Pore Analysis[11,45,50-52]

We adapted the method described by Durbin et al[48] to estimate the pore radii and the relative fractions of available pore area in bullfrog lung alveolar epithelium. Briefly, it can be shown that for a given population in a porous membrane,

$$PS = D (A_p/dx) f(x) \qquad (1)$$

where S = surface area
   A_p = pore area
   dx = pore length
   x = a/r
   a = solute molecular radius
   r = radius of equivalent, water-filled, cylindrical pores

and the function f(x) is a correction factor which includes the effects of competition of solutes for entry into the pores and restriction offered by the pore wall.[53,54] In order to eliminate the unknowns A_p and dx, PS ratios can be used to obtain

$$P/P' = (D/D') f(x)/f(x') \qquad (2)$$

where ' denotes the values for the reference solute, 2-deoxyglucose.[45] A large pore radius (r_l) is estimated by generating a theoretical curve using equation (2) which best fits the observed values of P/P' for those solutes that appear to primarily traverse the large-pore pathway (2-deoxyglucose to raffinose). By extending the theoretical P/P' for the large pores to smaller molecular radii, the fraction of small solute P/P' due to restricted diffusion through the large pores can be determined and subtracted from the total observed P/P'. The small pore radius (r_s) is then determined using these "corrected" P/P' and equation (2) by finding the best-fit

Table 4-1
Normal Alveolar Epithelial Permeability Properties (Mean ± SE)

Solute	P,cm/s × 10^{-7}	D,cm^2/s × 10^{-6}	a,nm	P/P′	D/D′
Water	369.9 ± 47.0	24.4	0.15	106.2 ± 19.3	3.396
Formamide	190.8 ± 22.7	16.1	0.21	51.04 ± 9.70	2.241
Acetamide	154.2 ± 18.5	14.1	0.24	41.26 ± 7.87	1.957
Urea	17.89 ± 2.36	13.8	0.24	4.785 ± 0.950	1.918
Ethylene glycol	96.18 ± 6.13	11.5	0.25	25.73 ± 4.15	1.594
Glycerol	23.07 ± 6.10	9.40	0.30	6.171 ± 1.871	1.308
Erythritol	7.519 ± 1.069	8.00	0.35	2.011 ± 0.413	1.114
2-Deoxyglucose	3.738 ± 0.553	7.18	0.36	1.000 ± 0.209	1.000
Mannitol	3.395 ± 0.342	6.82	0.43	0.908 ± 0.163	0.949
Sucrose	2.381 ± 0.272	5.23	0.52	0.637 ± 0.119	0.727
Raffinose	1.771 ± 0.160	4.34	0.61	0.474 ± 0.082	0.604

theoretical relationship for those solutes that primarily traverse the small pore pathway (water to erythritol). Figure 4-4 shows the theoretical (solid line) and observed solute and water permeabilities plotted against molecular radius for normal bullfrog lung alveolar epithelium. Theoretical permeabilities were calculated using equation (2), while the squared error between theoretical and observed permeabilities was minimized to obtain the best-fit pore radii. The large pore radius is about 5.15 nm in the normal lung, where these pores occupy only 4% of the total pore area. The small pore radius is approximately 0.5 nm, occupying the remaining pore area (96%). The ratio N_s/N_1 (number of small pores/number of large pores) calculated from these pore radii and fractional pore areas is 2680. Our findings can be compared with several reports of heteropore characteristics in other epithelial barriers. Frog and canine gastric mucosae are functionally equivalent to a membrane possessing a major population (93% of total pore area) of small pores (r = 0.25 nm) and a small population of larger pores (radius 6.0 nm).[48] Small intestine,[55] gallbladder,[56,57] urinary bladder,[57] and choroid plexus[57] have been reported to exhibit similar heteropore properties. These heteropore characteristics are not confined to epithelia alone, since they have also been demonstrated in capillaries.[58]

Passive Water Fluxes[11,52]

Hydrostatically and osmotically driven water fluxes across bullfrog alveolar epithelium have been measured. Water fluxes were determined under control conditions and under three experimental conditions (metabolic inhibition by 1 mmol/L DNP; low temperature (2°C), and half-isosmotic media in the pleural bath) that would be expected to cause increases in intracellular volume in the alveolar epithelium. A summary of the effects of the three experimental maneuvers on hydrostatic (L_{ph}) and osmotic (L_{po}) hydraulic conductivities is as follows. The control values

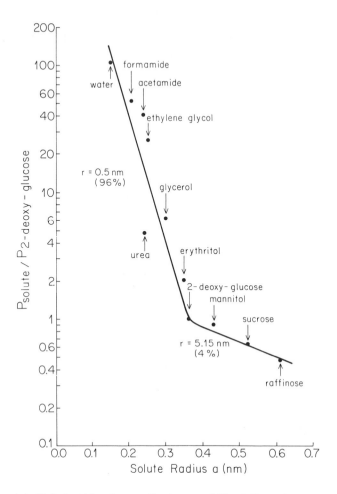

Figure 4-4 Relationship of normalized permeability P/P′ and molecular radius a for water and hydrophilic solutes in normal bullfrog lung alveolar epithelium. Lines shown are those obtained theoretically using r values that lead to minimum squared error between observed and theoretical permeabilities. Small pores occupy 96% of available pore area. Large pores occupy 4% of available pore area. (Reproduced with permission from *J Appl Physiol.*[45])

of L_{ph} and L_{po} are 2.14×10^{-10} mL/dyne-s and 3.65×10^{-12} ml/dyne-s, respectively. Decreasing temperature to 2°C had the greatest effect, reducing L_{ph} by 92.4% of the control value. One mmol/L DNP and hyposmotic media had approximately the same effect; control L_{ph} was decreased by 76.7% and 83.0%, respectively. Similar to the hydrostatic pressure experiments, decreased temperature diminished L_{po} to the greatest extent. However, the cold environment led to a decrease in L_{po} of 58.7%, a reduction which was less than the 92.4% reduction in L_{ph}. The percent decrease in L_{po} caused by 1 mM DNP and hyposmolality were also smaller than the corresponding decrease in L_{ph}, and were 55.5% and 33.6%, respectively.

The finding that L_{ph} always decreased more than L_{po} when the lungs were exposed to all three of the experimental conditions suggests that increased cell volume primarily causes increased resistance to water flow in the paracellular pathway, with a smaller effect taking place in the transcellular pathway. An increase in epithelial cell volume would cause increased path length and increased resistance to osmotically driven water flow. However, increased epithelial cell volume would also likely lead to altered (narrowed or more tortuous) lateral intercellular spaces and increased resistance to hydrostatically driven water flow. Consistent with these speculations are recent morphologic findings of major alterations in the anatomy of lateral intercellular spaces of gallbladder (with relatively minor changes in other cell characteristics) after short term (less than 60 minutes) exposure to hypotonic media.[59]

Interestingly, L_{ph} is always two to three orders of magnitude greater than L_{po}. This phenomenon has been observed previously in a number of tissues, including squid axon,[60] gastric mucosa,[61] and goat rumen.[62] The most likely explanation is that hydrostatically and osmotically driven water fluxes utilize different pathways when biological tissues have a heterogeneous population of pores. Hydrostatically driven water flux would utilize larger pores effectively, whereas a small pore population would be more important for osmotically driven water flux. Recently, van Os et al[63] suggested, based on data obtained using very small Δp across gallbladder, that hydrostatic water flow occurs predominantly through a paracellular pathway whereas osmotic water flow takes place primarily transcellularly. These observations that $L_{po} \neq L_{ph}$ suggest that the use of Starling's equation for fluid flux across biological barriers is not generally applicable.

The results for exposure to hyposmotic fluid may be of particular importance in relation to changes in the alveolar epithelial barrier following near-drowning in fresh water. In previous studies,[64,65] it was found that intratracheal instillation of fresh water leads to morphologic changes in the alveolar epithelium, including swelling of the epithelial cells. It has also been reported that adult respiratory distress syndrome[66,67] and pulmonary edema[67] frequently develop after fresh water near-drowning. These findings make it attractive to speculate that, after near-drowning in fresh water, swelling of the alveolar epithelial cells may slow fluid absorption and help to prevent vascular overload. As a consequence, however, cell swelling could also retard clearance of the alveolar fluid and perhaps lead to prolonged impairment of gas exchange.

Passive Ion Permeability Characteristics
of Bullfrog Alveolar Epithelium[68]

It has been shown[10] that the bullfrog alveolar surface (apical) is slightly anion-selective ($P_{Na}+/P_{Cl}- = 0.53$). Biionic potential measurements[68] performed on inactive tissues (2 mmol/L ouabain) yielded permeability sequences of the apical surface of the bullfrog lung alveolar epithelium. The anionic sequence is $SCN^- : NO_3^- : Br^- : I^- : Cl^- : ClO_4^- :$ isethionate$^- $: gluconate$^- = 1.12 : 1.07 : 1.05 : 1.05 : 1 : 0.89 : 0.29 : 0.25$. The cationic sequence is $K^+ : Rb^+ : Cs^+ : Na^+ : Li^+ = 1.51 : 1.46 : 1.42 : 1 : 0.82$. The data suggest that passive cation flux occurs via sites with intermediate field strength.[69] The anions, on the other hand, traverse the barrier in a relatively nonselective fashion, except for slow permeation by gluconate and isethionate ions.

Pathways for Transport Across Bullfrog
Alveolar Epithelium[45,70]

The presence of multiple pathways in bullfrog alveolar epithelium has major implications for the bulk flow of water across this barrier. If we assume that laminar flow occurs through both large and small pores in response to a hydrostatic pressure gradient (Δp), the ratio of hydrostatically driven water flow (J_{vh}) through the large pores to that through the small pores is:

$$J_{vh,l}/J_{vh,s} = N_l r_l^4/N_s r_s^4 = 4.2 \qquad (3)$$

where l and s represent large and small pores, respectively. Thus, for bullfrog alveolar epithelium, about 80% of the hydrostatically driven flow normally takes place through the 5.15 nm pores, even though they account for only 4% of the total available pore area. Under these circumstances, the measured hydraulic conductivity reflects primarily the effect of the large pores in the alveolar epithelium.

In order to estimate the distribution of osmotically driven water flow across the alveolar epithelium, we must first estimate the reflection coefficients (σ) for an osmotically active particle for both the large and small pores. These reflection coefficients can be estimated using the theoretical relationship[54,71]:

$$\sigma = 5.333 \, x^2 - 6.667 \, x^3 + 2.333 \, x^4 \qquad (4)$$

where $x = a/r$ as above. Using equation (4), $\sigma_{raffinose} = 0.99$ and 0.06 for $r = 0.5$ and 5.15 nm, respectively. Then, if water flow (J_{vo}) due to an osmotic pressure gradient ($\Delta \pi$) is also laminar:

$$J_{vo,l}/J_{vo,s} = N_l r_l^4 \sigma_l/N_s r_s^4 \sigma_s = 0.25 \qquad (5)$$

As can be seen, under these assumptions, the dominant pathway for hydrostatically driven water flow is the large pore population, while osmotically driven water flow occurs predominantly through the small pores in the bullfrog alveolar epithelium.

One implication resulting from the considerations above is that the two apparent overall hydraulic conductivities (L_{ph} and L_{po}) may be markedly different in heteroporous biological tissues. Using a modification of an equation given by Vargas,[60] we can show that:

$$L_{ph}/L_{po} = \sigma_c(1 + [N_l r_l^4/N_s r_s^4])/\{\sigma_s(1 + [N_l r_l^4 \sigma_l/N_s r_s^4 \sigma_s])\} = 3.6 \quad (6)$$

where σ_c ($= 0.866$) is the apparent composite reflection coefficient for the tissue.[47] Such inequality of L_{ph} and L_{po} has been observed experimentally in numerous biological tissues,[4,60-62] although the magnitude of the ratio is greater than that predicted theoretically. It becomes apparent from this discussion that, depending upon the specific definitions of the various parameters and the solutes used, application of Starling's equation, $J_v = L_p (\Delta p - \sigma \Delta \pi)$, to biological tissue barriers should be undertaken only with considerable caution.

Effects of Lung Inflation[51]

We measured the transport of solutes and water across bullfrog lungs at different volumes. In some experiments, two lungs from the same animal were used simultaneously (5 mL and 50 mL). In other experiments, one lung was studied at 50 mL and the other lung was overstretched by inflation to greater than 80 mL for 15 minutes before emptying and reinflation to 50 mL. The results of these studies revealed no differences in both bioelectric and permeability properties between the 5 mL lungs and the 50 mL lungs. However, there were large increases in permeability for overinflated lungs as compared to control lungs. Our speculation is that the lung alveolar epithelium depleats as it is inflated within the physiologic range,[72] after which tight junctions and perhaps cell membranes are irreversibly damaged by increasing tension within the plane of the epithelium. These results suggest that alveolar epithelial leakiness is not likely to be increased by the use of positive end-expiratory pressure (PEEP) in vivo.

Effects of Acid Exposure[45,50]

$P_{acid}/P_{control}$ v time of exposure to pH 2.0 is plotted in Figure 4-5. Water permeability did not change significantly even after up to 60 minutes of exposure. Exposure to pH 2 for 60 minutes leads to an apparent single pore radius of 27 nm in bullfrog alveolar epithelium.[45] The increases in P_{solute} after acid exposure are generally comparable to mammalian lung data.[73-76] There is a remarkable similarity in the threshold pH (below

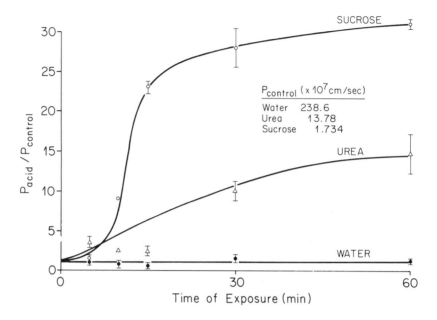

Figure 4-5 $P_{acid}/P_{control}$ of solutes and water v time of acid exposure of bullfrog alveolar epithelium to pH 2.0. P_{acid} denotes permeability after lung was exposed to acid; $P_{control}$ represents permeability of paired control lung. Note that $P_{acid}/P_{control}$ for urea and sucrose appear to reach steady values after about 45 to 50 minutes of acid exposure. $P_{acid}/P_{control}$ for water did not change with acid exposure for up to 60 minutes. pH of serosal fluid remained approximately 8.0 throughout experiments. (Reproduced with permission from *J Appl Physiol.* [50])

which changes in P occur) in the mammalian lung preparations and in our studies on bullfrog alveolar epithelium.

The initial alteration in alveolar epithelial transport properties after acid contacts the alveolar surface appears to be damage to its active transport mechanisms.[50] The increase in tissue conductance and solute permeability with time of exposure to acid suggests increasing leakiness of the intercellular tight junctions, such that at 60 minutes of exposure to pH 2, no effective barrier to solute flow remains. However, the diffusion of water did not increase after acid exposure. This rather peculiar result may be due to the fact that the normal small pore population (r = 0.5 nm) remains more or less intact, while the large pore population (r = 5.15 nm) increases to 27 nm. Our observation of progressive leakiness of the acid-damaged alveolar epithelium may be related to the development of alveolar flooding after aspiration of gastric contents.

Unidirectional Fluxes of Macromolecules
Across Alveolar Epithelium

We have performed preliminary measurements of radiolabel flux after ^{14}C-bovine serum albumin is placed on one side of the tissue. Flux data[25] across the short-circuited bullfrog lung are as follows. The apparent permeability of albumin estimated for the alveolar to the pleural direction is 2.3 (± 3.2) $\times$ 10^{-7} cm/s, about an order of magnitude greater than that for a much smaller polysaccharide, methylhydroxy inulin (3.1 $\times$ 10^{-8} cm/s). The apparent permeability in the pleural to alveolar direction, 5.23 (± 1.4) $\times$ 10^{-8} cm/s, is slightly larger than that for inulin. For comparison, in a typical leaky epithelium such as rabbit gallbladder, the albumin permeability is less than 10^{-8} cm/s, while inulin permeability is 2.9 $\times$ 10^{-6} cm/s, and the permeability for a dextran (molecular weight range 15,000 to 17,000) is 1.02 $\times$ 10^{-6} cm/s.[77] Inulin (5000 daltons) permeability has been reported as 1.2 $\times$ 10^{-7} cm/s and dextran (60,000 to 90,000 daltons) has been found to have a permeability of 8 $\times$ 10^{-8} cm/s in the saline-filled dog lung.[24]

Preliminary data on radiolabel flux indicate that there are no significant differences among apparent permeability values obtained with any given transepithelial voltage (-20, 0, $+20$ mV) imposed across the tissue.[78] On the other hand, there are significant differences among the apparent permeability values in the two different directions at any given clamping voltage. These data suggest that the transport process for albumin translocation across the alveolar epithelium is not dependent on transepithelial electrical gradient and does not occur by simple restricted diffusion of radiolabeled albumin.

The mechanisms for these large and asymmetric fluxes of bovine serum albumin across the alveolar epithelial barrier remain to be determined. These preliminary findings suggest that there is a specialized transport pathway for the translocation of radiolabel across the barrier. The presence of asymmetric and large flows of plasma protein may play a significant role in the pathogenesis and resolution of alveolar pulmonary edema.

REFERENCES

1. Olver RE, Davis B, Marin MG, et al: Active transport of Na^+ and Cl^- across the canine tracheal epithelium *in vitro*. *Am Rev Respir Dis* 1975;112:811–815.
2. Ussing HH, Zerahn K: Active transport of sodium as the source of electric current in the short-circuited isolated frog skin. *Acta Physiol Scand* 1951; 23:110–127.
3. Knowles MR, Buntin WH, Bromberg PA, et al: Measurements of transepithelial electric potential differences in the trachea and bronchi of human subjects *in vivo*. *Am Rev Respir Dis* 1982;126:108–112.

4. Widdicombe JH, Ueki IF, Bruderman I, et al: The effects of sodium substitution and ouabain on ion transport by dog tracheal epithelium. *Am Rev Respir Dis* 1979;120:385-392.

5. Boucher RC, Stutts MJ, Gatzy JT: Regional differences in bioelectric properties and ion flow in excised canine airways. *J Appl Physiol* 1981;51:706-714.

6. Olver RE: Fetal lung liquids. *Fed Proc* 1977;36:2669-2675.

7. Olver RE, Ramsden CA, Strang LB: Adrenaline induced changes in net lung liquid volume flow across the pulmonary epithelium of the foetal lamb: evidence for active sodium transport, abstracted. *J Physiol* 1981;319:38P.

8. Adamson TM, Boyd RDH, Platt HS, et al: Composition of alveolar liquid in the foetal lamb. *J Physiol* 1969;204:159-168.

9. Olver RE, Strang LB: Ion fluxes across the pulmonary epithelium and the secretion of lung liquid in the foetal lamb. *J Physiol* 1974;241:327-357.

10. Gatzy JT: Bioelectric properties of the isolated amphibian lung. *Am J Physiol* 1967;213:425-431.

11. Crandall ED, Kim K-J: Transport of water and solutes across bullfrog alveolar epithelium. *J Appl Physiol* 1981;50:1263-1271.

12. Goodman BE, Crandall ED: Dome formation in primary cultured monolayers of alveolar epithelial cells. *Am J Physiol* 1982;243:C96-C100.

13. Mason RJ, Williams MC, Widdicombe JH, et al: Transepithelial transport by pulmonary alveolar Type II cells in primary culture. *Proc Natl Acad Sci USA* 1982;79:6033-6037.

14. Brown SES, Goodman BE, Crandall ED: Type II alveolar epithelial cells in suspension: separation by density and velocity. *Lung* 1984;162:271-280.

15. Misfeldt DS, Hamamoto ST, Pitelka DR: Transepithelial transport in cell culture. *Proc Natl Acad Sci USA* 1976;73:1212-1216.

16. Cereijido M, Robbins ES, Dolan WJ, et al: Polarized monolayers formed by epithelial cells on a permeable and translucent support. *J Cell Biol* 1978;77:853-880.

17. Goodman BE, Fleischer RS, Crandall ED: Evidence for active Na^+ transport by cultured monolayers of pulmonary alveolar epithelial cells. *Am J Physiol* 1983;245:C78-C83.

18. Goodman BE, Brown SES, Crandall ED: Regulation of transport across pulmonary alveolar epithelial cell monolayers. *J Appl Physiol* 1984;57:703-710.

19. Field M: Ion transport in rabbit ileal mucosa II. Effects of cyclic AMP. *Am J Physiol* 1971;221:992-997.

20. Beck NP, Reed SW, Murdough HV, et al: Effects of catecholamines and their interaction with other hormones on cAMP of kidney. *J Clin Invest* 1972;51:939-944.

21. Sugahara K, Caldwell JH, Mason RJ: Electrical currents flow out of domes formed by cultured epithelial cells. *J Cell Biol* 1984;99:1541-1546.

22. Goodman BE, Crandall ED: Permeability of cultured monolayers of Type II alveolar epithelial cells to inulin, abstracted. *Fed Proc* 1984;43:829.

23. Matthay MA, Widdicombe JH, Staub NC: Clearance of alveolar fluid in sheep may involve an active transport process, abstracted. *Fed Proc* 1982;41:1244.

24. Theodore J, Robin ED, Gaudio R, et al: Transalveolar transport of large polar solutes (sucrose, inulin and dextran). *Am J Physiol* 1975;229:989-996.

25. Kim K-J, LeBon TR, Shinbane JS, Crandall ED: Asymmetric ^{14}C-albumin transport across bullfrog alveolar epithelium. *J Appl Physiol* 1985, in press.

26. Crandall ED, Heming TA, Palombo RL, Goodman BE: Effects of terbutaline on sodium transport in isolated perfused rat lung. *J Appl Physiol* 1985, in press.

27. Crandall ED, Palombo RL, Goodman BE: Transport of sodium across the alveolocapillary barrier is increased by terbutaline, abstracted. *Clin Res* 1984;32:528A.
28. Normand ICS, Reynolds EOR, Strang LB: Passage of macromolecules between alveolar and interstitial spaces in foetal and newly ventilated lungs of the lamb. *J Physiol* 1970;210:151–164.
29. Taylor AE, Gaar KA: Estimation of equivalent pore radii of pulmonary capillary and alveolar membranes. *Am J Physiol* 1970;218:1133–1140.
30. Chinard FP, Enns T, Nolan MF: The permeability characteristics of the alveolar capillary barrier. *Trans Assoc Am Physicians* 1962;75:253–262.
31. Egan EA, Nelson RM, Olver RE: Lung inflation and alveolar permeability to non-electrolytes in the adult sheep *in vivo*. *J Physiol* 1976;260:409–424.
32. Taylor AE, Guyton AC, Bishop VS: Permeability of the alveolar membrane to solutes. *Circ Res* 1965;16:353–362.
33. Schneeberger-Keeley EE, Karnovsky MJ: The ultrastructural basis of alveolar-capillary membrane permeability to peroxidase used as a tracer. *J Cell Biol* 1968;37:781–793.
34. Pietra GG, Szidon JP, Leventhal MM, et al: Hemoglobin as a tracer in hemodynamic pulmonary edema. *Science* 1969;166:1643–1646.
35. Schneeberger EE, Karnovsky MJ: The influence of intravascular fluid volume on the permeability of newborn and adult mouse lungs to ultrastructural protein tracers. *J Cell Biol* 1971;49:319–334.
36. Marinkovich VA, Klein RG: Immunologic characterization of a lung surfactant preparation. *Am Rev Respir Dis* 1972;105:229–235.
37. Hurst DJ, Kilburn KH, Lynn WS: Isolation and surface activity of soluble alveolar components. *Respir Physiol* 1973;17:72–80.
38. King RJ, Klass DJ, Gikas EG, et al: Isolation of apoproteins from canine surface active material. *Am J Physiol* 1973;224:788–795.
39. Klass DJ: Immunochemical studies of the protein fraction of pulmonary surface active material. *Am Rev Respir Dis* 1973;107:784–789.
40. Reifenrath R, Zimmerman I: Blood plasma contamination of the lung alveolar surfactant obtained by various sampling techniques. *Respir Physiol* 1973;18:238–248.
41. Scarpelli EM, Wolfson DR, Colacicco G: Protein and lipid protein fractions of lung washing. Immunological characterization. *J Appl Physiol* 1973;34:750–753.
42. Tuttle WC, Westerberg SC: Alpha$_1$ globulin trypsin inhibitor in canine surfactant protein. *Proc Soc Exp Biol Med* 1974;146:232–235.
43. Bignon J, Chahinian P, Feldman G, et al: Ultrastructural immunoperoxidase demonstration of autologous albumin in the alveolar capillary membrane and in the alveolar lining material in normal rats. *J Cell Biol* 1975;64:503–509.
44. Bignon J, Jaurand MC, Pinchon MC, et al: Immunoelectron microscopic and immunochemical demonstrations of serum proteins in the alveolar lining material of the rat lung. *Am Rev Respir Dis* 1976;113:109–120.
45. Kim K-J, Crandall ED: Heteropore populations of bullfrog alveolar epithelium. *J Appl Physiol* 1983;54:140–146.
46. Dainty J: Water relations of plant cells. *Adv Bot Res* 1963;1:279–326.
47. House CR: *Water Transport in Cells and Tissues*. Monograph of the Physiological Society (No. 24), London, Edward Arnold, 1974.
48. Durbin RP, Frank H, Solomon AK: Water flow through frog gastric mucosa. *J Gen Physiol* 1956;39:535–551.

49. Hays RM: Independent pathways for water and solute movement across the cell membrane. *J Membr Biol* 1972;10:367-371.
50. Kim K-J, Crandall ED: Effects of exposure to acid on alveolar epithelial water and solute transport. *J Appl Physiol* 1982;52:902-909.
51. Kim K-J, Crandall ED: Effects of lung inflation on alveolar epithelial solute and water transport properties. *J Appl Physiol* 1982;52:1498-1505.
52. Schaeffer JD, Kim K-J, Crandall ED: Effects of cell swelling on fluid flow across alveolar epithelium. *J Appl Physiol* 1984;56:72-77.
53. Renkin EM: Filtration, diffusion, and molecular sieving through porous cellulose membranes. *J Gen Physiol* 1954;38:225-243.
54. Levitt DG: General continuum analysis of transport through pores. *Biophys J* 1975;15:533-551.
55. Loehry CA, Axon ATR, Hilton PJ, et al: Permeability of the small intestine to substances of different molecular weight. *Gut* 1970;11:466-470.
56. Smulders AP, Wright EM: The magnitude of nonelectrolyte selectivity in the gall bladder epithelium. *J Membr Biol* 1971;5:297-318.
57. Wright EM, Pietras RJ: Routes of nonelectrolyte permeation across epithelial membranes. *J Membr Biol* 1974;17:293-312.
58. Parker JC, Parker RE, Granger DN, et al: Vascular permeability and transvascular fluid and protein transport in the dog lung. *Circ Res* 1981;48:549-561.
59. Bundgaard M, Zeuthen T: Structure of necturus gallbladder epithelium during transport at low external osmolarities. *J Membr Biol* 1982;68:97-105.
60. Vargas FF: Filtration coefficient of axon membranes as measured with hydrostatic and osmotic methods. *J Gen Physiol* 1968;51:13-27.
61. Moody FG, Durbin RP: Water flow induced by osmotic and hydrostatic pressure in the stomach. *Am J Physiol* 1969;217:255-261.
62. Engelhardt WV: Movement of water across the rumen epithelium, in Phillipson AT (ed): *Physiology of Digestion and Metabolism in the Ruminant.* Newcastle, Oriel Press, 1970, pp 132-146.
63. Van Os CH, Wiedner G, Wright EM: Volume flow across gall bladder epithelium induced by small hydrostatic and osmotic gradients. *J Membr Biol* 1979;49:1-20.
64. Reidboard HE: An electron microscopic study of the alveolar-capillary wall following intratracheal administration of saline and water. *Am J Pathol* 1966;50:275-289.
65. Reidboard HE, Spitz WU: Ultrastructural alterations in rat lungs: changes after intratracheal perfusion with freshwater and sea water. *Arch Pathol* 1966; 81:103-111.
66. Rivers JF, Orr G, Lee HA: Drowning: its clinical sequelae and management. *Br Med J* 1970;2:157-161.
67. Van Harrington JR, Blokzijl EJ, Van Dyl W, et al: Treatment of the respiratory distress syndrome following nondirect pulmonary trauma with positive-end-expiratory pressure, with special emphasis on near-drowning. *Chest* 1974; 66:305-345.
68. Kim K-J, Shinbane JS, Crandall ED: Permeability of apical surface of bullfrog alveolar epithelium to monovalent ions, abstracted. *Fed Proc* 1983;42:1283.
69. Eisenman G: On the elementary atomic origin of equilibrium ionic specificity, in Kleinzeller A, Kotyk A (eds): *Membrane Transport and Metabolism.* New York, Academic Press, 1961, p 163.
70. Kim K-J, Crandall ED: Analysis of distribution of water flow across alveolar epithelium. *AIChE Symposium Ser* 1984;79:70-74.

71. Drake R, Davis E: A corrected equation for the calculation of reflection coefficients, letter. *Microvasc Res* 1978;15:259.
72. Gil J, Bachofen H, Gehr P, et al: Alveolar volume-to-surface area relationship in air- and saline-filled fixed by vascular perfusion. *J Appl Physiol* 1979;47:990-1001.
73. Awe WC, Fletcher WS, Jacob SW: Pathophysiology of aspiration pneumonia. *Surgery* 1966;60:232-239.
74. Glauser FL, Miller JE, Falls R: Effects of acid aspiration on pulmonary alveolar epithelial membrane permeability. *Chest* 1979;76:201-205.
75. Jones JG, Berry M, Hulands GH, et al: The time course and degree of change in alveolar-capillary membrane permeability induced by aspiration of hydrochloric acid and hypotonic saline. *Am Rev Respir Dis* 1978;118:1007-1013.
76. Jones JG, Grossman RF, Berry M, et al: Alveolar capillary membrane permeability: correlation with functional, radiographic, and post-mortem changes after fluid aspiration. *Am Rev Respir Dis* 1979;120:399-410.
77. Van Os CH, de Jong MD, Slegers JFG: Dimensions of polar pathways through rabbit gallbladder epithelium. *J Membr Biol* 1974;15:363-382.
78. Crandall ED, Kim K-J: Net albumin flux out of alveolar fluid due to asymmetric transport across alveolar epithelium, abstracted. *Am Rev Respir Dis* 1984;129:A345.

5 Assessment of Permeability of the Distal Pulmonary Epithelium

Richard M. Effros
Gregory R. Mason

The structure of the mammalian alveolar-capillary barrier must be considered one of the most remarkable products of biological evolution. Gas exchange has been optimized by reducing the thickness of the cells which constitute this barrier to what may well be an absolute minimum, particularly among smaller mammals.[1] Less appreciated is the effectiveness with which these membranes resist the movement of solutions. For example, Wangensteen et al[2] estimated that the permeability of the rabbit alveolar epithelium to sucrose is 1.3×10^{-8} cm/s, and there is reason to believe that this estimate is excessive by a factor of four (see below). This suggests that despite its attenuated structure, the pulmonary epithelium of this species is 100 times less permeable to this extracellular solute than the epithelium of the frog lung[3] or turtle lung.[4] Kim and Crandall[5] found evidence for a population of large pores 5.15 nm in diameter in normal frog lungs which do not seem to be present in prenatal lambs, before birth, or newborn lambs at 12 hours after birth.[6] The resistance of the epithelium of the alveoli to the movement of extracellular solutes presumably inhibits the flow of fluids into the alveolar spaces, an event which would imperil gas exchange.

Development of methods for measuring pulmonary epithelial permeability has been motivated by the recognition that noncardiogenic pulmonary edema and interstitial lung disease are frequently associated with a variety of injuries to this membrane. Over the past decade, these procedures have progressed from experimental techniques in animals to a clinically useful tool for detecting alterations in the integrity of the pulmonary epithelium (see recent review[7]). Although measurements are made in these studies of the movement of indicators across the interstitium and endothelium as well as the epithelium, there is good reason to believe that it is primarily the epithelium which resists the movement of extracellular, lipophobic solutes, including most ions, sugars, and macromolecules.[7] In distinct contrast to gases, such substances penetrate cellular membranes very slowly and must presumably diffuse along the same intercellular and perhaps pinocytotic routes through which solutes and water flow during edema formation.

Procedures for measuring pulmonary epithelial permeability can be conveniently divided into those which require instillation of labeled solutions into the airway and those which are based upon inhalation of radioaerosols. Some of the advantages and disadvantages of these approaches are briefly reviewed in this chapter, with emphasis upon recent studies conducted in our laboratory.

INSTILLATION PROCEDURES

Advantages and Disadvantages

In these procedures, fluid containing a variety of indicators is directly instilled into the airways and the disappearance of these indicators from the airway fluid or their subsequent appearance in the blood is monitored. Blood concentrations of indicators are more difficult to interpret than airway concentrations because indicators can diffuse out of the systemic vessels into the peripheral tissues or be lost in urine, bile or other secretions. This problem can be solved if (1) the lungs are isolated and perfused, (2) a second indicator with the same properties as that introduced into the airway fluid is injected directly into the perfusion fluid and its subsequent loss is determined, or (3) the appearance of the indicators in the pulmonary vein is determined before recirculation. The diffusion of extracellular indicators is much too slow to permit the last approach and most of these experiments have been conducted with the first, and, to a lesser extent, with the second procedure.

Among the advantages of the instillation approach are the following features: (1) multiple indicators can be readily incorporated into the instillate, (2) most of the fluid should enter the exchange area of the lungs, and (3) radioactive exposure can be kept to a minimum. On the other hand, (1) the procedure may interfere with gas exchange or produce lung injury and/or infection, (2) it would be difficult to determine regional permeability in this way, and (3) the movement of indicators across the alveolar surface could be influenced by diffusion within the instillate. Although the first two problems may to some extent be unavoidable, the third can be resolved through the use of a simple model which can also be used to derive an estimate of the alveolar surface area involved in exchange.

A Model of Alveolar Exchange

Diffusion of indicators through unstirred layers is a common problem in studies of epithelial permeability. For example, when epithelial membranes are mounted in Ussing chambers, consideration must be given to the delay associated with diffusion through the relatively stagnant layer of fluid immediately adjacent to the membrane surface.[8] Mixing is considerably more difficult to attain in a structure as complex as the mammalian lung and studies within Ussing chambers have been confined to amphibian lungs, which are much less intricate but may have different permeability properties. Because mixing is probably negligible in the alveoli of fluid-filled mammalian lungs, delivery of solute molecules to the alveolar walls is probably dependent upon diffusion rather than convection. By considering diffusion in a comparable theoretical model, some insight can be gained concerning the potential delay in exchange which may be imposed by diffusion through the alveolar fluid. These calculations suggest that even in the absence of convection, solute concentrations within individual alveoli remain uniform.

Since the alveoli contain two thirds of the lung volume,[9] it is likely that much of the fluid instilled into the lungs comes into contact with the alveolar epithelium. Exchange between fluid within the alveoli and the surrounding blood can be modeled by assuming that the alveolus is shaped like a sphere with radius a. Solutes diffuse from this sphere through a thin epithelial barrier into the bloodstream which surrounds the membrane. The model does not take into account the fact that the capillary phase is not continuous but estimates of the capillary density are not far from this. For example, it has been estimated that as much as 90% of the alveolar wall is covered with capillaries.[10] Nor does this model permit solute concentrations in the blood to increase. This problem can be minimized by studying transport at an early time, before blood levels have increased appreciably.

Expressed mathematically, if C_i is the concentration of the indicator initially placed within the alveolus, $C_s(t,a)$ is the concentration at the alveolar surface and $C(t,r)$ the concentration at a distance, r, from the center of the sphere at time, t, then

$$\frac{\partial C(t,r)}{\partial t} = D\left[\frac{\partial^2 C(t,r)}{\partial r^2} + \frac{2\partial C(t,r)}{r\partial r}\right] \qquad (1)$$

$$-D\frac{\partial C(t,a)}{\partial r} = PC_s(t,a) \qquad (2)$$

where P is the permeability (cm/s) of the alveolar wall. The analytical solution of this set of partial differential equations is provided by Crank[11]:

$$\frac{C(t,r)}{C(i)} = \frac{2La}{r} \sum_{n=1}^{\infty} \frac{\exp{(-Db_n^2 t/a^2)} \sin{(b_n r/a)}}{[b_n^2 + L(L-1)] \sin{b_n}} \tag{3}$$

where each value of b_n is a root of the equation:

$$b_n \cot b_n + L - 1 = 0 \tag{4}$$

and

$$L = aP/D \tag{5}$$

If $P = 9.5 \times 10^{-8}$ cm/s (pulmonary epithelial permeability of rabbit epithelium to sodium 22 cations [^{22}Na$^+$] estimated by Wangensteen et al[2]), $a = 4 \times 10^{-3}$ cm (radius of rabbit alveolus),[12] and $D = 1.3 \times 10^{-5}$ cm^2/s,[13] the ratios $C(t,r)/C(i)$ shown in Figure 5-1A are obtained. It will be noted that the concentration remains quite uniform throughout the alveolus because the rate of diffusion of ^{22}Na$^+$ through the epithelium is slow compared to the rate of diffusion in the alveolar fluid. Only when the ratio P/D is increased by approximately 10^4 would a concentration gradient become significant. Thus, the absence of mixing should be of little importance for extracellular solutes such as ^{22}Na$^+$, though it would presumably be of importance for gases dissolved in alveolar fluid, since these rapidly cross the epithelial membranes.

Intuitively, it might be expected that concentration gradients within the alveolus might appear if its dimensions were increased. As indicated in Figure 5-1D, increasing the alveolar radius by a factor of 100 did not result in the appearance of a concentration difference within the alveolus if P/D is constant. This reflects the fact that the surface/volume ratio of the sphere decreases with its size and overall diffusion of the solute into the blood is consequently slowed. Only if both the alveolar diameter and P/D increased could a concentration gradient be expected.

Of course some of the structures into which the fluid is instilled might not be spherical in shape and as a general case, it is instructive to consider exchange with a flat membrane. If s is the thickness of the unstirred layer which is assumed to be present on only one side of the membrane, P_a and P_i are the apparent and real permeabilities of the membrane to the solute and D is the free water diffusion coefficient of the solute, then[8]:

$$\frac{1}{P_a} = \frac{1}{P_i} + \frac{s}{D} \tag{6}$$

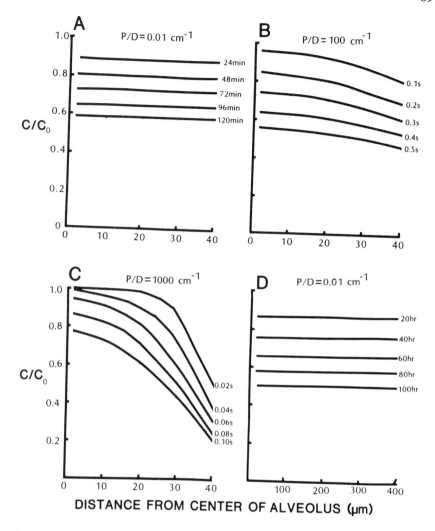

Figure 5-1 Spherical model of solute exchange in a fluid-filled lung. Values of solute concentration (C) at various distances from the center of the alveolus are divided by the original concentration in the instilled fluid (C_0). **A** The value of $P/D = 0.01 \text{ cm}^{-1}$ was calculated from the data of Wangensteen et al[2] for $^{22}Na^+$. Note that concentrations of $^{22}Na^+$ should remain uniform throughout the alveolus. **B** and **C** A decrease in C/C_0 would only become evident if the permeability of the alveolar wall to the solute were increased by a factor of 10,000. **D** Increasing the diameter of the alveolus by a factor of 10 without increasing the epithelial permeability would slow diffusion out of the alveolus and concentrations would remain uniform.

Assuming that P_i for Na^+ is 10^{-7} cm/s and that D of Na^+ is 10^{-5} cm²/s, then the unstirred layer would have to reach 11 cm before the value of P_a would fall to 10% below that of P_i. Thus, even in the absence of mixing, the value of P_i for Na^+ is so small compared to D that concentrations of Na^+ within any collection of fluid in the lung should remain very uniform.

An important advantage of the spherical alveolar model is that measurements of the total surface area of the exchange area of the lungs become unnecessary. All that would be needed is an estimate of average alveolar radius. Since the concentrations of extracellular indicators remain uniform within the alveoli, the calculation of permeability becomes greatly simplified.

$$-PS_a c = V_a \, dc/dt \qquad (7)$$

where S_a and V_a are the surface and volume of the alveolus and c is the concentration of indicator in the alveolar fluid. Since

$$S_a = 4\pi r^2 \qquad (8)$$

$$V_a = (4/3)\pi r^3 \qquad (9)$$

$$c/c_o = \exp(-3Pt/r) \qquad (10)$$

and

$$P = (-r/3t)\ln(c/c_o) \qquad (11)$$

measurements of c must be made before plasma concentrations become significant, but this is generally not a problem since diffusion rates are relatively slow and these experiments are usually terminated within a few hours to avoid deterioration of the preparation.

Another advantage of the alveolar model is that there is no need to assume filling of the entire lobe or lung with fluid. It is only necessary to assume that the alveoli which receive the fluid are completely filled, an assumption which seems to be true in pulmonary edema[14] and may be checked histologically.

We have used equation (11) to analyze some recent studies of $^{22}Na^+$ exchange in fluid-filled rabbit lungs. Sodium 22 cation concentrations in the air-space fluid decreased by approximately 6% over the course of an hour. If an alveolar radius of 40 μm is assumed, then $P = 2.2 \times 10^{-8}$ cm/s. This value is only 25% of that obtained by Wangensteen et al[2] who estimated the total surface area of the rabbit lung by adjusting the total surface area obtained morphometrically in men on the basis of the relative weights of the rabbit and man. Since the alveoli of rabbits are significantly smaller than those in man, this would probably lead to an underestimate of the surface area and a corresponding overestimate of the value of P.

It should be added that more sophisticated models of the shape of a fluid-filled alveolus could be used and a morphometric analysis of a fluid-filled lung would permit derivation of a distribution of alveolar sizes in those regions of the lung which contain fluid.

Are Alveolar Fluid and Solutes Actively Absorbed by the Epithelium?

Evidence has appeared over the past few years suggesting that active transport by the pulmonary epithelium may influence the movement of fluid and electrolytes from the lungs. Data indicating transport of ions and/or fluid from the lungs have been reported in (1) fetal lungs,[15] (2) mammalian airways,[16-20] (3) amphibian lungs,[3,21,22] and (4) cultures of alveolar type II cells.[3,23]

Since active epithelial transport could play a role in the resolution of pulmonary edema, we undertook a study to determine whether ionic fluxes into the air spaces of fluid-filled lungs were different from the corresponding fluxes out of the air-space fluid.[24] These studies were conducted by perfusing in situ rabbit lungs with a buffered 0.1 g/dL albumin solution in a modified Ringer's lactate solution. The air spaces were filled with the same solutions and indicators were placed in either the vascular or air-space fluids. Samples were then taken at intervals from the perfusion solution and at the end of an hour, fluid was pumped from the air spaces into serial sample tubes. The latter procedure permitted us to distinguish between the more proximal fluid which was presumably obtained from the larger airways, and the more distal fluid which was assumed to represent the exchange region of the lung.

Iodine 125 (^{125}I) albumin, $^{22}Na^+$, chlorine 36 anions ($^{36}Cl^-$) and/or carbon 14–urea (^{14}C-urea) were placed in either the perfusion or airway fluid. After instillation into the air spaces, concentrations of ^{125}I albumin rose by an average of about 5%. Since this indicator exchanged across the pulmonary epithelium very slowly, this increase was presumably due to a corresponding absorption of fluid. Transport of solutes was calculated in terms of clearance on the basis of a two-compartment model to compensate for differences in the vascular and airway volumes and changes in compartmental concentrations (see Figure 5-2).[2,25] It will be noted that $^{22}Na^+$, $^{36}Cl^-$, and ^{14}C-urea are cleared from the perfusate at about twice the rate at which they leave the air-space fluid. Furthermore, only about half of the indicators lost from the perfusate could be found in the airway fluid. These observations suggest that when the indicators are placed in

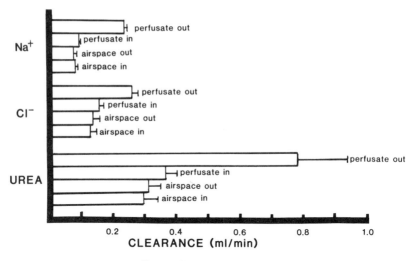

Figure 5-2 Diffusion of $^{22}Na^+$, $^{36}Cl^-$, and ^{14}C-urea between the vascular and alveolar compartments of fluid-filled, in situ lungs. The rate of diffusion was calculated in terms of the clearance of a two-compartment model of exchange.[2,23] For each of these indicators, the rate at which the label left the vascular compartment (perfusate out) exceeded those at which they entered the compartment (perfusate in) or either left or entered the air space volume (air space out and air space in). This suggests that the endothelium is more permeable to these solutes than the epithelium, resulting in the selective diffusion of these solutes from the vasculature into the interstitium. The epithelium was more permeable to urea than to Cl^- and more permeable to Cl^- than to Na^+. The rates at which $^{22}Na^+$ and $^{36}Cl^-$ left the perfusate were similar.

the perfusate, they diffuse into the tissue compartments more readily than when they are placed in the airway fluid. It is obvious that the standard two-compartment model of an air space and a vascular volume is inadequate to describe these experiments — at least one tissue compartment must also be assumed.

More rapid access of indicators from the vascular space to the tissue than from the air-space fluid could mean that either the endothelium is more permeable than the epithelium or the surface area to volume relationship was more favorable in the vasculature than in the airways of these lungs. One finding which suggests that the epithelium is "tighter" than the endothelium is the observation that whereas $^{36}Cl^-$ appears to cross the pulmonary epithelium more rapidly than $^{22}Na^+$, losses of $^{36}Cl^-$ and $^{22}Na^+$ from the perfusate occur at about the same rate. This suggests that the endothelium is less selective to the movement of these ions than the epithelium.

Although losses of $^{22}Na^+$ and $^{36}Cl^-$ from the vasculature were similar after an hour of perfusion, more of the $^{36}Cl^-$ reached the air-space fluid than ^{22}Na$^+$. This also suggests that the epithelium is more selective than the endothelium. When transport across the entire endothelial-epithelial membrane was considered, we could find no evidence that any ion was being transported more in one direction than the other, a phenomenon observed in some epithelial membranes which actively transport ions. Nor was there any tendency for significant changes in the concentrations of unlabeled Na$^+$ or Cl$^-$ in fluid-filled, isolated lungs (see Figure 5-3; a slight concentration of each ion in each compartment may have been related to some evaporation of water from the preparation).

Fluid transport out of the air space of the rabbit lung (as judged by concentration of T-1824 bound to protein) remained very slow even when 10^{-5} molL terbutaline sulfate was added to the preparation. However, when isolated rat lungs were studied in the same fashion, we found evidence for fluid transport out of the air spaces with more substantial increases

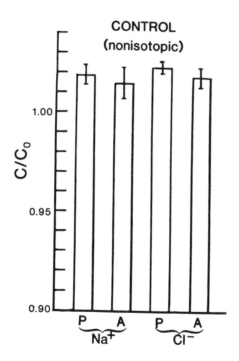

Figure 5-3 Changes in Na$^+$ and Cl$^-$ concentrations of fluid instilled into isolated rabbit lung after one hour of perfusion. In these studies (n = 5), concentration of both Na$^+$ and Cl$^-$ may have increased slightly by about the same extent in both the airway fluid and perfusate (note expanded scale). This may indicate a modest amount of evaporation in the study or generation of osmoles within the tissue and uptake of water from these solutions. No gradients of either ion were measurable across the epithelial barrier.

in concentrations of T-1824 over the course of an hour. Only a small fraction of the fluid leaving the air spaces was found in the perfusate (as judged by the decline in T-1824 in the perfusate) and it seems likely that much of the fluid was retained in the interstitium. This implies that it is the epithelium rather than the endothelium which is responsible for transport. Terbutaline significantly increased the loss of fluid from the air spaces. Since Na^+ and Cl^- concentrations remained unchanged in the air-space fluid, transport of fluid from the rat lung presumably involves the flow of isosmotic fluid across the epithelium. Sodium ions may be actively transported across the epithelium and the resulting positive potential in the interstitium could then drive Cl^- into this compartment. Fluid would then flow into the interstitium in response to the osmotic gradient between the interstitium and air-space fluids. Differences found between the rabbit and rat lungs may presumably be related to differences in the numbers or properties of the type II cells in these organs.

Potential Clinical Applications

Although the instillation procedure of measuring epithelial permeability has been used almost exclusively in animal models, there is no reason it cannot be applied clinically. With the increasing popularity of bronchoalveolar lavage, it should be possible to instill fluid containing as many as four or five indicators of different molecular weight into the bronchus. The loss of each might provide a good index of the integrity of the pulmonary epithelium, would have no effect on cytologic or enzymatic studies and would require minimal radioactive exposure, since the sample recovered from the airways could be counted for long intervals.

RADIOAEROSOL PROCEDURES

Development and Application

The radioaerosol approach to measuring pulmonary epithelial permeability was derived from earlier studies of the distribution of ventilation. Taplin and Hayes and their colleagues[26,27] showed that if the radioaerosol droplets were sufficiently small, they could be used in place of radioactive gases such as xenon 133 (^{133}Xe) to determine the regional distribution of inhaled air within the lungs. The aerosol generated from a simple nebulizer was introduced into a balloon in which settling of larger droplets occurred. More recently a variety of commercial devices have become available which require no balloon and the procedure has become increasingly popular.[28,29] The radioaerosol technique for measuring the distribution of ventilation has two important advantages over gaseous procedures: (1) following deposition, the distribution of radioactivity in the lungs remains relatively constant, permitting multiple views, and (2) the same isotope, technetium 99m (^{99m}Tc), can be used sequentially in both the perfusion and ventilation scans, thereby avoiding artifacts related to different tissue penetration of eg, ^{99m}Tc and ^{133}Xe.

Taplin also suggested to us that if ^{99m}Tc diethylenetriamine pentaacetate (DTPA) were used in the aerosol, pulmonary emboli might be detected without the need for a perfusion scan. He reasoned that if ventilation to a region of the lung were intact, the droplets would be deposited on the pulmonary epithelium. The ^{99m}Tc DTPA would then diffuse into the vasculature from which it would be washed out of the lung by the pulmonary blood flow. If the flow were obstructed by an embolism, then the ^{99m}Tc DTPA would remain near the site of deposition and the presence of an embolism would be signaled by a hot spot. The hot spot could only appear if (1) ventilation to the region was intact and (2) there was no blood flow to the region. This mismatch would be comparable to that characteristically obtained with perfusion and ventilation scans in the presence of pulmonary embolic disease but would require only one scan and the appearance of a hot spot might be more easily visualized than a perfusion cold spot.

Early studies in our laboratory soon showed that this procedure was relatively insensitive to pulmonary embolism because transport of ^{99m}Tc DTPA out of the lung was limited primarily by the time it took for this radionuclide to diffuse across the pulmonary epithelium. The rate of transport was so slow, that even a very much reduced flow rate was sufficient to wash the indicator out of the lungs. Significant reduction in the rate of solute clearance would only be expected if both pulmonary and bronchial blood flows were nearly arrested.[30]

We realized that ^{99m}Tc DTPA radioaerosols might provide an index of pulmonary epithelial permeability and initially studied a group of patients with chronic interstitial lung disease. We expected that thickening of the alveolar capillary membranes would slow solute diffusion but were surprised to find quite the contrary: apparently the characteristic morphologic changes such as replacement of type I cells with type II cells[31] were accompanied by an increase in epithelial permeability. Accelerated clearances of ^{99m}Tc DTPA have been documented in many patients with a variety of chronic interstitial diseases including idiopathic pulmonary fibrosis, progressive systemic sclerosis and some pneumoconioses.[32-34]

It was subsequently shown by Jones and Minty and their colleagues[35,36] that the clearance of ^{99m}Tc DTPA was accelerated by smoking. Rather than using a scintillation camera these investigators utilized a single probe and were able to correct for accumulation of the indicator in the bloodstream by monitoring the appearance of radioactivity over the thigh. We were able to document a diffuse increase in the clearance of radionuclide from the lungs in smokers and confirmed that this abnormality was rapidly reversed when smoking was discontinued.[37]

More recently we have found that the clearance of ^{99m}Tc DTPA is accelerated in most patients with adult respiratory distress syndrome (ARDS) whereas clearances are usually within normal limits in patients with pulmonary edema due to congestive heart failure[38,39]; Royston et al have also found increased clearance rates in patients with noncardiogenic pulmonary edema.[40] Studies by Jeffries et al[41] in neonatal respiratory distress indicate that this disorder is also accompanied by increases in the clearance of ^{99m}Tc DTPA.

Methodologic Considerations

Although the radioaerosol technique has been described in previous articles, a number of technical matters which can improve the quality of these studies are worth stressing:

1. The radioaerosol droplets should be kept below 2 or 3 μm in diameter to minimize central deposition.

2. Because radionuclide clearance tends to slow with time, the loading interval during which the patient inhales the radioaerosol should be no longer than two minutes to minimize overlap of the more rapid with the slower phases of clearance.

3. Slowing of clearance could be due to (a) accumulation of the radionuclide in the blood and interstitium of the lung and chest wall or (b) the presence of a heterogeneous pulmonary epithelium. When the time-concentration curves of ^{99m}Tc DTPA are corrected for accumulation in blood, the curves become more linear suggesting that the first factor is responsible for some of the multiexponential appearance of the uncorrected data.[35,36] It should be understood, however, that it is unlikely that blood concentrations ever become sufficiently high to slow diffusion of the ^{99m}Tc DTPA from the aerosol droplets into the blood since the activity in these droplets is so great. The apparent slowing merely represents accumulation in compartments (blood and interstitium) which are monitored by the scintillation camera.

4. If a specific procedure for correcting for blood and tissue accumulation of ^{99m}Tc DTPA is not employed, the early disappearance of the indicator should be stressed since this will minimize the contribution of counts from activity in the interstitium and blood of the lungs and chest wall.

5. Gamma markers should be placed on the chest to rule out movement artifacts which are particularly likely to be severe at the margins of the lung fields.

6. Radionuclide clearance is best expressed in terms of percentage clearance per minute rather than half-time of clearance. This tends to decrease the variability in the control data.

The term "clearance" is generally used to indicate loss of indicators from the lungs. Strictly speaking, this is not appropriate since the dimensions of clearance are conventionally volume per unit time (mL/min) whereas those of radioaerosol indicator loss are percentage per unit time (%/min). However, convenience and custom will probably prevail and the term will be retained.

Some uncertainty persists regarding the effect of surface area upon aerosol clearances. This is related in part to the question of whether the surfaces reached by the inhaled droplets are wet or dry. As indicated in a previous review,[7] if there is a continuous and uniform layer of fluid covering the epithelium, then the clearance rate would be influenced by the thickness of this layer but not by the fraction of the epithelial surface area reached by the solute. To the extent that acute distention of the alveoli increases the surface area of the lung, the thickness of the fluid layer would presumably become more attenuated and clearance would be increased. Pulmonary distention with positive end-expiratory pressure (PEEP) does increase solute clearance[33] but this could also be related to tension exerted on the interendothelial junctions. In seated patients, clearances are greater in the upper lung regions[33,34] where alveolar dimensions are greater than in inferior regions, but this observation may be influenced by the accumulation of radioactivity in the blood. Since there is more blood in the dependent lung regions of these subjects, apparent solute clearances will be slowed more in the lower lobes when the radioactivity of the blood rises. If the surfaces of the lung are dry, then clearances will presumably be governed by the dimensions of the aerosol droplets deposited on the epithelial membrane (which could be relatively constant) and by whether the droplet had access to an interepithelial junction. The probability of the latter event would be increased if the number of junctions or the diameter of the droplet were increased.

The presence or absence of fluid on the surfaces reached by the aerosol droplets could play an important role in determining whether active transport of fluid and electrolytes by the epithelium would influence the clearance of an indicator molecule such as ^{99m}Tc DTPA. If there is little or no fluid in the region on which the droplet is deposited, then active absorption of the fluid within the droplet would tend to carry the radionuclide molecules across the epithelium ("solvent drag"). If the fluid left the alveolus more rapidly than the radionuclide, radionuclide concentrations would increase and diffusion of the radionuclide out of the air spaces would be enhanced. On the other hand, if the droplet were deposited in a relatively large pool of fluid which remained at a relatively constant volume, then the ability of the epithelium to transport fluid out of the air space would have little effect upon clearance of the radionuclide.

Perhaps the most important advance that could be made in the radioaerosol approach would be the introduction of a second indicator with a molecular weight different from that of ^{99m}Tc DTPA, which was preferably labeled with an alternative isotope. By comparing the clearance of these indicators, it might be possible to obtain information concerning "pore" size that cannot be surmised from data derived from use of a single indicator. Technetium 99m-pertechnetate (^{99m}TcO$_4^-$) has been used for this purpose and as expected, this lower molecular weight indicator is cleared more rapidly than ^{99m}Tc DTPA.[33,34] Furthermore, discrimination between the radionuclides appeared to be decreased in the presence of lung injury, suggesting that the pores were widened and readily accommodated both the small and large indicators.[34] However, we have recently found evidence that some cells in the lungs concentrate the ^{99m}TcO$_4^-$, a factor which could influence the rate of clearance. Selection of an alternative chelate with a different radionuclide would permit data to be obtained with a single procedure and might prove even more helpful in detecting lung injury than the single radionuclide radioaerosol approach.

ACKNOWLEDGMENTS

This study was supported by grants from the National Institutes of Health (NH HL18606) and the Los Angeles Affiliate of the American Heart Association.

REFERENCES

1. Weibel ER: Oxygen demand and the size of the respiratory structures in mammals, in Wood SC, Lenfant C (eds): *Evolution of Respiratory Processes. A Comparative Approach.* New York, Marcel Dekker, Inc, 1979, pp 289–346.
2. Wangensteen OD, Wittmers LE Jr, Johnson JA: Permeability of the mammalian blood-gas barrier and its components. *Am J Physiol* 1969;216:719–727.
3. Crandall ED: Water and nonelectrolyte transport across alveolar epithelium. *Am Rev Respir Dis* 1983;127:S16–S24.
4. Deitchman D, Paganelli CV: Solute movement across the alveolar-capillary membrane of the turtle. *Physiologist* 1964;7:154.
5. Kim JJ, Crandall ED: Heteropore population of bullfrog alveolar epithelium. *J Appl Physiol* 1983;54:140–146.
6. Egan EA: Fluid balance in the air-filled alveolar space. *Am Rev Respir Dis* 1983;127:S37–S39.
7. Effros RM, Mason GR: Measurements of pulmonary epithelial permeability *in vivo. Am Rev Respir Dis* 1983;127:S59–S65.
8. House CR: *Water Transport in Cells and Tissues.* London, E Arnold Ltd, 1974, pp 104–113.
9. Weibel ER: Morphometrics of the lung, in Fenn WO, Rahn H (eds): *Handbook of Physiology. Respiration.* Washington, American Physiological Society, 1964, vol 1, section 3, pp 285–307.
10. Sobin SS, Fung YCB, Tremer AM, et al: Elasticity of the pulmonary alveolar microvascular sheet in the cat. *Circ Res* 1972;30:440–490.

11. Crank J: *The Mathematics of Diffusion,* ed 2. London, Oxford University Press, 1975, p 96.
12. Tenney SM, Remmers JE: Comparative quantitative morphology of mammalian lungs: diffusing areas. *Nature* 1983;197:54-56.
13. Wang JH, Miller S: Tracer diffusion in liquids II. The self-diffusion of sodium ion in aqueous sodium chloride solution. *J Am Chem Soc* 1952;74:1611-1612.
14. Staub NC, Gee M, Vreim C: Mechanism of alveolar flooding in acute pulmonary edema. *Ciba Found Symp 38 (new series): Lung Liquids,* 1976;255-272.
15. Olver RE: Fluid balance across the fetal alveolar epithelium. *Am Rev Respir Dis* 1983;127:S33-S35.
16. Matthay MA, Landolt CC, Staub NC: Differential liquid and protein clearance from the alveoli of anesthetized sheep. *J Appl Physiol* 1982;53:96-104.
17. Marin MG, Davis B, Nadel JA: Effect of acetylcholine on Cl^- and Na^+ fluxes across dog tracheal epithelium in vitro. *Am J Physiol* 1976;231: 1546-1549.
18. Al-Bazzaz FJ, Al-Awqati Q: Interaction between sodium and chloride transport in canine tracheal mucosa. *Am J Physiol* 1979;46:111-119.
19. Frizzell RA, Welsh MJ, Smith PL: Hormonal control of chloride secretion by canine tracheal epithelium: an electrophysiological analysis. *Ann NY Acad Sci* 1981;372:558-569.
20. Boucher RC, Narvarte J, Cotton C, et al. Sodium absorption in mammalian airways, in Quinton PM, Martinex JR, Hofer U (eds): *Fluids and Electrolyte Abnormalities in Exocrine Glands in Cystic Fibrosis.* San Francisco, San Francisco Press, 1982, pp 271-288.
21. Gatzy JT: Bioelectric properties of isolated amphibian lung. *Am J Physiol* 1967;213:425-431.
22. Gatzy JT: Ion transport across excised bullfrog lung. *Am J Physiol* 1975;228:1162-1171.
23. Mason RJ, Williams MC, Widdicombe JH: Fluid and electrolyte transport across monolayers of alveolar type II cells *in vitro. Am Rev Respir Dis* 1983;127:S24-S28.
24. Mason GR, Effros RM: Diffusion of anions and cations between rabbit airways and vessels. *Fed Proc* 1984;43:1028.
25. Taylor AE, Guyton AC, Bishop VS: Permeability of the alveolar membrane to solutes. *Circ Res* 1965;16:353-362.
26. Taplin GV, Chopra SK: Inhalation lung imaging with radioactive aerosols and gases, in Guter M (ed): *Progress in Nuclear Medicine.* Basel, S Karger, 1978, vol 5, pp 119-143.
27. Hayes M, Taplin GV, Chopra SK, et al: Improved radioaerosol administration system for routine inhalation lung imaging. *Radiology* 1979:131-258.
28. Coates G, Dolovich M, Newhouse MT: Evaluation of pulmonary epithelial permeability with submicronic Tc-99mDTPA aerosols. *Radiology* 1983; 149:149(P).
29. Alderson PO, Biello DR, Gottschalk A, et al: Tc-99m-DTPA aerosol and radioactive gases compared as adjuncts to perfusion scintigraphy in patients with suspected pulmonary embolism. *Radiology* 1984;153:515-521.
30. Huchon GJ, Little JW, Murray JF: Assessment of alveolar-capillary membrane permeability of dogs by aerosolization. *J Appl Physiol* 1981;51:955-962.
31. Crystal RJ, Fulmer JD, Roberts W, et al: Idiopathic pulmonary fibrosis. *Ann Intern Med* 1976;85:769-788.
32. Rinderknecht J, Krauthammer M, Uszler JM, et al: Solute transfer across

the alveolar capillary membrane in pulmonary fibrosis. *Am Rev Respir Dis* 1977;115:156.

33. Rinderknecht J, Shapiro L, Krauthammer M, et al: Accelerated clearance of small solutes from the lungs in interstitial lung disease. *Am Rev Respir Dis* 1980;121:105-117.

34. Chopra SK, Taplin GV, Tashkin DP, et al: Lung clearance of soluble radioaerosols of different molecular weight in systemic sclerosis. *Thorax* 1979;34:63-67.

35. Jones JG, Lawler P, Crawley JCW, et al: Increased alveolar epithelial permeability in cigarette smokers. *Lancet* 1980;1:66-67.

36. Minty BD, Jordan C, Jones JG: Rapid improvement in abnormal permeability after stopping smoking. *Br Med J* 1981;282:1184-1186.

37. Mason G, Effros RM, Uszler JM, et al: Rapidly reversible alterations of pulmonary epithelial permeability induced by smoking. *Chest* 1983;83:6-11.

38. Mason G, Uszler JM, Effros RM: Differentiation between hemodynamic and nonhemodynamic pulmonary edema by a scanning procedure. *Am Rev Respir Dis* 1981;123:238.

39. Mason GR, Effros Rm, Uszler JM, et al: Small solute clearance from the lungs of patients with cardiogenic and non-cardiogenic pulmonary edema. *Chest,* in press.

40. Royston D, Minty BD, Lockwood G, et al: An index of the permeability factor (Kep) and pulmonary oedema in man. *Br J Anesth* 1983;55:246P.

41. Jeffries AL, Coates G, O'Brodovich H: Pulmonary epithelial permeability in hyaline-membrane disease. *N Engl J Med* 1984;311:1075-1079.

6 Pulmonary Vasoreactivity in Acute Lung Injury

Charles A. Hales

Adult respiratory distress syndrome (ARDS) describes a clinical and pathologic picture that follows acute lung injury in a variety of settings. Recent evidence has suggested that several of these seemingly diverse modes of lung injury actually have a final common pathway involving complement activation, pulmonary leukostasis, oxygen-free radical release, and stimulation of the arachidonic acid cascade.[1-11] Experimental acute lung injuries that seem to use this sequence are endotoxemia, gram-negative bacteremia, scald burns, exposure of blood to artificial membranes, pulmonary embolism, or activation of leukocytes with phorbol myristate acetate.[1,3-9,14-18] The outcome of this chain of events is changes in both pulmonary vasoreactivity and permeability. This chapter will focus on the changes in vasoreactivity and will primarily examine the changes in acute lung injury occurring in endotoxemia since that is the setting where pulmonary vasoreactivity has been most extensively characterized.

The normal adult lung performs two physiologically important vasomotor functions:

1. It maintains a low pulmonary vascular resistance which largely seems to be related to its anatomy but to some extent is due to the endogenous production of an eicosanoid vasodilator since cyclo-oxygenase inhibition will raise resting tone modestly.[19-21] Possibly other dilators such as adenosine may play a role in maintaining the normal low pulmonary vascular resistance but this is unknown.[22,23] Autonomic fibers traveling with the vagus are also vasodilators but seem to have little influence on resting pulmonary vascular tone.[24]

2. It vasoconstricts locally in response to regional alveolar hypoxia to shift blood flow from poorly ventilated to better ventilated alveoli, thus enhancing ventilation to perfusion ($\dot{V}/\dot{Q}$) balance and gas exchange. Hypercapnia and acidosis also cause pulmonary vasoconstriction but in particular potentiate alveolar hypoxic pulmonary vasoconstriction.[25] The lung can also vasoconstrict to many humoral agonists and it can increase

vascular tone mildly in response to sympathetic discharge as occurs with systemic hypotension.[24] Only alveolar hypoxic vasoconstriction, though, has been found to perform an important physiologic role since loss of alveolar hypoxic vasoconstriction, as occurs in the presence of the vasodilator nitroglycerin, can worsen $\dot{V}/\dot{Q}$ balance and lower arterial oxygen tension (PaO_2) in normal humans over the age of 30 and in subjects with small airways dysfunction by 14 ± 2 mmHg.[26]

The endogenous production of a pulmonary vasodilator eicosanoid may normally be helpful in maintaining a low pulmonary vascular tone, so that right heart work is minimized and the ability of alveolar hypoxic vasoconstriction in a small lung zone is maximized in diverting blood flow to better ventilated, low-resistance, and highly compliant lung vessels elsewhere. At times, however, the production of this eicosanoid vasodilator can become excessive and inhibit hypoxic vasoconstriction as well. Hales et al[19] and Ahmed et al[27] have found in acutely catheterized dogs and sheep, respectively, that cyclo-oxygenase blockade turns poor or weak vasoconstrictors to alveolar hypoxia into vigorous ones. Furthermore, the isolated perfused lung, which necessarily undergoes considerable trauma in preparation, is a poor reactor to alveolar hypoxia in contrast to the in vivo lung. Cyclo-oxygenase blockade will turn it into a vigorous reactor, however, suggesting that either the lung or, less likely its blood perfusate, was the source of the dilator eicosanoid and that the process of preparing the isolated lung turns on the dilator eicosanoid production.[19]

It is also apparent that some of the weak alveolar hypoxic vasoconstriction in different animals apparently due to excessive production of an eicosanoid vasodilator may represent side effects of the experimental procedures involved in measuring alveolar hypoxic vasoconstriction. Dogs with weak alveolar hypoxic vasoconstriction of the kind that can be enhanced with cyclo-oxygenase blockade will spontaneously become vigorous reactors to alveolar hypoxia over four hours' time after line placement and anesthesia.[28] This suggests the excess vasodilator eicosanoid is not continuously present in the weak reactors but is elicited on occasion by the trauma of the experimental protocol or some other unexplained event in the animal's existence that day. Thus, in the noninvaded and nontraumatized animal, the variability in alveolar hypoxic vasoconstriction may or may not be due to excess vasodilator eicosanoid production and may be due to genetics[29] or other factors. Nevertheless, it is apparent that in certain circumstances, endogenous production of a vasodilator eicosanoid, such as prostacyclin, can blunt or prevent alveolar hypoxic vasoconstriction.

Prostacyclin is the major candidate to be the eicosanoid vasodilator as it is a potent pulmonary vasodilator produced from arachidonic acid in the lung as well as in most other organs.[30] In addition, prostacyclin is produced by the lung when it vasoconstricts to hypoxia or other agonists.[31,32] Prostaglandin E$_1$ is the only other known strong lung vasodilator but it is a product of dihomo-γ-linoleic acid and is relatively sparse in the body.[33] Prostaglandin E$_2$ has been reported to be a weak pulmonary vasodilator in man although it is not clear that this effect is not secondary to a rise in cardiac output with passive recruitment of lung vessels.[34,35] In dogs and cats prostaglandin E$_2$ is a weak vasoconstrictor.[35] Thus, the best candidate to be the eicosanoid responsible for blunting pulmonary vasoreactivity is prostacyclin. We therefore correlated arterial levels of 6-keto-prostaglandin F$_{1\alpha}$ (PGF$_{1\alpha}$), the stable metabolite of prostacyclin (as measured by Drs. Myron Peterson and David Watkins) with the *strength* of regional alveolar hypoxic vasoconstriction in anesthetized dogs.

Figure 6-1 is a perfusion scan of a dog lung performed with the positron-emitting isotope nitrogen 13 (^{13}N). The dog is intubated with a double-lumen endotracheal tube which allows independent ventilation of each lung. In the left image both lungs are ventilated wth air. After clearance of the ^{13}N the right lung was ventilated with O$_2$ to maintain systemic normoxia while the left lung was ventilated with nitrogen as a hypoxic challenge. Seven minutes later the perfusion scan on the right was taken. It shows a dramatic decrease in perfusion to the hypoxic lung which occurred in spite of a PaO$_2$ of 89 mmHg and a mixed venous O$_2$ tension

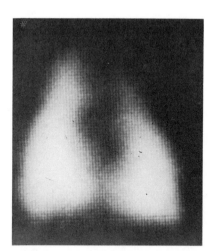 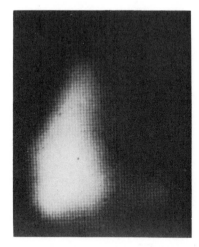

Figure 6-1 Perfusion scans done with nitrogen 13 (^{13}N) and a positron camera in a supine dog with a double-lumened endotracheal tube in place. The scan at left is done while both lungs are ventilated with air while the scan at right is taken seven minutes after ventilation of one lung with N$_2$ and the other with O$_2$ to maintain systemic oxygenation. The decrease in ^{13}N in the hypoxic lung represents less distribution of perfusion to that lung during alveolar hypoxia. (Reproduced with permission from Hales et al.[57])

(PvO$_2$) of 34 mmHg. In most dogs the decrease in perfusion to the hypoxic lung is less dramatic and averages about a 30% reduction compared to the room air perfusion distribution. There are, however, occasional animals with 14% or less decrease in perfusion to the hypoxic lung and these are the ones made more vigorous by cyclo-oxygenase blockage.[19]

Unfortunately, a very poor correlation exists between circulating levels of the metabolite of prostacyclin with the strength of regional hypoxic vasoconstriction (Figure 6-2). The scatter was impressive. However, upon further analysis it is apparent that much of the scatter is in animals with circulating levels of prostacyclin below the limits of detection, which is 50 pg/mL. Indeed in the six dogs wth measurable prostacyclin levels there was a weak or absent reaction to hypoxia in five dogs whereas in the animals with a decrease in perfusion of more than 14% to the hypoxic lung (strong reactors), there was a nondetectable level of the prostacyclin metabolite in all but one ($P < .05$ by Fisher exact test). In addition, in serial studies on three dogs the reactivity of the vessels correlated with

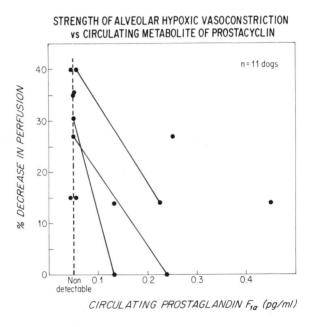

STRENGTH OF ALVEOLAR HYPOXIC VASOCONSTRICTION
vs CIRCULATING METABOLITE OF PROSTACYCLIN

Figure 6-2 Relationship of circulating levels of 6-keto-prostaglandin F$_{1\alpha}$, the stable metabolite of the vasodilator prostacyclin, to the strength of hypoxic pulmonary vasoconstriction. The dashed line represents the lower limits of detection of the radioimmunoassay.[3] In all but one animal with detectable circulating levels of the metabolite of prostacyclin, there is weak alveolar hypoxic vasoconstriction as shown by a ≤14% decrease in perfusion to the hypoxic lung. The three dual points connected by solid lines represent values obtained in the three animals at different times on the same day.

the appearance or disappearance of detectable levels of prostacyclin in the plasma. It is thus possible to see some association between the circulating levels of the prostacyclin metabolite with pulmonary vasoreactivity.

This experience, however, highlights the difficulty in associating any random circulating prostacyclin level with pulmonary vasoreactivity. First, prostacyclin may be much more effective locally where it is produced and thus the overflow into the systemic circulation has a poor correlation with local vasoreactivity. Second, circulating prostacyclin may be physiologically active at levels below the 50 pg/mL level of present reliable detection. Third, any given eicosanoid may be exerting its influence with another simultaneously produced eicosanoid of opposite vasoreactivity. Fourth, prostacyclin itself has a short half-life and thus it is not assayed directly. It is monitored through its metabolite 6-keto-$PGF_{1\alpha}$ which is not vasoactive but has a long half-life. Therefore, a high level of the prostacyclin metabolite 6-keto-$PGF_{1\alpha}$ may reflect ongoing production of active prostacyclin vasodilator but may also reflect persistence of the metabolites without ongoing prostacyclin formation. Prostacyclin is also unique in having another major metabolite besides 6-keto-$PGF_{1\alpha}$ that is an active vasodilator. Nevertheless, it is apparent our understanding of the role of prostacyclin in pulmonary vasoreactivity in acute lung injury requires at least preselected animals with vigorous alveolar hypoxic vasoconstriction and thus likely to have initially low levels of circulating prostacyclin.

With this as a background, we turned to acute lung injury with endotoxin because we were intrigued with the variations in pulmonary vasoreactivity that could be seen with different doses of endotoxin and because of previous demonstrations that shock doses of endotoxin released some of the classic prostaglandins.[37-40] Endotoxin, even at doses of 15 μg/kg, can convert vigorous hypoxic pulmonary vasoconstriction into weak hypoxic vasoconstriction and this conversion has variably been prevented by pretreatment of the animals with cyclo-oxygenase inhibitors.[37-39] Thus, endotoxin seems capable of inducing a vasodilator eicosanoid such as prostacyclin and thus inhibiting alveolar hypoxic vasoconstriction. Indeed, an increase in circulating levels of the prostacyclin metabolite was readily demonstrable when animals with vigorous alveolar hypoxic vasoconstriction and low or nondetectable levels of 6-keto-PGF_1 were treated with endotoxin (Figure 6-3). This rise in prostacyclin metabolite was not associated with any fall in pulmonary vascular resistance perhaps because near maximum vasodilation was already present. It was, however, associated with marked loss of pulmonary vasoconstriction to hypoxia or to the agonists $PGF_{2\alpha}$ or angiotensin II (AII) (Figure 6-4). Indomethacin blocked the appearance of the circulating metabolite of prostacyclin after endotoxin and prevented the loss of vasoreactivity, thus strongly suggesting prostacyclin is indeed the endotoxin-induced eicosanoid responsible for blunting

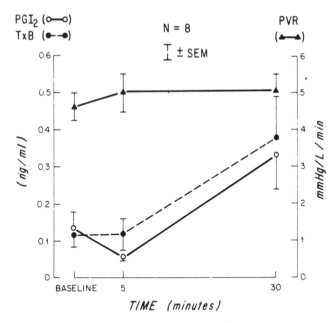

Figure 6-3 The time relationship of circulating levels of prostacyclin (PGI$_2$) and thromboxane (TxB$_2$) with pulmonary vascular resistance before (base line) and at five and 30 minutes after a dose of 15 μg/kg endotoxin. (Reproduced with permission from Hales et al.[3])

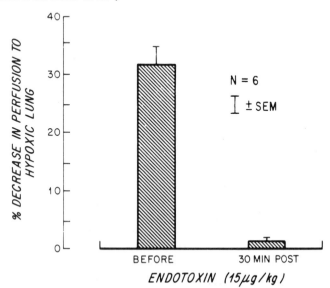

Figure 6-4 Percent decrease in perfusion to the hypoxic lung during unilateral alveolar hypoxia as in Figure 6-1 before and after a minute dose of endotoxin. There is a complete loss of alveolar hypoxic vasoconstriction after endotoxin. (Reproduced with permission from Hales et al.[3])

pulmonary vasoreactivity.[3] This does not prove that prostacyclin is the vasodilator eicosanoid, but it does show its potential to be so. It does show that in response to acute lung injury such as endotoxemia, prostacyclin is released and is probably producing flaccid pulmonary vessels.

After 15 μg/mL of endotoxin, thromboxane B_2 (TxB$_2$), the metabolite of the putative pulmonary vasoconstrictor TxA$_2$, but not the vasoconstrictor PGF$_{2\alpha}$, also rose to a level similar to 6-keto-PGF$_1$ (Figure 6-3). The physiologic effect, however, favored the vasodilator prostacyclin.

When larger doses of endotoxin (150 μg/kg) were given to dogs, there was a transient pulmonary vasoconstriction lasting one to ten minutes followed by up to four hours of persistent pulmonary vascular hyporesponsitivity to hypoxia, as well as to PGF$_{2\alpha}$ and angiotensin II (Figure 6-5). The transient rise in pulmonary vascular resistance (PVR) was associated with a marked outpouring of the vasoconstrictor thromboxane and to a lesser degree of the less powerful vasoconstrictor PGF$_{2\alpha}$. The rise in pros-

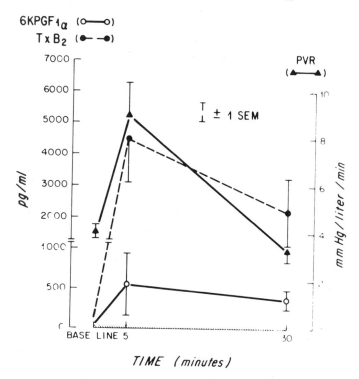

Figure 6-5 Pulmonary vascular resistance and associated circulating levels of the metabolites of thromboxane and prostacyclin after 150 μg/kg of endotoxin given after base line. The transient rise in pulmonary vascular resistance correlates with the rise in the vasoconstrictor thromboxane. At 30 minutes after endotoxin the vessels were hypoactive to hypoxia and other agonists, suggesting a predominant influence by prostacyclin. (Reproduced with permission from Hales et al.[3])

tacyclin, however, was not dissimilar to that seen with lower dose endotoxin. As opposed to thromboxane and $PGF_{2\alpha}$, which fell toward normal 30 minutes after endotoxin, the level of prostacyclin remained elevated. At this point, the pulmonary vessels were flaccid favoring an effect of prostacyclin even though the absolute levels of thromboxane exceeded those of prostacyclin. Pretreatment with indomethacin again prevented any change in PVR or pulmonary vasoreactivity.[3]

The source of the eicosanoids responsible for the pulmonary vasomotor changes after endotoxin may be systemic as well as pulmonary. However, the lung alone is capable of producing these eicosanoids; increases in arteriovenous differences across the lung are seen when early repeated sampling is done after the insult, and lung lymphatic levels of eicosanoids are elevated after endotoxin injury.[5-7,41,42]

The specific eicosanoids responsible for the pulmonary vasoconstriction have not been fully delineated and indeed there may be a complex interaction among several of them. Certainly at higher doses of endotoxin, other eicosanoids such as the vasoconstrictor $PGF_{2\alpha}$ are released.[40] Indeed, even at lower doses $PGF_{2\alpha}$ may be released but in quantities that the lung can degrade in a single passage. Pretreatment with inhibitors specific for thromboxane synthetase do prevent the rise in thromboxane and in pulmonary vascular resistance after acute lung injury from endotoxin,[3,6] but levels of the vasodilator prostacyclin are also higher, probably because the released arachidonic acid is diverted into prostacyclin synthesis due to blocking of the thromboxane synthetase pathway. It is thus not resolved how much of the lack of a rise in PVR after thromboxane synthetase inhibition plus endotoxin is due to the absence of a rise in thromboxane or to an excess of the potent vasodilator prostacyclin. It is, however, apparent that some eicosanoid, and it may well be thromboxane, does mediate pulmonary hypertension after a bolus of endotoxin.[3] This is also true after infusion of gram-negative organisms, after a bolus of activated complement, or during cardiopulmonary bypass, all of which produce transient pulmonary hypertension and an increase in circulating thromboxane levels.[1-15,18]

When endotoxin stimulates the release of arachidonic acid, the arachidonic acid likely enters the lipoxygenase pathway as well as the cyclo-oxygenase pathway, releasing the vasoactive and edema-producing leukotrienes. Since cyclo-oxygenase blockade prevents the pulmonary vasomotor changes after endotoxin injury, it indicates that leukotrienes are either not necessary for the acute vasomotor changes after endotoxin or if they are involved, they are vasoactive indirectly through release of cyclo-oxygenase–mediated products. Precedence has been found for this in airways[43] and in pulmonary vessels.[44] This also does not negate a possible role for leukotrienes in the late-phase permeability pulmonary edema that follows endotoxemia or gram-negative sepsis.

Indeed, because leukotrienes might be injurious to the lung, and may well be released after endotoxemia and cannot be measured readily in vivo, we investigated the potential for high-dose steroids to prevent their release. High-dose steroids have been reported by some to help in animal and man in gram-negative sepsis or endotoxemia.[45-49] High-dose steroids in vitro have been shown to inhibit the release of arachidonic acid from cell membranes through the induction of a factor that inhibits phospholipase A_2.[50,57] Thus, high-dose steroids might be working to help endotoxic shock by shutting off the lipoxygenase as well as the cyclo-oxygenase pathway. However, pretreatment of dogs with 40 mg/kg methylprednisolone intravenously failed to stop the increase in circulating levels of thromboxane or prostacyclin after endotoxin.[52,53] Thus, the protective effect of steroids in clinical endotoxemia, if it exists, is not via inhibition of the arachidonic acid cascade.

The relevance of the acute lung injury models to pulmonary vasoreactivity in ARDS is unclear. Pulmonary vascular resistance is usually high in ARDS when measured[54] but often this is many hours to days after the original insult. Some pulmonary vasoconstriction may be present at that time as isuprel hydrochloride and nifedipine will decrease PVR[55] but undoubtedly considerable architectural change in the lung vessels is also present.[56,57] Correlation of pulmonary vasoreactivity with circulating levels of eicosanoids may also be difficult in particular since for prostacyclin and thromboxane it is not the vasoactive products themselves but their long-lasting and only weakly vasoactive metabolites that are measured. Finally, some eicosanoids dilate and some constrict. Thus, turning them off with a cyclo-oxygenase inhibitor will likely eliminate the good as well as the bad effects.

The acute changes in pulmonary vasoreactivity in multiple forms of lung injury in animals are at least to some degree due to eicosanoid production. Does this acute period in humans now pass before ARDS is recognized and do other factors account for the high pulmonary vascular resistance? Could damage to the lung endothelium eliminate the local production of the vasodilator prostacyclin and thus predispose to vasoconstriction? Are eicosanoids such as thromboxane still actively producing the pulmonary hypertension? Are leukotrienes at fault? These factors, coupled with the problem in correlating circulating eisosanoid levels with pulmonary vasoreactivity, becloud our understanding of the effect of eicosanoids on lung vessels in ARDS.

ACKNOWLEDGMENTS

This research was supported by the Burn Trauma Center (NIH GM21700-7) and a grant from the Shriners Burn Institute.

REFERENCES

1. Cooper JD, McDonald WD, Ali M, et al: Prostaglandin production associated with the pulmonary vascular response to complement activation. *Surgery* 1980;88:215-221.
2. Brigham KL, Meyrick B: Interactions of granulocytes with the lungs. *Circ Res* 1984;54:623-635.
3. Hales CA, Sonne L, Peterson M, et al: Role of thromboxane and prostacyclin in pulmonary vasomotor changes after endotoxin in dogs. *J Clin Invest* 1981;68:497-505.
4. Perkowski SZ, Havill AM, Flynn JT, et al: Role of intrapulmonary release of eicosanoids and superoxide anion as mediators of pulmonary dysfunction and endothelial injury in sheep with intermittent complement activation. *Circ Res* 1983;53:574-583.
5. Garcia-Szabo RR, Peterson MB, Watkins WD, et al: Thromboxane generation after thrombin. Protective effect of thromboxane synthetase inhibition on lung fluid balance. *Circ Res* 1983;53:214-222.
6. Watkins WD, Huttemeier PC, Kong D, et al: Thromboxane and pulmonary hypertension following *E. coli* endotoxin infusion in sheep: effect of an imidazole derivative. *Prostaglandins* 1982;23:273-285.
7. Peterson MB, Huttemeier PC, Zapol WM, et al: Thromboxane mediates acute pulmonary hypertension in sheep extracorporeal perfusion. *Am J Physiol* 1982;243:H471-H479.
8. Demling RH: Role of prostaglandins in acute pulmonary microvascular injury. *Ann NY Acad Sci* 1982;384:517-534.
9. Nerlich M, Flynn J, Demling RH: Effect of thermal injury on endotoxin-induced lung injury. *Surgery* 1983;93:289-296.
10. Proctor RA: Endotoxin in vitro interactions with human neutrophils: depression of chemiluminescence, oxygen consumption, superoxide production and killing. *Infect Immun* 1979;25:912-921.
11. Fine D: Activation of classic and alternate pathways by endotoxin. *J Immunol* 1974;112:763-769.
12. Shasby M, Fox R, Harada R, et al: Reduction of the edema of acute hyperoxic lung injury by granulocyte depletion. *J Appl Physiol* 1982;52:1237-1244.
13. Staub NC, Schultz EL, Albertine KH: Leukocytes and pulmonary vascular injury. *Ann NY Acad Sci* 384:332-342.
14. Johnson D, Ward P: Acute and progressive lung injury after contact with phorbol myristate acetate. *Am J Pathol* 1982;107:29-35.
15. Loyd J, Newman J, English D, et al: Lung vasculature effects of phorbol myristate acetate in awake sheep. *J Appl Physiol* 1983;54:267-276.
16. Meyrich B, Brigham K: Effect of a single infusion of zymosan activated plasma on the pulmonary microcirculation of sheep: Structure-function relationships. *Am J Pathol* 1984;114:32-45.
17. Sacks T, Moldow C, Craddock P, et al: Oxygen radicals mediate endothelial cell damage by complement-stimulated granulocytes: an in vitro model of immune vascular damage. *J Clin Invest* 1978;61:1161-1167.
18. Till G, Johnson K, Kunkel R, et al: Intravascular activation of complement and acute lung injury: Depending on neutrophils and toxic oxygen metabolites. *J Clin Invest* 1982;69:1126-1135.
19. Hales CA, Rouse ET, Slate JL: Influence of aspirin and indomethacin on variability of alveolar hypoxic vasoconstriction. *J Appl Physiol* 1978;45:33-39.

20. Kadowitz PJ, Chapnick BM, Joiner PD, et al: Influences of inhibitors of pro-staglandin synthesis on the canine pulmonary vascular bed. *Am J Physiol* 1975;299:941-946.

21. Hales CA, Rouse ET, Buchwald IA, et al: Role of prostaglandins in alveolar hypoxic vasoconstriction. *Respir Physiol* 1977;29:151-162.

22. Hellewell PG, Pearson JD: Metabolism of circulating adenosine by the porcine isolated perfused lung. *Circ Res* 1983;53:1-7.

23. Husted S, Nedergaard OA: Inhibition of adrenergic neuroeffector transmission in rabbit pulmonary artery and aorta by adenosine and adenine nucleotides. *Acta Pharmacol Toxicol* 1981;49:334-353.

24. Shoukas AA, Brunner MJ, Frankle AE, et al: Carotid sinus baroreceptor reflex control and the role of autoregulation in the systemic and pulmonary arterial pressure-flow relationships of the dog. *Circ Res* 1984;54:674-682.

25. Fishman AP: Vasomotor regulation of the pulmonary circulation. *Ann Rev Physiol* 1980;42:211-220.

26. Hales CA, Westphal D: Hypoxemia following the administration of sublingual nitroglycerin. *Am J Med* 1978;65:911-918.

27. Ahmed T, Oliver W Jr, Wanner A: Variability of hypoxic pulmonary vasoconstriction in sheep: role of prostaglandins. *Am Rev Respir Dis* 1983;127:59-62.

28. Miller MA, Hales CA: Stability of alveolar hypoxic vasoconstriction with intermittent hypoxia. *J Appl Physiol* 1980;49:846-850.

29. Weir EK, Will DH, Alexander AF, et al: Vascular hypertrophy in cattle susceptible to hypoxic pulmonary hypertension. *J Appl Physiol* 1979;46:517-521.

30. Gryglewski RJ, Korbut R, Ocetkiewicz A: Generation of prostacyclin by lungs in vivo and its release into the arterial circulation. *Nature* 1978;273:765-767.

31. Voelkel NF, Gerber JG, McMurtry IF, et al: Release of vasodilator prostaglandin, PGI_2, from isolated rat lung during vasoconstriction. *Circ Res* 1981;48:207-213.

32. Ellsworth ML, Gregory TJ, Newell JC: Pulmonary prostacyclin production with increased flow and sympathetic stimulation. *J Appl Physiol* 1983;55:1225-1231.

33. Hyman AL, Mathe AA, Lippton HL, et al: Prostaglandins and the lung. *Med Clin North Am* 1981;65:789-807.

34. Secher NJ, Thayssen P, Arnsbo P, et al: Effect of prostaglandin E_2 and F_2 on the sytemic and pulmonary circulation in pregnant anesthetized women. *Acta Obstet Gynecol Scand* 1982;61:213-218.

35. Ekland B, Carlson LA: Central and peripheral circulatory effects and metabolic effects of different prostaglandins given I.V. to man. *Prostaglandins* 1980;20:333-347.

36. Kadowitz PJ, Gruetter CA, Spannhake EW, et al: Pulmonary vascular responses to prostaglandins. *Fed Proc* 1981;40:1991-1996.

37. Reeves JT, Grover RF: Blockade of acute hypoxic pulmonary hypertension by endotoxin. *J Appl Physiol* 1974;36:328-332.

38. Weir EK, Miczoch J, Reeves JT, et al: Endotoxin and prevention of hypoxic pulmonary vasoconstriction. *J Clin Med* 1976;88:975-983.

39. Miczoch J, Weir EK, Grover RF, et al: Pulmonary vascular effects of endotoxin in leukopenic dogs. *Am Rev Respir Dis* 1978;118:1097-1099.

40. Anderson FL, Jubiz W, Tsagaris TJ, et al: Prostaglandin F and E levels during endotoxin-induced pulmonary hypertension in calves. *Am J Physiol* 1975;228:1479-1482.

41. Berti F, Folco G, Giachetti A, et al: Atropine inhibits thromboxane A_2 generation in isolated lungs of the guinea pig. *Br J Pharmacol* 1980;68:467–472.

42. Sun FF, Chapman JP, McGuire JC: Metabolism of prostaglandin endoperoxide in animal tissues. *Prostaglandins* 1978;14:1055–1074.

43. Samuelsson B: Leukotrienes: mediators of immediate hypersensitivity reactions and inflammation. *Science* 1983;220:568–575.

44. Lee CW, Lewis RA, Jung W, et al: Cardiopulmonary responses to leukotriene B_4 in the guinea pig. *Am Rev Resp Dis* 1985;131:A2.

45. Thomas CS, Brockman SK: The role of corticosteroid therapy in *Escherichia coli* endotoxin shock. *Surg Gynecol Obstet* 1968;126:61–69.

46. Kadowitz PJ, Yard AC: Circulatory effects of hydrocortisone and protection against endotoxin shock in cats. *Eur J Pharmacol* 1970;9:311–318.

47. Schumer W: Steroids in the treatment of clinical septic shock. *Ann Surg* 1976;184:333–334.

48. Demling RH, Smith M, Gunther R, et al: Endotoxin-induced lung injury in unanesthetized sheep: effect of methylprednisolone. *Circ Shock* 1981;8:351–360.

49. Brigham KL, Bowers RE, McKeen CR: Methylprednisolone prevention of increased lung vascular permeability following endotoxemia in sheep. *J Clin Invest* 1981;67:1103–1110.

50. Flower RJ, Blackwell GJ: Anti-inflammatory steroids induce biosynthesis of a phospholipase A_2 inhibitor which prevents prostaglandin generation. *Nature* 1979;278:456–459.

51. Conde G, Garcia-Barrens P, Muncio AM, et al: In vitro and in vivo activity of *Escherichia coli* endotoxin on mitochondrial phospholipase A_2 activity. *FEBS Lett* 1981;127:115–120.

52. Hales CA, Brandstetter RD, Peterson M, et al: Influence of solumedrol on pulmonary and systemic vasomotor changes following endotoxin induced release of eicosanoids. *Am Rev Respir Dis* 1983;127:3030.

53. Neely C, Brandstetter RD, Peterson M, et al: Methylprednisolone fails to prevent release of prostanoids after endotoxin. *Circulation* 1983;68:III-34.

54. Zapol WM, Snider MT: Pulmonary hypertension in severe acute respiratory failure. *N Engl J Med* 1977;296:476–480.

55. Snider MT, Rie MA, Lauer J, et al: Normoxic pulmonary vasoconstriction in ARDS: detection by sodium nitroprusside (N) and isoproterenol (I) infusions. *Am Rev Resp Dis* 1980;121:191.

56. Snow RL, Davies P, Pontoppidan H, et al: Pulmonary vascular remodeling in adult respiratory distress syndrome. *Am Rev Respir Dis* 1982;126:887–892.

57. Zapol WM, Kobayashi K, Snider MT, et al: Vascular obstruction causes pulmonary hypertension in severe acute respiratory failure. *Chest* 1977;71:306–307.

58. Hales CA, Ahluwalia B, Kazemi H: Strength of pulmonary vascular response to regional alveolar hypoxia. *J Appl Physiol* 1975;38:1082–1087.

7 Mechanisms of Pulmonary Edema

Norman C. Staub

Nearly all types of pulmonary edema reduce to two forms: increased pressure edema and increased permeability edema, as specified by the Starling equation:

$$\dot{Q} = K[(Pmv - Ppmv) - \sigma(\pi mv - \pi pmv)]$$

where

$\dot{Q}$ = the net transvascular liquid filtration rate
K = the liquid conductance of the microvascular barrier
P = the hydrostatic pressure in the microvascular (mv) lumen and in the perimicrovascular (pmv) interstitial liquid space, respectively
σ = the reflection coefficient (a number between 0 and 1 representing the resistance of the microvascular barrier to protein leakage)
π = the protein osmotic pressure in the microvascular and perimicrovascular liquid, respectively

There is one other form of pulmonary edema due to obstruction of lymphatic outflow, such as occurs after lung transplantation[1] or adjacent to tumors, where the local lymphatics are blocked.[2] This type of edema is due to primary lymphatic insufficiency and will not be considered further. But it is worth remembering that, in a sense, all forms of edema are due to inability of the lymphatic system to remove excess interstitial liquid as rapidly as it accumulates.[3]

Figure 7-1 illustrates the effect of increasing microvascular pressure on liquid filtration for the two principal forms of edema. In the normal lung, as microvascular pressure rises (eg, congestive heart failure), there is a slow but steady increase in the rate of liquid filtration. The rate accelerates at high pressures.[4] When the lung is injured (eg, after sepsis),

93

net liquid filtration is augmented, as shown by the vertical line at "normal" microvascular pressure. That is, even normal microvascular pressure is too high in terms of liquid filtration, when the lung is injured. There is an increased filtration at every pressure. In addition, the rate of increase (slope of the line representing the injured lung) is greater than for the normal lung. This is due to failure of the protein osmotic feedback mechanism, which protects the normal lung.[4,5]

The cardinal point to remember about clinical pulmonary edema is that *all* forms of edema are pressure-dependent. All forms are exacerbated by an increase in microvascular hydrostatic pressure, and all forms are alleviated by a decrease in microvascular hydrostatic pressure.

ANIMAL MODELS

The unanesthetized sheep or goat preparation for studying lung liquid and solute exchange has been available for 15 years[6] and has become the

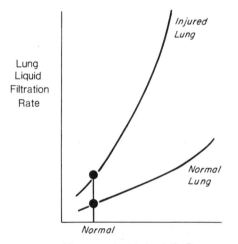

Figure 7-1 Graphic representation of the Starling equation for normal and injured lungs. The net liquid filtration (Y-axis) is a function of microvascular hydrostatic pressure. In the normal lung there is a net (outward) liquid filtration, even at normal microvascular pressures (vertical line and lower dot). When microvascular pressure is elevated, as in increased pressure edema, there is a steady increase in liquid filtration, which tends to accelerate at high pressures because of the exhaustion of the osmotic feedback control mechanism.[4] When the lungs are injured (upper curve) there is increased filtration at all pressures, even at normal microvascular pressures (upper dot on vertical line). Even more important is the fact that the rate of increase filtration (the slope of the upper line) is greater than for the normal lung.

main research tool for studying the pathophysiology of pulmonary edema. The rapid acceleration of investigations and of our knowledge of the basic pathophysiologic processes involved in acute lung injury are examples of how satisfactory development of an animal model of disease can be. Figure 7-2 shows a fully instrumented sheep during an experiment on lung liquid and solute exchange.

The value of large animal investigations in biological research cannot be overemphasized. No matter how many cell culture dishes or tubes of chemicals are tested, there can be no successful extrapolation to man, except through the intermediary of whole-animal investigations. There is no other way to understand the interactive controls, responses, and defense mechanisms that are involved.

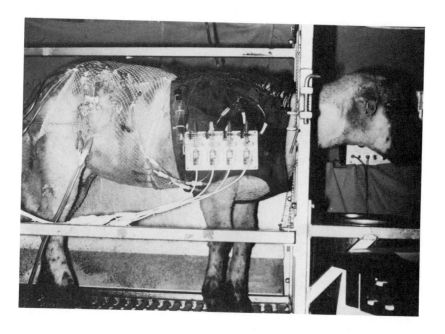

Figure 7-2 Instrumented, unanesthetized sheep with long-term lung lymph fistula. Because the preparation and care of these animals is time-consuming and expensive, we cater to their comfort. Each sheep lives in a mobile metabolism cage to which it adapts easily. They have free access to food and water, and the cages are cleaned daily. The white rectangular plate contains four disposable pressure transducers. There are numerous plastic tubes which connect to the catheters in the femoral and carotid arteries and the femoral and jugular veins. Above and to the left of the pressure transducer plate on the sheep's protective vest, one can see a tapered centrifuge tube. It is into this tube that the long-term lung fistula drains.

MICROEMBOLISM MODEL
OF REVERSIBLE ACUTE LUNG INJURY

Following Saldeen's landmark review of the microembolism syndrome,[7] we began to use microemboli in sheep. Although we used several different types of emboli (glass beads, mineral oil, fibrin microclots), we have found it more convenient to use air microemboli because we can control the amount of embolization and the injury is completely reversible and can be repeated many times.[8]

Figure 7-3 shows the time course of an air embolism experiment in an unanesthetized sheep. Note the increase in pulmonary arterial pressure during the three-hour air infusion. During embolization lung lymph flow increased to a high level and remained elevated for many hours after embolization had ended. The protein concentration of the lung lymph also remained high, indicating a large increase in protein flow across the microvascular barrier. The recovery required about 48 hours.

In studying the mechanism of this acute injury, we followed Saldeen's lead and first examined the clotting system. But we were unable to find that the clotting cascade, specifically fibrinogen, was necessary for the

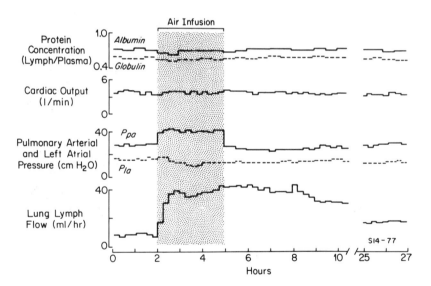

Figure 7-3 Time course of acute air microembolism injury in an unanesthetized sheep. During three hours of air embolization, the pulmonary arterial pressure was elevated and lung lymph flow rose to a high level and remained elevated even after pulmonary arterial pressure decreased. Recovery was not complete at 24 hours. The lymph protein concentration (shown as the separate lymph/plasma protein concentration ratios for albumin and "globulin") remained high throughout the experiment indicating an increase in protein leakage in parallel to the rising lymph flow. (Reproduced with permission from Crandall et al.[9])

lung injury in sheep.[10] Nor could we demonstrate an essential role for platelets.[11]

But when we made the sheep neutropenic, we saw a marked attenuation of the air embolism injury.[12] Figure 7-4 shows an example of the response in an unanesthetized sheep. For the same amount of embolization, the lymph flow and protein flow response were markedly reduced, when the animal was leukopenic. Several investigators have implicated circulating granulocytes (neutrophils) in acute lung injury.[13-15]

PATHOLOGY OF MICROEMBOLISM LUNG INJURY

Figures 7-5, 7-6, and 7-7 show the specific pathology of the injury and Table 7-1 summarizes the quantitative data we have obtained. At the

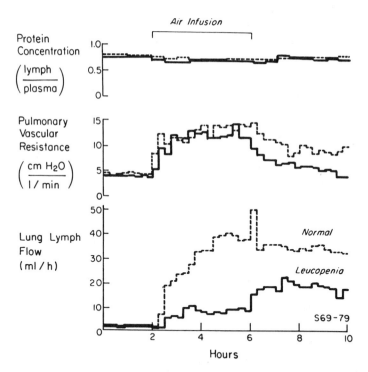

Figure 7-4 Time course of acute lung embolization response in an unanesthetized sheep under control conditions (normal, dashed line) and during chemically induced leukopenia (solid line). During the four-hour air infusion [2 to 3 ml/(kg × h)] pulmonary vascular resistance was increased equally in both experiments. But there was a marked disparity in the lymph flow response. Also, the lymph protein concentration tended to be lower during the leukopenic experiment. (Reproduced with permission from Flick et al.[12])

interface between the air bubbles and blood there are a large number of polymorphonuclear leukocytes (Figure 7-5). When the bubbles become lodged in the small pulmonary arteries, these neutrophils are brought into close relationship with the microvascular endothelium. Damage to the microvascular endothelium is evident (Figures 7-6 and 7-7).

As Table 7-1 shows, the injury visible by ultrastructural analysis is confined to the small muscular pulmonary arteries and arterioles. From the quantitative micropathology, we believe the neutrophils are producing damage to the microvascular endothelium as a result of the activation of one or more of their potent scavenger processes. One can argue that liquid and protein leakage may be due to some change in the microvascular barrier that cannot be detected by ultrastructural analysis. That may be so, but I tend to agree with Hurley[15] who claims there is a close correlation between observable microvascular damage and increased microvascular permeability.

There is evidence that the most likely process is that of superoxide radical generation,[17,18] although other processes have not been ruled out. It is likely that one or more oxygen radical scavengers will soon become available for clinical testing in patients with neutrophil-mediated lung in-

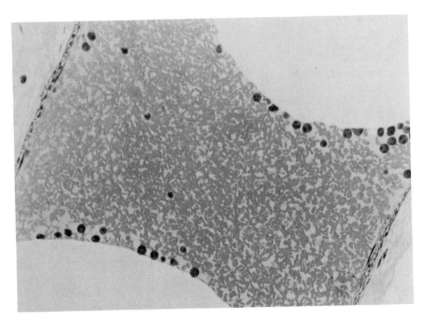

Figure 7-5 Low power light microscopic section of a sheep lung following air embolization. Two emboli are shown lodged in a small muscular pulmonary artery. At the blood-air interface there are many leukocytes, mostly polymorphonuclear leukocytes. (Reproduced with permission from Ohkuda et al.[8])

jury. But in order to make good use of such an approach, it is necessary to distinguish among different types of injury.

TYPES OF ACUTE LUNG MICROVASCULAR INJURY AND TREATMENT

There are two general types of injury to the microvascular endothelium of the lung: *direct* (the inciting agent causes the damage), and *indirect* (the inciting agent alone is not injurious but interacts with some component of blood).[16] The injury caused by air microemboli is of the indirect type because it requires, for its full manifestation, the presence of circulating polymorphonuclear leukocytes.

The first step in the rational management of acute lung microvascular injury ought to be identification of the causative factor to determine

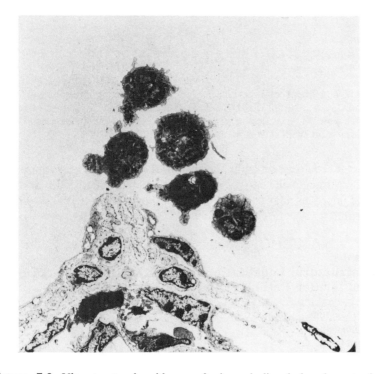

Figure 7-6 Ultrastructural evidence of air embolism-induced acute lung microvascular injury. The figure shows five leukocytes (four neutrophils and one lymphocyte) clustered at the bifurcation of a pulmonary arteriole. The neutrophils are polarized (showing pseudopod formation), which is not seen normally in intravascular neutrophils. There are vacuoles in the intact portions of the endothelium and for a distance of approximately 0.5 μm immediately adjacent to the neutrophils the endothelium is absent. (Reproduced with permission from Albertine et al.[23])

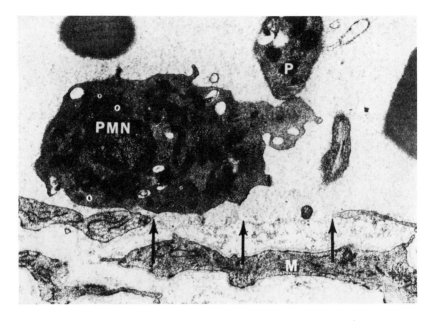

Figure 7-7 Ultrastructural evidence of lung microvascular injury during air embolization. A neutrophil (PMN), lies adjacent to a denuded section (arrow) of arteriolar wall. M = arteriolar smooth muscle cell; P = platelet. (Reproduced with permission from Albertine et al.[23])

whether it requires neutrophil mediation. If neutrophils are required, the proper treatment will be to prevent the activation of neutrophils or to protect the microvascular endothelium from the toxic products of activated neutrophils.

Table 7-1
Ultrastructural Localization of Air Microembolism Lung Microvascular Pathology in Sheep*

Vascular Segment[†]	Vessels Injured (%)
Pulmonary	
Arterioles	100
Capillaries	0
Venules	4
Bronchial	
Microvessels	0

*Two sheep following one- and four-hour air embolization, respectively. Two control sheep (not shown) showed no lesions in any vessels.

[†]Stratified random sampling was used to ensure that the entire lung was sampled. Arterioles include muscularized vessels of up to 500-μm diameter; venules of up to 200-μm diameter.[22]

An example of this treatment policy is the effect of high-dose corticosteroids. Whether corticosteroid treatment will prove useful in any particular patient depends on knowing the type of injury and the timing of the therapy. Protective effects have been found in the sheep model of endotoxic lung injury.[19,20] There is also evidence that high-dose corticosteroids are helpful, both as protection against and treatment of microembolic lung injury.[21,22]

Figure 7-8 shows an air embolus in a small pulmonary artery of an animal that had been treated with high-dose corticosteroids (methylprednisolone, 30 mg/kg) prior to infusion of the air emboli. The most striking difference is the absence of neutrophils attached to the air-blood interface. Table 7-2 shows quantitative data as to the number of lesions detected in the lungs of sheep protected by high-dose corticosteroids. Compared to animals receiving air emboli alone, the number of lesions in the arteriolar endothelium is greatly reduced.

We believe that the beneficial effect of the high-dose corticosteroids is nonspecific and consists of modifying neutrophil surface receptors in such a way that they do not bind to the blood-embolus interface or become

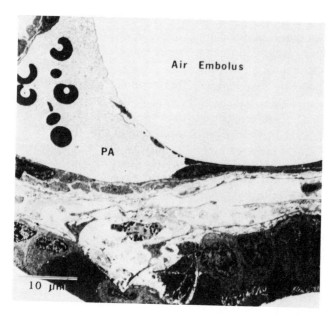

Figure 7-8 Ultrastructurally normal pulmonary arteriole in a sheep protected by high-dose corticosteroids given before air embolization. No neutrophils are seen at the plasma-air interface. (Photomicrograph courtesy of Albertine et al, unpublished data, 1983.)

Table 7-2
Ultrastructural Evidence for Protection by High-Dose Corticosteroids Against Neutrophil-Mediated Acute Lung Microvascular Injury in Sheep

Condition*	Arteriolar Injury (%)[†]
Control	0
Air embolism	100
Corticosteroids	28

*One control and one air embolism sheep (different animals from Table 7-1). Two sheep were treated by 30 mg/kg intravenous bolus of methylprednisolone one hour before embolization began.
[†]Arterioles of up to 500-μm diameter. No other category of vessel showed injury. See also Table 7-1.[20]

activated. The blood-embolus interface appears to contain plasma components (probably denatured proteins or lipids), which form a thin layer that can be seen on electron microscopy (Figure 7-8).[23,24] We suggest that the sequence of events in the pathophysiology of air microembolism injury is the attachment of the neutrophils to the blood-embolus interface, then activation of the neutrophils either by complement or by some substance produced in the material at the interface. An alternate view is that the emboli modify the microvascular endothelial surface, which then binds and activates the neutrophils.[25]

One difficulty with therapy is that it is not usually feasible to protect against injury, although that may be possible in selected high-risk patients. It is important, therefore, to determine whether high-dose corticosteroids can be beneficial *after* the onset of injury. Although I would like to report that the injury is reversed by treatment, this does not appear to be the case. But at whatever time the corticosteroid is given, it may be able to stop progression of the injury. Figure 7-9 shows the average lymph flow response to air microemboli in a group of seven unanesthetized sheep. The steady-state lung lymph flow is shown before and during air embolization for three conditions, namely, air emboli alone, corticosteroids (30 mg/kg intravenous bolus) given prophylactically before embolization and the same dose of corticosteroids given one to 1½ hours after the beginning of embolization.

When the animals were given the corticosteroids as treatment, the effect was not to reverse the increased lymph flow but to stop further increase. In other words, the corticosteroid acted as if it prevented additional injury during embolization. Sibbald et al[26] have presented a clinical study indicating that septic lung injury can be ameliorated by early treatment with high-dose corticosteroids.

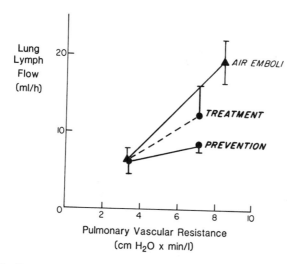

Figure 7-9 Summary of effects of high-dose corticosteroids in the prevention and treatment of acute air embolization lung injury. Each symbol and vertical bar represents the mean and standard deviation of a group of seven unanesthetized sheep. All three experiments were done in each animal. Steady-state lung lymph flow during the base-line period is compared with steady-state lung lymph flow during the last two hours of air embolization. Air emboli caused a threefold rise in lung lymph flow. Prophylactic corticosteroids (30 mg/kg intravenous bolus one hour before air embolization) almost completely prevented the rise in lung lymph flow. Treatment of the sheep by the same dose of corticosteroids after 1.5 hours of embolization also reduced the final steady-state lymph flow indicating significant partial protection. (Figure courtesy of Culver et al, unpublished data, 1983.)

ACKNOWLEDGMENTS

Most of the work was supported by US Public Health Service Grant HL25816 (Program Project). Some of this material was also presented at the Thirteenth Tromsø Seminar in Medicine, University of Tromsø, Norway, June 20–23, 1984. Ms Bernie Baccay and Ms Judy White prepared the manuscript. The Upjohn Corporation, Kalamazoo, Mich, supplied the methylprednisolone.

REFERENCES

1. Cowan GSM, Staub NC, Edmunds LH: Changes in the fluid compartments and dry weights of reimplanted dog lungs. *J Appl Physiol* 1976;962–970.
2. Staub NC: Pulmonary edema. *Physiol Rev* 1974;54:678–811.
3. Rusznyak J, Fold M, Szabo G: *Lymphatics and Lymph Circulation: Physiology and Pathology.* Oxford, Pergamon Press, Inc, 1967.

4. Staub NC: The pathogenesis of pulmonary edema. *Prog Cardiovasc Dis* 1980;28:53-80.

5. Erdmann JA, Vaughan TR, Brigham KL, et al: Effect of increased vascular pressure on lung fluid balance in unanesthetized sheep. *Circ Res* 1975;37: 271-284.

6. Staub NC: Steady state pulmonary transvascular water filtration in unanesthetized sheep. *Circ Res* 1971;28/29:135-139.

7. Saldeen T: The microembolism syndrome. *Microvasc Res* 1976;11:227-259.

8. Ohkuda K, Nakahara K, Binder A, et al: Venous air emboli in sheep: reversible increase in lung microvascular permeability. *J Appl Physiol* 1981; 51:887-894.

9. Crandall ED, Staub NC, Goldberg HS, et al: Recent developments in pulmonary edema. *Ann Intern Med* 1983;99:808-822.

10. Binder AS, Nakahara K, Ohkuda K, et al: Effect of heparin or fibrinogen depletion on lung fluid balance in sheep after emboli. *J Appl Physiol* 1979; 47:213-219.

11. Binder AS, Kageler W, Perel A, et al: Effect of platelet depletion on lung vascular permeability after microemboli in sheep. *J Appl Physiol* 1980;48: 414-420.

12. Flick MR, Perel A, Staub NC: Leucocytes are required for increased lung microvascular permeability after microembolization in sheep. *Circ Res* 1981; 48:344-351.

13. Craddock PR, Fehr J, Brigham KL, et al: Complement and leukocyte-mediated pulmonary dysfunction in hemodialysis. *New Engl J Med* 1977;296:769-774.

14. Johnson A, Malik AB: Pulmonary edema after glass bead microembolization—protective effect of granulocytopenia. *J Appl Physiol* 1982;52:155-161.

15. Heflin AC, Brigham KL: Prevention by granulocyte depletion of increased vascular-permeability of sheep lung following endotoxemia. *J Clin Invest* 1981;68:1253-1260.

16. Hurley JV: Current views on mechanisms of pulmonary edema. *J Pathol* 1978;125:59-79.

17. Fantone JC, Ward PA: Role of oxygen-derived free radicals and metabolites in leucocyte-dependent inflammatory reactions. *Am J Pathol* 1982;107: 397-418.

18. Flick MR, Hoeffel JM, Staub NC: Superoxide-dismutase with heparin prevents increased lung vascular permeability during air emboli in sheep. *J Appl Physiol* 1983;55:1284-1291.

19. Brigham KL, Bowers RE, McKeen CR: Methylprednisolone prevention of increased lung vascular permeability following endotoxemia in sheep. *J Clin Invest* 1981;64:1103-1110.

20. Demling RH, Smith M, Gunther R: Endotoxin-induced lung injury in unanesthetized sheep: effect of methylprednisolone. *Circ Shock* 1981;8: 351-360.

21. Albertine KA, Culver PC, Rao WH, et al: Methylprednisolone protects the lung's microcirculation from ultrastructural damage during air embolization in awake sheep. *Physiologist* 1983;26:A56.

22. Perel A, Flick A, Staub NC: Methylprednisolone partially protects against microemboli-induced permeability injury in lungs of awake sheep. *Am Rev Respir Dis* 1980;121:442.

23. Albertine KA, Wiener-Kronish JP, Koike K, et al: Quantification of damage by air emboli to lung microvessels in anesthetized sheep. *J Appl Physiol* 1984;57:1360-1368.

24. Philp RB, Inwood MJ, Warren BA: Interactions between gas bubbles and components of the blood: implications in decompression sickness. *Aerospace Med* 1972;43:946–953.
25. Brigham KL, Meyrick B: Granulocyte-dependent injury of pulmonary endothelium—a case of miscommunication. *Tissue Cell* 1984;16:137–155.
26. Sibbald WJ, Anderson RR, Reid B, et al: Alveolocapillary permeability in human septic adult respiratory distress syndrome. Effect of high dose corticosteroid therapy. *Chest* 1981;79:133–142.

8 Leukocytic Oxygen Radicals and Acute Lung Injury

Peter A. Ward
Kent J. Johnson
Gerd O. Till

The use of immune complex–induced injury, either in cutaneous blood vessels or in the lung of rats, has been a useful model because this is an acute and intense type of tissue injury that can be precisely quantitated with the end-point being four hours in time. The pathogenesis of this type of injury is known to be associated with the chemotactic activation of the complement system, resulting in the formation of the C5a chemotactic peptide and perhaps other mediators with the eventual accumulation of large numbers of neutrophils at the sites of immune complex deposition and complement activation.[1-3] It is also known that the development of injury is totally dependent upon the participation and recruitment of neutrophils since neutrophil depletion totally protects the tissues from injury in spite of the presence of immune complexes and evidence of complement activation products.[2-4] Our recent studies of immune complex injury involving dermal venules and the lungs of rats have indicated that oxygen radicals play a pivotal role in the development of tissue injury. This has been demonstrated by the fact that immune complex–induced injury in the lung can be almost totally prevented by the pretreatment of rats with catalase which is mixed with the antibody as it is instilled into the airways, followed by the intravenous (IV) injection of antigen. Approximately 80% of the injury can be prevented by this manipulation.[5] The specificity of this reaction has been demonstrated by the fact that chemically inactivated catalase fails to protect against the lung injury (Figure 8-1). In attempting to determine additional details of this mechanism of injury, studies with either catalase or superoxide dismutase (SOD) were carried out in rats. As the data in Figure 8-2 show, catalase has a continued and sustained protective effect, especially in the lung, whereas treatment of rats with SOD is time-limited in terms of protective

108

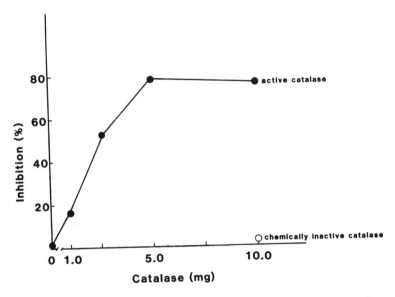

Figure 8-1 Catalase-induced inhibition of immune complex–mediated tissue injury. The degree of injury is assessed by leakage into the lung of radiolabeled albumin. Catalase with intact enzymatic activity will suppress up to 80% of the tissue injury while inactivated catalase has no effect.

effects and within three hours no additional protection by SOD alone is found.[5,6] The reasons for these differential effects of catalase and SOD will be described below.

In recent studies of immune complex–induced injury of cutaneous vessels of rat skin, evidence has been obtained that iron and hydroxyl radical ($\cdot$OH) may be involved in the pathogenesis of the injury.[7] As summarized in Figure 8-3, neutrophil depletion almost totally averts the development of tissue injury while treatment of rats systemically with apolactoferrin also is markedly protective providing approximately 55% reduction of vascular injury. The specificity of this effect has been demonstrated by the fact that companion experiments employing iron-saturated apolactoferrin failed to show any significant evidence of protection. Underlying the likely role of iron in these reactions, treatment of rats with nanomolar concentrations of iron in its fully oxidized state markedly potentiates the injury, causing a greater than 60% increase in the extent of vascular injury (Figure 8-3). Prior treatment of the animals with dimethyl sulfoxide (DMSO), a potent scavenger of the hydroxyl radical, also provides a high degree of protection against immune complex–induced vascular injury of rat skin.

A general provisional summary of the events associated with immune complex–induced injury of tissues is shown in Figure 8-4, where deposi-

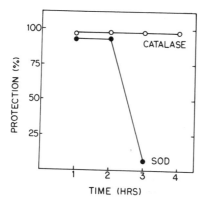

Figure 8-2 Duration of the protective effects of SOD and catalase in immune complex induced tissue injury. Note that SOD is initially protective but that its inhibitory effects are overcome with time. In contrast, catalase achieves a continued sustained high level of suppression of the tissue injury.

tion of immune complexes leads to complement activation with the generation of the C5a peptide which results in the initial recruitment of neutrophils. The production of superoxide anion (O_2^-) and the demonstrated ability of this radical in vitro to bring about conversion of arachidonic acid to a chemotactic lipid[8,9] may result in the appearance of a lipid mediator which amplifies the initial inflammatory reaction, resulting in increased recruitment of neutrophils to the sites of immune complex deposits. Understandably, treatment of the animals with SOD precludes this initial amplification step. Increased activation of complement in the presence of the complexes may produce more C5a with time, overriding the amplification process associated with the formation of chemotactic lipid mediated by O_2^- generation. It would appear that the generation of hydrogen peroxide in the presence of iron salt and perhaps also in the presence of (O_2^- results ultimately in the formation of the hydroxyl radical[10,11] which has been shown in recent studies to be associated with lung vascular injury–associated intravascular activation of the complement system.[12] In immune complex–induced tissue injury, similar pathways may be operating. This would explain the persistent protective effects either of catalase or of hydroxyl radical scavengers such as dimethyl sulfoxide in protecting against immune complex–induced tissue damage. It is also possible that hydrogen peroxide in the presence of leukocytic myeloperoxidase and of a halide results in a toxic halide product such as either hypochlorous acid (HOCl) or a stable chloramine.[13] At present it is difficult to rule out the development of toxic products via the myeloperoxidase pathway, but there is some evidence at least suggesting that hydroxyl radical formation is probably an important pathway of oxygen radical pro-

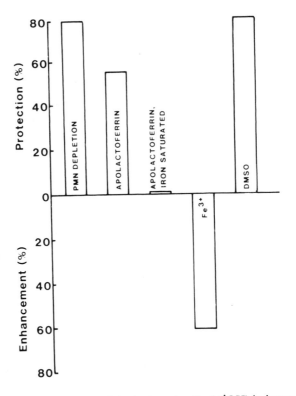

Figure 8-3 Postulated role of the hydroxyl radical ($^.$OH) in immune complex-induced tissue injury. As expected prior neutrophil (PMN) depletion leads to virtually complete protection from tissue injury. The postulated role of the neutrophil-generated hydroxyl radical is shown by the fact that the administration of iron chelators (apolactoferrin) or hydroxyl radical scavengers (DMSO) markedly protects against tissue injury. Conversely, the administration of excess iron (Fe^{3+}), which should increase hydroxyl radical formation, markedly augments the degree of tissue injury.

duction leading to tissue damage. It is also possible that other iron radicals such as either the perferryl or the ferryl radicals are being produced[14] but the strongly protective effects of catalase in the immune complex model of tissue injury suggests that the chief role of iron may be to bring about conversion of hydrogen peroxide (H_2O_2) to hydroxyl radical. A more definitive definition of the relevant pathways awaits further work.

Oxygen radical production by phagocytic cells of the lung can also result in not only acute but also progressive lung injury. When small amounts (10 μg) of phorbol myristate acetate (PMA) are instilled into rat lung, acute and intensive lung injury occurs, resulting in extensive intra-alveolar hemorrhage, edema, and fibrin deposition.[15] There is extensive injury of both alveolar lining cells as well as lung vascular endothelial cells.

So intense is the injury that the alveolar spaces are virtually denuded of all alveolar lining cells. These events can be largely prevented by coinstillation of catalase with the PMA. Similar intervention with SOD has little, if any, protective effects. This model of lung injury has also been demonstrated to be independent of the role of neutrophils since neutrophil depletion with antibody prior to lung instillation of PMA has little, if any, protective effects against the lung injury. There is little known about what conversion products of H_2O_2 may be largely responsible for the injury in the PMA model. Whether hydroxyl radical or halide-dependent products mediated via myeloperoxidase might be involved is not known at the present time.

The PMA model also results in progressive injury with the rapid onset of an interstitial pulmonary fibrotic response and parenchymal collapse beginning as early as the third to fourth day and being complete by the seventh or eighth day. Again, this outcome is prevented if the animals are initially pretreated with catalase at the time of phorbol instillation into the lung. What is responsible for this rapid progressing interstitial reaction with extensive collagen deposition as demonstrated histopathologically is unknown, but the rapid progression and catastrophic outcome appear to be related to the virtual complete denuding of the alveolar compartment by alveolar lining cells, precluding epithelial cell regeneration during the first five days. It is also possible that the oxygen radicals have a direct stimulatory effect on the interstitial fibroblasts but this is largely an unknown possibility at the present time.

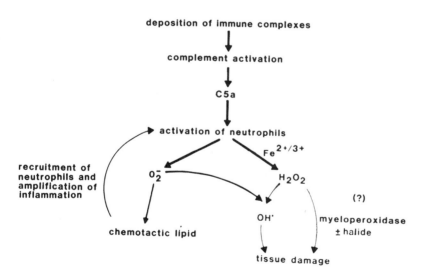

Figure 8-4 Postulated sequence of events occurring in immune complex–induced tissue injury.

As the mechanisms of oxygen radical–induced damage of tissues becomes better understood, it is not surprising that a series of protective interventions have been developed experimentally and that these may ultimately have clinical applicability. The current mechanisms and various points of intervention are summarized in Figure 8-5. Tissue injury associated with oxygen radical involvement can be brought about either by leukocyte activation as the models above emphasize or also by activation of tissue xanthine oxidase via its conversion by proteases from xanthine dehydrogenase, as demonstrated by McCord and coworkers.[16,17] The xanthine oxidase pathway has been demonstrated to be operative in ischemic tissue injury involving both the myocardium as well as the small bowel.[16-19] Irrespective of the mechanism of oxygen radical formation, ultimately O_2^- is formed, followed by its dismutation to H_2O_2 or by alternative pathways converging and bringing about H_2O generation. As has been suggested before, hydrogen peroxide may be converted either via the myeloperoxidase and halide system to the toxic products such as HOCl or H_2O_2 may be converted in the presence of partly reduced iron to the hydroxyl radical, resulting ultimately in evidence of lipid peroxidation and other examples of oxidant effects.[13,14] If the oxygen radical pathway has been initiated by the xanthine oxidase system, pretreatment with allopurinol will block this pathway. Both in the case of ischemic injury of the myocardium and the small bowel, this type of intervention has been demonstrated to be effective.[16-19] In leukocyte-dependent systems, interventions that block leukocyte activation may be protective. Lipoxygenase pathway inhibitors and steroids as well as any number of other drugs have been demonstrated to block activation of both neutrophils and other phagocytic cells diminishing or preventing the production of toxic oxygen products.[20,21] There is also considerable evidence in the literature that certain cyclo-oxygenase inhibitors are protective, but it is not at all clear if their effects are to diminish the output of oxygen radicals or otherwise interfere with activation of phagocytic cells.[20,22,23] The next step in these pathways for intervention is the step involving O_2^- produc-

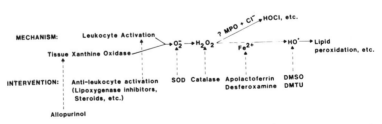

Figure 8-5 Possible therapeutic interventions in oxygen radical–induced tissue injury.

tion in which treatment of animals with SOD in certain instances may be protective.[6,24] It should be pointed out that in general SOD per se is not especially effective in providing sustained protection against tissue injury initiated by oxygen radicals from activated phagocytic cells. However, catalase is a potent protective agent, as emphasized above, and intercepts any further oxygen product formation beyond the point of H_2O_2 formation.[5,15,25] As was also described above, there is at least some evidence that treatment with iron chelators such as apolactoferrin or deferoxamine will provide protective interventions but this has not been studied extensively experimentally.[7,12] Finally, scavengers which will interrupt hydroxyl radical generation, including DMSO or dimethyl thiourea (DMTU) provide significant protection against injury as demonstrated both in the model of acute lung injury following systemic activation of complement or in immune complex–induced vasculitis.[7,12] As more information becomes available regarding the various pathways leading to tissue injury, more selective interventions will become available. There is substantial evidence to indicate that some of these interventions may have some clinical applicability. Additional studies in animal models as well as further definition of human diseases in which oxygen radicals are likely to participate, as has been demonstrated recently with the adult respiratory distress syndrome,[26,27] will provide the information that will make effective therapeutic interventions possible.

REFERENCES

1. Cochrane CG, Aiken BS: Polymorphonuclear leukocytes in immunologic reactions. *J Exp Med* 1966;124:733–752.
2. Johnson KJ, Ward PA: Acute immunologic pulmonary alveolitis. *J Clin Invest* 1974;54:349–357.
3. Cochrane CG: Immune complex mediated tissue injury, in Cohen S, Ward PA, McCluskey RT (eds): *Mechanisms of Immunopathology*. New York, John Wiley & Sons, 1974.
4. Cochrane CG, Janoff A: The Arthus reaction: A model of neutrophil and complement-mediated injury, in Zweifach BW, Grant L, McClusky RT (eds): *The Inflammatory Process*, ed 2. New York, Academic Press, 1974, vol 2, pp 86–162.
5. Johnson KJ, Ward PA: Role of oxygen metabolites in immune complex injury of lung. *J Immunol* 1981;126:2365–2369.
6. McCormick JR, Harkin MM, Johnson KJ, et al: Suppression of superoxide dismutase in immune-complex-induced pulmonary alveolitis and dermal inflammation. *Am J Pathol* 1981;102:55–61.
7. Fligiel SEG, Ward PA, Johnson KJ, et al: Evidence for the role of hydroxyl radical in immune complex induced vasculitis. *Am J Pathol* 1984;115:375–382.
8. Perez HD, Goldstein JM: Generation of a chemotactic lipid from arachidonic acid by exposure to a superoxide generating system, abstracted. *Fed Proc* 1980;34:1170.

114

9. Petrone WF, Englis DK, Wong K, et al: Free radicals and inflammation: The superoxide dependent activation of a neutrophil chemotactic factor in plasma. *Proc Natl Acad Sci USA* 1980;77:1159-1163.
10. McCord JM, Day ED Jr: Superoxide dependent production of hydroxyl radical catalyzed by iron-EDTA complex. *FEBS Lett* 1978;86:139-142.
11. Halliwell B: Superoxide-dependent formation of hydroxyl radicals in the presence of iron chelates: Is it a mechanism for hydroxyl radical production in biochemical systems? *FEBS Lett* 1978;92:321-326.
12. Ward PA, Till GO, Kunkel R, et al: Evidence for role of hydroxyl radical in complement and neutrophil dependent tissue injury. *J Clin Invest* 1983; 72:789-801.
13. Klebanoff S-J: Oxygen metabolism and the toxic properties of phagocytes. *Ann Intern Med* 1980;93:480-489.
14. Aust SD, Slinger BA: The role of iron in enzymatic lipid peroxidation, in Pryor WA (ed): *Free Radicals in Biology.* New York, Academic Press, 1982, vol 5, pp 1-28.
15. Johnson KJ, Ward PA: Acute and progressive lung injury after contact with phorbol myristate acetate. *Am J Pathol* 1982;107:29-35.
16. Granger DN, Rutili G, McCord JM: Superoxide radicals in feline intestinal ischemia. *Gastroenterology* 1981;81:22-29.
17. Parke DA, Bulkley GB, Granger DN, et al: Ischemia injury in the cat small intestine: Role of superoxide radicals. *Gastroenterology* 1982;82:9-15.
18. Rao PS, Evans RG, Val-Mejias J, et al: The role of superoxide dismutase in reducing CK depletion of infarcted myocardium in the rat, abstracted. *Clin Res* 1978;26:262A.
19. Bailie MB, Jolly SR, Lucchesi BR: Reduction of myocardial ischemic injury by superoxide dismutase plus catalase, abstracted. *Fed Proc* 1982;41:1736.
20. Ward PA, Sulavik MC, Johnson KJ: Rat neutrophil activation and effects of lipoxygenase and cyclooxygenase inhibitors. *Am J Pathol* 1984;116:223-233.
21. Kunkel SL, Chensue SW, Mouton C, et al: Role of lipoxygenase products in murine pulmonary granuloma formation. *J Clin Invest* 1984;74:514-524.
22. Metz S, VanRollins M, Strife R, et al: Lipoxygenase pathway in islet endocrine cells: Oxidative metabolism of arachidonic acid promotes insulin release. *J Clin Invest* 1983;71:1191-1205.
23. Perkowski SZ, Hamill AM, Flynn JT, et al: Role of intrapulmonary release of eicosanoids and superoxide anion as endothelial injury in sheep with intermittent complement activation. *Circ Res* 1983;53:574-583.
24. Fridovich I: Superoxide radical: An endogenous toxicant. *Annu Rev Pharmacol Toxicol* 1983;23:239-257.
25. Johnson KJ, Fantone JC III, Kaplan J, et al: In vivo damage of rat lungs by oxygen metabolites. *J Clin Invest* 1981;67:983-993.
26. McGuire WW, Spragg RG, Cohen AB, et al: Studies on the pathogenesis of the adult respiratory distress syndrome. *J Clin Invest* 1982;69:543-553.
27. Cochrane CG, Spragg RC, Revak SD: Pathogenesis of the adult respiratory distress syndrome: Evidence of oxidant activity in bronchoalveolar lavage fluid. *J Clin Invest* 1983;71:754-761.

9 Oxygen Radicals and Pulmonary Edema

Aubrey E. Taylor
Denis Martin

EDEMA FORMATION IN LUNG

The formation of excess fluid in the interstitial spaces can be classified into two categories: (1) Those which result from increased microvascular pressures (usually referred to as capillary pressure) or decreased plasma colloids osmotic pressure, ie, *hydrostatic edema;* or (2) Those which result from alterations in the ability of the microcirculation to prevent the escape of plasma proteins into the tissues, ie, the microvascular membrane becomes excessively permeable to plasma proteins, *permeability edema.*[1,2]

The equation that describes the process of edema formation is the following[3,4]:

$$J_V = K_{F,C}[(P_C - P_T) - \sigma_d(\pi_P - \pi_T)]$$

Hydrostatic Factors (above)

Permeability Factors (below)

(1)

where

J_V = the net volume flow occurring across the microvessel walls into the interstitium

P_C and P_T = the hydrostatic pressures in the microvessels (capillaries) and interstitial spaces, respectively

π_P and π_T = the colloid osmotic pressure of the plasma and tissues, respectively

$K_{F,C}$ = the hydraulic conductance of the microvascular wall and is a function of the total surface area available at the microvessel walls, and, if flow occurs through the microvessel wall in a laminar fashion, is proportional to the fourth power of pore radius

σ_d = the reflection coefficient of the plasma proteins at the microvascular wall

115

If the molecule is not able to escape the circulation, $\sigma_d = 1.0$, but if it crosses the microvascular wall as easily as water, then $\sigma_d = 0$.[4] For many years, physiologists thought that $\sigma_d = 1.0$ in many vascular beds. It is now known that σ_d is between 0.75 and 0.9 for total plasma proteins in many vascular beds that possess both continuous and fenestrated endothelial microvessel barriers.[5] The ability of the lung's microvasculature to reflect plasma proteins may be less than other vascular beds, since the plasma protein σ_d is probably about 0.8 in lung microvessels. This means that 80% of the calculated osmotic pressure of plasma proteins is actually exerted across capillary walls.[6,7]

Hydrostatic Edema

Equation (1) also indicates which parameters are hydrostatic and which are permeability factors. Any increase in P_C will tend to cause more fluid to move from the vascular system into the interstitium. Alterations in P_T can also be caused by lung inflation; in fact, P_T becomes more negative as transpulmonary pressures are increased.[8] P_T also becomes more positive as edema fluid accumulates.[9,10] Table 9-1 shows

Table 9-1
Factors Producing Fluid Accumulation in the Tissues*

Hydrostatic Factors	Permeability Factors
Increased Vascular Pressures	*Capillary Walls*
Heart failure	Endotoxin shock?
Histamine	Sepsis?
Serotonin	Complement activation
Prostaglandins	Oxygen radicals (O_2^-, H_2O_2, OH˙)
Leukotrienes	ANTU
Norepinephrine	Alloxan
Epinephrine	Microemboli
	Activation of Neutrophils?
Decreased Plasma Colloids	Activation of macrophages
Nephrotic syndrome	Ca^{++} removal from plasma (EDTA)
Burns	Oleic acid
Protein synthesis deficiencies	Fat emboli
Liver loss (ascites formation)	High vascular pressures?
Protein degradation increases	Alveolar hypoxia?
Insufficient protein in diets	High airway pressures
Gastrointestinal protein-losing	Paraquat
problems	Hyperoxia
Renal disease	
	Alveolar Membrane
	High airway pressures
	Oxygen radicals
	High tissue pressures

*Modified from Taylor and Parker.[1]

many conditions that can alter the pulmonary microvascular pressure.[11] Left atrial pressure elevations caused by heart failure, hormones such as norepinephrine, epinephrine, serotonin, histamine, arachidonic acid products, etc, all produce an increase in pulmonary microvascular pressure either by increasing the venous outflow resistance or by increasing both inflow and outflow resistances in the face of increased pulmonary arterial pressures. Histamine acts in the former fashion and norepinephrine and serotonin in the latter.[12] The other component of the volume flow equation which is a hydrostatic factor that can be altered clinically is the plasma colloid osmotic pressure.[13] If this pressure is decreased, the tendency for fluid to accumulate in the tissues increases because it normally acts to oppose the hydrostatic capillary pressures. π_P can be decreased by protein deficiencies in diets, plasma loss associated with renal loss (nephrotic syndrome), loss into the peritoneal cavity (associated with cirrhosis), loss through the gastrointestinal (GI) tract, loss through denuded skin (burns), excess fluid retention (renal disease), excessive plasma dilution in the clinical setting, and problems with either albumin or globulin synthesis and catabolism.[11]

Permeability Edema

Also shown in equation (1) are the factors responsive to changes in the ability of the capillary wall to restrict the passage of plasma proteins. The colloid osmotic pressure of the tissues will be larger when the vascular wall is more permeable to plasma proteins. Consequently, $\pi_P - \pi_T$ will be smaller and provide less opposition to increases in P_C. σ_d will be smaller when the capillary wall is leakier to plasma proteins so that $\sigma_d(\pi_P - \pi_T)$ will be even smaller. Consider the following examples: For normal capillaries: If

$$\sigma_d = 0.8,\ \pi_P = 25\ \text{mmHg, and}\ \pi_T = 10\ \text{mmHg}$$

then

$$\sigma_d\Delta\pi = 0.8(25-10) = 0.8(15) = 12\ \text{mmHg}$$

For leaky capillaries: If

$$\sigma_d = 0.4,\ \pi_P = 25\ \text{mmHg, and}\ \pi_T = 20\ \text{mmHg}$$

then

$$\sigma_d\Delta\pi = 0.4(25-20) = 0.4(5) = 2\ \text{mmHg}$$

Thus, with leaky capillaries the change in the effective colloid osmotic gradient, $\sigma(\pi_P - \pi_T)$, is not simply additive but decreases drastically because of the multiplicity effect of σ on $\Delta\pi$, ie, the change in colloid osmotic gradient when capillaries become leakier to plasma proteins behaves as an amplifier factor because both σ and $\Delta\pi$ decrease.[1] These examples show dramatically how increased vascular permeability leads to a rapid accumulation of edema fluid. Considering that $Pc = 12$ mmHg, then for the normal lung example given above, $Jv = K_{F,C}(0) = 0$ (no tendency for fluid to move), but for the permeability type of edema $Jv = K_{F,C}(10)$. Therefore, fluid will accumulate in lung tissues at very low vascular pressures, because the imbalance in faces is 10 mmHg in this case. Therefore, it is clear that estimates of capillary pressure in the critically ill patient is a very crucial parameter in assessing the state of lung fluid balance.[14]

Finally, $K_{F,C}$ will also increase if the capillary walls become more permeable to plasma proteins and for a given change in capillary pressure a greater amount of edema fluid will tend to accumulate in the lung interstitium. Table 9-1 shows a partial list of compounds which may cause pulmonary capillaries to become more permeable to plasma proteins. In some species, the various conditions do not always result in measurable endothelial damage. Sepsis appears to damage sheep lung capillaries, but the same challenge hardly effects dog lungs; the effect of sepsis on human lungs is not known.[15,16] However, it is now becoming clear that oxygen radicals will cause the pulmonary microvessel walls to become abnormally leaky to plasma proteins. Curiously, high airway pressures appear to also disrupt the endothelial barrier of the lung.[17]

Alveolar Membrane

Table 9-1 also shows the effects of different compounds on the alveolar membrane. Although little is known about the factors that disrupt the integrity of this barrier, it is known that once disrupted, fluid moves out of the interstitium into the air spaces, proteins are not restricted to any significant degree, and interstitial fluid simply spills over into the airways (perhaps the large plasma proteins such as β-lipoprotein are restricted).[18] Some conditions are known to disrupt this important biological barrier, such as the presence of oxygen radicals[19] and high airway pressures (>10 cmH$_2$O).[20] Since airway pressures affect the alveolar membrane, then high tissue pressures should also increase the alveolar epithelial membrane permeability to plasma proteins.[3] It is of interest to note that a pressure gradient of only 4 mmHg acting across the intestinal epithelium disrupts that membrane which is similar in structure and passive permeability characteristics to the alveolar membrane (pores with 5 to 8 nm radii).[21-23] In addition, plasma proteins leak into the intestinal lumen without any sieving at the mucosal barrier, ie, tissue fluid and luminal fluid are identical.[22] Therefore, only small gradients in hydrostatic pressures operating across the alveolar walls should cause them to become extremely leaky to plasma proteins. It should be emphasized that the exact location of the leakage sites are not presently known. They are most likely located at the junction of the alveolar ducts and alveoli, since alveolar epithelial cells appear to migrate in that direction as they age and may be more susceptible to elevated tissue pressures. To carry the intestinal analogy further, the most aged mucosal epithelial cells are located at the villus tips and these cells are shed when pressure gradients between tissue and lumen exceed 4 mmHg, producing a very leaky mucosal membrane.[24] It is likely that epithelial cells at the alveolar duct region behave similarly and are shed from the alveolar surface when tissue pressure exceeds alveolar fluid pressure by 4 mmHg. Much more research needs to be done relative to alveolar damage before we can understand alveolar flooding, but the following equation does describe fluid movement ($J_{V,A}$) across this important barrier:

$$J_{V,A} = K_{F,t}(P_T - P_{AL}) - \sigma_{AL}(\pi_T - \pi_{AL}) \tag{2}$$

where

P_{AL} = the alveolar fluid pressure
P_T and π_T = the tissue hydrostatic and colloid osmotic pressures respectively
π_{AL} = the colloid osmotic pressure in the alveolar fluid

It appears that $\sigma_{AL} \rightarrow 0$ when intra-alveolar edema develop such that

$$J_{V,A} = K_{F,t}(P_T - P_{AL}) \tag{3}$$

and the volume flow occurring across this barrier is a function of $K_{F,t}$, which is related to the filtration properties of both the capillary and alveolar membranes, and the differences between the tissue hydrostatic pressure and alveolar fluid pressures acting across the airway, similar to flow occurring in a pipe.[25]

The effect of the oxygen radicals in producing alveolar membrane disruption appears to be a promising experimental model.[19] Many forms of edema and ARDS may be related to the characteristics of this membrane barrier rather than to problems associated with changes in the selective nature of the capillary walls.

OXYGEN RADICAL DAMAGE

It has become clear that oxygen radicals derived from either damaged tissues or neutrophils may explain many of the seemingly divergent causes

120

of pulmonary edema shown in Table 9-1.[1,26,27]

Figure 9-1 shows how damaged tissues form superoxide radicals (O_2^-).[26] In the presence of superoxide dismutase (SOD), the superoxide radical is reduced to hydrogen peroxide (H_2O_2), which, in the presence of catalase or glutathione reductase, is reduced to water and O_2. In addition, O_2^- and H_2O_2 can combine to form the hydroxyl radical (OH$^.$). Both H_2O_2 and OH$^.$ are highly reactive in lung tissues and destroy membrane components on contact. Neutrophils can also produce superoxides through the reduction of nicotinamide adenine dinucleotide phosphate (NADPH) to nicotinamide adenine dinucleotide (NADH), and use this compound (or some subsequently formed oxygen radical) to kill bacteria that invade the body.[22]

Figure 9-2 is a flow diagram which describes how tissue damage causes the release of arachidonic acid products (block 19) and the subsequent formation of O_2^- as prostaglandin G_2 (PGG$_2$) is converted to prostaglandin H_2 (PGH$_2$). In addition, O_2^- attracts neutrophils (block 8) to the

FREE RADICAL GENERATION

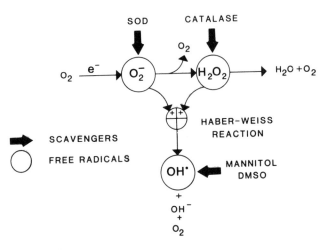

Figure 9-1 Schematic representation of how oxygen radicals are formed. O_2 is reduced to the superoxide radical (O_2^-) and superoxide dismutase (SOD) converts the superoxide to hydrogen peroxide (H_2O_2). H_2O_2 can be converted to H_2O and O_2 in the presence of catalase. Both O_2^- and H_2O_2 combine to form the hydroxyl radical (OH$^.$). The oxygen radicals are shown in circles and the scavengers and enzymes are shown as solid arrows. (Reproduced with permission from Taylor and Martin.[26])

tissues which also produce more O_2^-. Tissue hypoxia also produces O_2^- when xanthine oxidase converts xanthine to hypoxanthine. These sum to produce the total O_2^- levels, which can then form either H_2O_2 (block 10) or OH· (Haber-Weiss reaction). If the levels are sufficiently high, then capillary endothelial damage results. Interestingly, some compounds stimulate the production of SOD by lung tissue and this enzyme acts in a negative feedback fashion to convert the O_2^- produced by damaged tissue to H_2O_2.[28] However, H_2O_2 can be converted to a very toxic compound, hypochlorous acid (HOCl, like laundry bleach) in the presence of myeloperoxidase.[29] In summary, Figure 9-2 shows that tissue damage produces O_2^- radicals which, in the presence of SOD, are converted to H_2O_2. The O_2^- and H_2O_2 can then combine to produce OH·. The oxygen radicals can then readily destroy lung tissue.

The numbers circled in Figure 9-2 show the sites where various scavengers or compounds can prevent the damage associated with these compounds by either blocking the formation of the toxic oxygen radicals or scavenging them once formed. For example, dimethylsulfoxide (DMSO), mannitol, and ethanol can scavenge OH· as shown at (18) and catalase and glutathione reductase can convert H_2O_2 to water and O_2 at (16) and (17), respectively.

α-Napthylthiourea (ANTU) Production of Oxygen Radicals

Table 9-2 shows the results of a study conducted in our laboratory in which the oxygen radical system was investigated relative to lungs damaged with α-napthylthiourea (ANTU).[30] Figure 9-3 shows the results using our experimental model. A small prenodal lymphatic was cannulated in dog lungs in order to measure lymph flow and its protein composition. Left atrial pressure could be manipulated in the model to increase lymph flow. Shown in Figure 9-3 are lymph flow (J_v) times control, the concentration of total plasma protein in lymph relative to plasma (C_L/C_P), and lung water (Q_w). When left atrial pressure is elevated in normal lungs, lymph flow increases two- to threefold and C_L/C_P decreases from 0.75 to 0.5. When left atrial pressure is increased following the ANTU challenge, lymph flow increases to 12 times normal flow, yet C_L/C_P does not decrease. In addition, following this maneuver the lungs always fill rapidly with protein-rich fluid and Q_w greatly increases. These findings indicate that ANTU causes a large increase in pulmonary vascular permeability to plasma proteins, which results in the rapid and fatal development of pulmonary edema.[31]

When lungs were pretreated with SOD, ANTU did not produce edema in 70% of the lungs. Catalase was equally protective, and DMSO also protected the lung but to a lesser extent than either SOD or catalase. Since

122

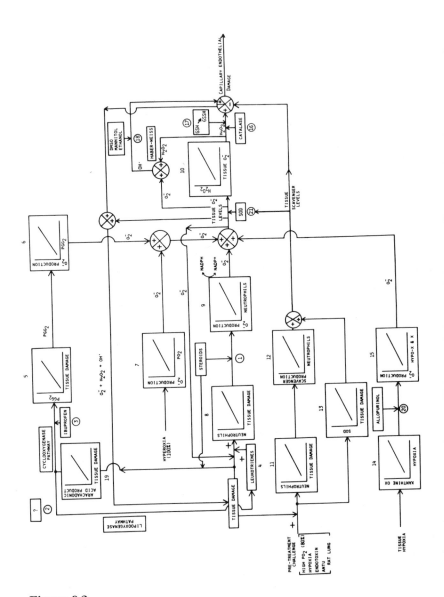

Figure 9-2

each blocked the damage equally, this implies that OH· radicals are responsible for producing the lung damage associated with ANTU challenge.[32]

How does ANTU bring about the production of the oxygen radicals? Table 9-2 shows that the presence of neutrophils are not required for the production of the lung damage since depletion of these cells to less than $20/mm^3$ using mustard, did not prevent the ANTU damage. Nor did pretreatment with allopurinol block the capillary damage. Thus, the oxygen radicals are not generated by the xanthine-xanthine oxidase system in this type of lung damage. But ibuprofen does protect the lung against the damage associated with ANTU indicating that this compound acts by disrupting the endothelial membranes, and releasing arachidonic acid products which lead to the formation of O_2^- when PGG_2 is converted to PGD_2.[32]

As a result of our studies and many others present in the literature, it seems likely that different oxygen radicals can severely damage lung tissues. Table 9-3 gives a partial listing of these studies. It will be noted that many challenges tend to produce O_2 radicals, but the particular radical responsible for the observed damage may be O_2^-, H_2O_2, OH· or HOCl. In some studies it is not clear as to which radical is responsible

Figure 9-2 Schematic model of the production scheme of oxygen radicals (O_2^-), hydroxyl radicals (OH·), and hydrogen peroxide (H_2O_2) in damaged lung tissue. Starting at the far left, tissue damage causes neutrophil infiltration into tissues with subsequent release of O_2^- formed by NADPH → $NADP^+$. These oxygen radicals combine with those produced by the formation of O_2^- by the arachidonic acid system (blocks 19, 5, and 6). In addition, the effects of hyperoxia on the generation of O_2^- is also shown (block 7). The effects of small challenges of superoxide dismutase (SOD) production and other free radical scavengers are shown in blocks 11, 12, and 13. The formation of H_2O_2 is shown at block 10, and above this block the formation of OH· in the Haber-Weiss reaction of O_2^- and H_2O_2. The free radicals, leukotrienes, and O_2^- feed back to cause further damage and neutrophil and/or macrophage activity. Finally, all radicals will cause vascular endothelial and alveolar epithelial damage. At several portions of the schematic (shown as circled numbers) different blockers or scavengers of the oxygen radicals are shown, eg, (1) the effect of steroids on membrane stabilization and neutrophil activity; (3) the effect of ibuprofen on blocking the cyclo-oxygenase pathway; (20) the effect of allopurinol on blocking xanthine oxidase activity; (21) the effect of SOD either from exogenous or endogenous sources on dismutation of O_2^- to H_2O_2; (16) the effects of catalase on converting H_2O_2 to H_2O; (11) the effects of the glutathione reductase system on detoxifying H_2O_2; and (18), which represents the scavenging of OH· radicals by dimethyl sulfoxide (DMSO), mannitol, etc. In order to simplify the schema, tissue macrophage activation can replace neutrophil activation to explain experimental findings at the appropriate point in the model. (Reproduced with permission from Taylor and Martin.[11,34])

124

for the lung damage; in fact, it may be a combination of all radicals but most likely OH· and H_2O_2 are the most toxic compounds formed that produce a positive feedback system with regard to producing further tissue damage.

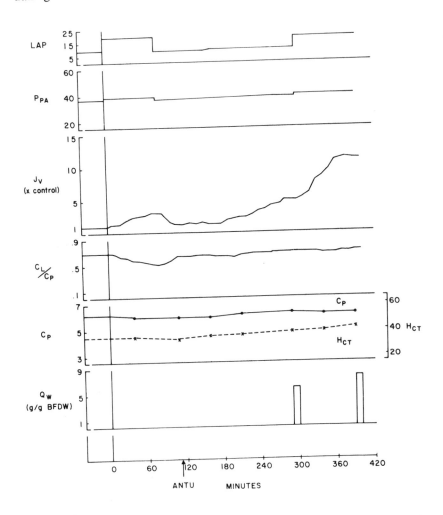

Figure 9-3 Plot of left atrial pressure (LAP) pulmonary atrial pressure (P_{PA}), lymph flow times control (Jv), concentration of total plasma proteins in lymph and plasma (C_L/C_P), and lung water (O_w) collected from a dog lung–lymphatic model.[34] Left atrial pressure was elevated and time was allotted for the system to attain a steady state in J_v and C_L/C_P. At the arrow α-naphthylthiourea (ANTU) was infused into the pulmonary artery and the parameters studied for another three hours, at which time LAP was again elevated. Note that J_v increases 12- to 14-fold but C_L/C_P was unchanged and the lung water indicates severe pulmonary edema. (Reproduced with permission from Rutili et al.[31])

Table 9-2
Hydroxyl Radical (OH·) Generation in α-Naphthylthiourea (ANTU)-Damaged Lungs*

Condition	Protection
ANTU	0
ANTU + superoxide dismutase	70%
ANTU + catalase	70%
ANTU + dimethyl sulfoxide	40%
Neutrophil depletion	0
Allopurinol	0
Ibuprofen	75%

*Modified from Martin et al.[32]

Table 9-3
Conditions Involving Free Radical Formation

Compound or Condition	Scavengers, Detoxifying Enzymes	Mechanism(s)
Thiourea[33]	DMSO, ethanol, mannitol catalase	OH· formation (no neutrophil requirement)
ANTU [26,32,34,35]	DMSO, SOD, catalase, ibuprofen	OH· formation Arachidonic acid products (no neutrophil requirement)
Microemboli, air bubbles [36,37]	SOD	OH· formation? O_2^-? (neutrophil requirement)
Hyperoxia [38]	SOD (intercellular)	OH·? O_2^- (no neutrophil requirement)
Irradiation [33]	Dimethylthiourea	OH· (no neutrophil requirement)
Endotoxin [39,40]	SOD caused more damage	H_2O_2 or HOCl (neutrophil requirement)
Complement activation [41]	Ibuprofen, SOD (capillary endothelial study)	OH· Arachidonic acid products (neutrophil requirement)?
Complement activation [42]	Catalase (capillary endothelial study)	H_2O_2, HOCl (neutrophil requirement)
Glucose-glucosidase, myeloperoxidase, or lactoperoxidase [19]	SOD (early), catalase (late) (alveolar epithelial study)	O_2^-? OH· (early), H_2O_2, HOCl (late) (neutrophil requirement)
Phorbal myristate acetate [43]	Catalase (alveolar epithelial study)	H_2O_2, HOCl, macrophage involvement (no neutrophil requirement)

Modified from Grimbert et al.[30]
ANTU = α-naphthylthiourea, DMSO = dimethyl sulfoxide, SOD = superoxide dismutase, OH· = hydroxyl radical, O_2^- = superoxide radical, H_2O_2 = hydrogen peroxide, HOCl = hypochlorous acid.

126

The mechanism by which these many forms of pathology initially produce the oxygen radicals is not known to any degree of certainty. It appears that both neutrophils and macrophages can produce tissue damage by the production of free radicals and both arachidonic acid products and the xanthine oxidase systems produce oxygen radicals in some types of tissue damage. Conditions which can easily occur in tissue, such as hypoxia, produce O_2^- radicals and various metals also appear to be involved in oxygen radical production.[44,45]

SUMMARY

Future research promises to produce new and exciting data relative to how the oxygen radicals are involved in lung pathology. Future studies will undoubtedly lead to improved care of critically ill patients who are prone to develop ARDS. It is important to emphasize that our ANTU studies demonstrate that the formation of fulminating pulmonary edema can be prevented by pretreatment of the animals with SOD, catalase or OH· scavengers. Perhaps compounds such as SOD, catalase, and others can be useful treatment regimens in the critically ill patient and will protect the lung against further oxygen radical damage, but more research is required before these experimental findings can be applied clinically.

REFERENCES

1. Taylor AE, Parker JC: The pulmonary interstitial spaces and lymphatics, in Fischman AP, Fisher AB (eds): *Handbook of Physiology. Pulmonary Circulation and Non-Respiratory Functions of the Lung.* Baltimore, Williams & Wilkins Co, 1985, vol 4, pp 167–230.
2. Staub, NC: Pulmonary edema. *Physiol Rev* 1974;54:687–811.
3. Taylor AE, Gibson WH, Granger HJ, et al: The interaction between intracapillary forces in the overall regulation of interstitial fluid volume. *Lymphology* 1973;6:192–208.
4. Kedem O, Kathcalsky A: Thermodynamic analysis of the permeability of biological membranes to non-electrolytes. *Biochim Biophys Acta* 1958;27: 229–246.
5. Taylor AE, Granger DN: Exchange of macromolecules across the circulation, in Renkin EM, Michel CG (eds): *Handbook of Microcirculation.* Baltimore, Williams & Wilkins Co, 1984, pp 467–520.
6. Parker JC, Parker RE, Granger DN, et al: Permeability of pulmonary capillaries. *Circ Res* 1981;48:549–561.
7. Parker RE, Rosseli RJ, Harris TR, et al: Effect of graded increases in pulmonary vascular pressure on lung fluid balance in unanesthetized sheep. *Circ Res* 1981;49:1164–1172.
8. Smith JC, Mitzner W: Analysis of pulmonary vascular interdependence in excised dog lobes. *J Appl Physiol* 1980;48:450–465.
9. Guyton AC, Granger HJ, Taylor AE: Interstitial fluid pressure. *Physiol Rev* 1971;51:527–563.

10. Parker JC, Guyton AC, Taylor AE: Pulmonary interstitial and capillary pressure estimates from intra-alveolar fluid pressures. *J Appl Physiol* 1978; 44:267–276.
11. Taylor AE, Martin D, Townsley MI: Oxygen radicals and pulmonary edema, in Said SI (ed): *The Pulmonary Circulation and Pulmonary Vascular Injury.* Futura Publishing Co, Mount Kisco, NY, 1985, pp 307–320.
12. Rippe B, Allison RC, Parker JC, et al: Effects of histamine, serotonin, and norepinephrine on the circulation of dog lung. *J Appl Physiol* 1984;57:223–232.
13. Taylor AE: Starling forces. *Circ Res* 1981;49:552–575.
14. Holloway H, Perry MA, Parker JC, et al: Estimation of pulmonary capillary pressures in intact dog lung. *J Appl Physiol* 1983;54:846–851.
15. Brigham KL, Bowers RE, Haynes J: Increased sheep lung vascular permeability caused by *E. coli* endotoxin. *Circ Res* 1979;45:292–297.
16. Kinnebrew PS, Parker JC, Taylor AE: Pulmonary microvascular permeability following *E. coli* endotoxin and hemorrhage. *J Appl Physiol* 1982;52:403–409.
17. Parker JC, Rippe B, Townsley M, et al: Effect of peak airway pressure (P_{aw}) on microvascular permeability in the lung. *Fed Proc* 1984;43:513.
18. Vreim CE, Snashall P, Staub NC: Protein composition of lung fluids in anesthetized dogs with acute cardiogenic edema. *Am J Physiol* 1976; 231:1466–1469.
19. Ward PA: Role of toxic oxygen products from phagocytic cells in tissue injury. *Adv Shock Res* 1983;10:27–34.
20. Egan EA: Response of alveolar epothelial solute permeability to changes in lung inflation. *J Appl Physiol* 1980;49:1032–1036.
21. Mortillaro NA, Taylor AE: Interaction of capillary and tissue forces in the cat small intestine. *Circ Res* 1976;39:348–357.
22. Yablonski ME, Lifson N: Mechanism of production of intestinal secretion by elevated venous pressure. *J Clin Invest* 1976;57:904–915.
23. Taylor AE, Gaar KA: Estimation of equivalent pore radii of pulmonary capillary and alveolar membranes. *Am J Physiol* 1970;218:1133–1140.
24. Granger DN, Cook BH, Taylor AE: Structural locus of transmucosal albumin efflux in canine ileum. A fluorescent study. *Gastroenterology* 1976;71: 1023–1027.
25. Drake RE, Gaar KA, Taylor AE: Estimation of the filtration coefficient of the pulmonary exchange vessels. *Am J Physiol* 1978;234:H266–H274.
26. Taylor AE, Martin D: Oxygen radicals and the microcirculation. *Physiologist* 1983;26:152–155.
27. Lewis DH, Del Maestro R, Arfors KE (eds): Free radicals in medicine and biology. *Acta Physiol Scand* 1980 (Suppl);492:1–168.
28. Frank L, Robert RL: Endotoxin protection against oxygen induced acute and chronic lung injury. *J Appl Physiol* 1979;47:577–581.
29. Del Maestro R, Bjork J, Arfors KE: Free radicals and microvascular permeability, in *Pathology of Oxygen.* New York, Academic Press, 1982, pp 157–173.
30. Grimbert FA, Parker JC, Taylor AE: Increased pulmonary vascular permeability following acid aspiration. *J Appl Physiol* 1981;51:335–345.
31. Rutili G, Parker JC, Taylor AE: Vascular permeability in dog lungs after ANTU. *J Appl Physiol* 1982;52:1444–1452.
32. Martin D, Korthuis RJ, Perry M, et al: Oxygen radical mediated lung damage associated with α-naphthylthiourea. *Acta Physiol Scand,* in press.
33. Fox RB, Harada RN, Tate RM, et al: Prevention of thiourea-induced pulmonary edema by hydroxyl-radical scavengers. *J Appl Physiol* 1983; 55:1456–1459.

34. Taylor AE, Martin D, Parker JC: The effects of oxygen radicals on pulmonary edema formation. *Surgery* 1983;94:433-438.
35. Parker JC, Martin DJ, Rutili G, et al: Prevention of free radical mediated vascular permeability increase in lung using superoxide dismutase. *Chest* 1983;83:525-528.
36. Flick MR, Hoeffel J, Staub NC: Superoxide dismutase prevents increased lung vascular permeability after microemboli. *Fed Proc* 1981;40:405.
37. Flick MR, Perel A, Staub NC: Leukocytes are required for increased lung microvascular permeability after microembolization in sheep. *Circ Res* 1981;48:344-351.
38. Crapo JD, Freeman BA, Barry BE, et al: Mechanisms of hyperoxic injury to the pulmonary microcirculation. *Physiologist* 1983;26:170-176.
39. Heflin AC, Brigham KL: Prevention by granulocyte depletion of increased vascular permeability of sheep lung following endotoxemia. *J Clin Invest* 1981;68:1253-1260.
40. Traber DL, Adams T, Sziebert L, et al: Potentiation of the lung vascular response to endotoxin by superoxide dismutase. *J Appl Physiol* 1985;58:1005-1009.
41. Perkowski SZ, Havill AW, Flynn JT, et al: Role of intrapulmonary release of eicosanoids and superoxide anion as mediators of pulmonary dysfunction and endothelial injury in sheep with intermittent complement activation. *Circ Res* 1983;53:574-583.
42. Till GO, Johnson KJ, Kunkel R, et al: Intravascular activation of complement and acute lung injury. *J Clin Invest* 1982;69:1126-1135.
43. Johnson KJ, Ward PA: Acute and progressive lung injury after contact with phorbol myristate acetate. *Am J Pathol* 1982;107:29-35.
44. Granger DN, Rutili G, McCord JM: Superoxide radicals in feline intestinal ischemia. *Gastroenterology* 1981;81:22-29.
45. Borg DC, Schaich KM: Cytotoxicity from coupled redox cycling of autoxidizing xenobiotics and metals. *Isr J Chem* 1984;24:38-53.

10 Erythrocyte (RBC) Antioxidants as Potential Protectors and/or Predictors of Oxidant-Induced Lung Injury

John E. Repine
Connie J. Beehler
Elaine M. Berger
Carl W. White
Karen M. Toth

NATURE AND SOURCES OF OXIDANTS CAUSING LUNG INJURY

Oxidants appear to be important causes of lung damage and other disorders.[1,2] The exact mechanisms responsible for the toxicity of oxidants are unknown but it is believed that key cell components, such as proteins, lipids, and/or nucleic acids are directly susceptible to oxidant injury. In addition, oxidants may initiate reactions which damage the lung in indirect ways. For example, reaction between oxidants and lung tissue can affect arachidonic acid metabolism, which in turn could alter pulmonary vasoconstriction and/or permeability.[3,4] Oxidants might also damage alveolar macrophages (or other lung cells) and in the process stimulate these cells to release factors which attract and activate neutrophils in the lung.[5] Recruited neutrophils may then further damage the lung by releasing toxic O_2 metabolites, proteolytic enzymes, arachidonic acid metabolites, and/or other products. The toxicity of the latter, especially neutrophil elastase, may be amplified if oxidants have previously inactivated circulating antiproteases or other protective mechanisms.[6]

Oxidants are generated from many sources. Externally derived oxidants include environmental toxins, such as nitrous oxide (NO_2), ozone, cigarette smoke, and hyperoxia. Within the body, extracellular oxidants include phagocytic cell products, such as superoxide anion (O_2^-), hydrogen peroxide (H_2O_2), hydroxyl radical ($\cdot OH$), and hypochlorous acid (HOCl).[7] Intracellularly derived oxidants include O_2 metabolite products from cellular oxidative metabolism.[8,9] In the latter situation, about 2% of the O_2 consumed by mitochondria may eventually be transferred into highly reactive O_2 intermediates. Moreover, cell perturbations following hyperoxia, radiation, or drugs may lead to excessive production of self-damaging O_2 metabolites by lung cells.[8,9] In addition, during reperfusion following ischemia, xanthine dehydrogenase may be converted to xanthine oxidase and generate O_2 metabolites.[10] The extent and importance of these O_2 metabolite-generating reactions, as well as the distance any of these "short-lived" O_2 metabolites can travel, especially in protein and lipid-rich milieus, remains unknown. Finally, other factors may modify the production, nature, and/or toxicity of oxidants in lung tissue. For example, iron, or other metals, may catalyze reactions which convert O_2^- and H_2O_2 to more toxic species, such as $\cdot OH$. Similarly, myeloperoxidase (MPO) may react with H_2O_2 to form HOCl and as a result, modify the type and/or location of injury.[7]

ENDOGENOUS AND EXOGENOUS LUNG ANTIOXIDANT DEFENSE MECHANISMS

The previous statements suggest that oxidants constitute a potent arsenal which can injure lung tissue. However, analogous to elastase-antiprotease lung balance mechanisms, there appears to be compensating antioxidant defenses which can counteract oxidant attacks on the lung. Relatively little is known about these antioxidant scavenger systems. In particular, it is unclear how their location, reaction rates, and/or specificities affect detoxification of various O_2 metabolites. This article will review briefly[11] these antioxidant defense mechanisms and then focus on new observations and speculations that RBC antioxidant enzymes may participate in lung antioxidant host-defense mechanisms.

Endogenous pulmonary antioxidant defense systems include cellular antioxidant enzymes and circulating antioxidants.[11] The best known cellular antioxidant is superoxide dismutase (SOD) which is a constituent of nearly all cells.[10] Superoxide dismutases are metal-containing enzymes which convert superoxide anion (O_2^-) to hydrogen peroxide (H_2O_2). The enzyme is present as a 32,000-dalton copper-zinc form in cell cytoplasm while an 86,000-dalton manganese form predominates in mitochondria. Other common cellular antioxidants are catalase, a scavenger of H_2O_2, and glutathione peroxidase (GPX) which can catalyze reduction of organic hydroperoxides and H_2O_2 to nontoxic compounds while oxidizing glutathione.[12] Catalase and glutathione peroxidase appear to complement each other in their intracellular locations and in their postulated relative abilities for scavenging higher and lower concentrations of H_2O_2, respectively. Independent of its role as cofactor for glutathione peroxidase, reduced glutathione (GSH) appears to be able to inhibit lipid peroxidation.

The evidence that any of the aforementioned cellular antioxidants protect the lung remains inferential. It is largely based on observations that a correlation exists between increases in lung antioxidant enzymes and protection against subsequent oxidant-induced lung injuries.[13] Although this intriguing correlation suggests that lung antioxidants are important in protection, the cause and effect relationship of this "tolerance" phenomenon is unproven. The potential contributions of circulating, extracellular antioxidant systems to lung host defense are even more unclear. Ceruloplasmin, which reduces O_2^- to H_2O_2, has been found to be elevated in rats which have been exposed to hyperoxia but the significance of this increase is unknown. Likewise, there has also been a recent report of a 134,000-dalton SOD in human lung alveolar spaces whose significance has not been determined.

Nutritional factors and administered antioxidants may also affect lung oxidant susceptibility. For example, vitamin E can terminate chain reaction lipid peroxidation in membranes in vitro but addition of greater than physiologic levels of vitamin E does not reduce oxidant injury in intact animals. β-Carotene is regarded as an effective scavenger of singlet oxygen and could prevent lipid peroxidation in animal tissues. The potential antioxidant role of another dietary factor, ascorbate, is debatable but theoretically ascorbate may act as an O_2 metabolite scavenger reducing tocopherols, lipid peroxides, and other radicals. Selenium is a needed component of the glutathione peroxidase enzyme system that reduces H_2O_2. As one might predict, rats with selenium deficiency have decreased pulmonary glutathione peroxidase activity and shortened survival in hyperoxia. The effect of fat or protein intake on oxidant-induced lung injury is also not entirely clear but rats fed a diet rich in saturated fats or low in protein are more susceptible to lung injury from hyperoxia than rats fed a standard diet.

Exogenous delivery of antioxidant enzymes may augment endogenous lung defense mechanisms. Unfortunately, the very short circulating half-lives of administered antioxidant enzymes have necessitated approaches designed to increase the half-lives of these enzymes. These approaches include entrapment of antioxidant enzymes in liposomes[14] and conjugation of antioxidant enzymes to polyethylene glycol.[15] Liposome-delivered catalase has been reported to decrease hydrogen peroxide-dependent injury of cultured pulmonary artery endothelial cells while liposome-delivered SOD protects cultured pulmonary endothelial cells against hyperoxic injury. Treatment with liposomes containing both SOD and catalase enhances survival of rats exposed to hyperoxia. However, in the latter case, the animals required preloading with latex beads, presumably to depress the rapid uptake of liposomes by phagocytic cells and/or the reticuloendothelial cell system. Because of this finding, it also seemed likely that liposomes containing antioxidant enzymes might impair O_2 metabolite-dependent phagocyte-mediated activities. Support for this premise includes observations that liposomes with or without SOD decrease extracellular release of O_2^- by neutrophils as well as intracellular killing of bacteria by neutrophils in vitro.[16] Administration of empty or SOD-containing liposomes also decreased the clearance of intravenously injected *Staphylococcus aureus* by rabbits in vivo.[16] Similar results have been found in assessments of the effects of liposomes on macrophages.[17]

Attachment to polyethylene glycol (PEG) greatly prolongs the circulation of exogenously administered antioxidant enzymes, diminishes lung injury, and increases survival of rats exposed to hyperoxia.[15] However, in contrast to liposomes, PEG antioxidants do not inhibit killing of bacteria by neutrophils in vitro or clearance of intravenously injected *S aureus*.[16]

Small, permeable chemical scavengers of oxygen metabolites could also decrease oxidant-induced lung injury. Dimethylthiourea (DMTU) is an effective O_2 metabolite scavenger which can decrease O_2 metabolite-dependent lung injury caused by phorbol myristate acetate–stimulated neutrophils in isolated perfused rabbit lungs and in vivo.[18,19] Dimethylthiourea also decreases lung edema of rats exposed to hyperoxia.[20] Dimethyl sulfoxide (DMSO)—a scavenger of hydroxyl radical—decreases lung injury in rats given cobra venom factor–induced oxidant insults.[21] Another scavenger, N-acetylcysteine, protects the lungs of animals given endotoxin.[22]

Theoretically, various chemical precursors of the tripeptide glutathione might be effective in increasing pulmonary glutathione. This could increase the rate of glutathione peroxidase–mediated reduction of H_2O_2 and resistance to oxidant stresses. The potential therapeutic effectiveness of augmenting glutathione synthesis may also depend on increasing pentose phosphate shunt activity to provide nicotinamide adenine dinucleotide phosphate (NADPH) for glutathione pathway activity.[23]

ERYTHROCYTE (RBC) ANTIOXIDANT ENZYMES AND OXIDANT-INDUCED LUNG INJURY

Recently, we found that RBC could decrease O_2 metabolite-induced damage in a number of lung injury models.[24] Because RBC contain vast amounts of antioxidant enzymes, this suggested that RBC might be an additional, intrinsic antioxidant host-defense mechanism. In support of this hypothesis, we found that addition of increasing concentrations of washed human RBC progressively decreased the weight gains and lavage albumin concentration increases in isolated lungs perfused with O_2 metabolites generated by hypoxanthine (HX) and xanthine oxidase (XO) (Table 10-1), lactate dehydrogenase (LDH) release from cultured pulmonary artery endothelial cells treated with hydrogen peroxide (H_2O_2) (Table 10-2), and oxidation of reduced cytochrome c by H_2O_2 in vitro (Table 10-3). The mechanisms of RBC protection appeared to involve scavenging of H_2O_2 by intracellular RBC antioxidant enzymes. This impression is based on the following observations. First, glutaraldehyde treated RBC—which did not release LDH when treated with H_2O_2 in vitro—protected as well as untreated RBC. Second, RBC treated with aminotriazole (AMT)—a catalase inhibitor—or dichloronitrobenzene (DCNB)—an inhibitor of glutathione—did not protect as well as untreated RBC.

Subsequently, it has been reported that RBC placed into the tracheobronchial tree improve the survival of rats exposed to hyperoxia.[25] These latter studies also suggest that recyclable glutathione is important in RBC protection in part because (1) RBC with cyanomethemoglobin were as beneficial as untreated RBC and (2) RBC with inhibited glutathione (following dichloronitrobenzene or N-ethylmalemide treatment) were less effective than untreated RBC.

Table 10-1
Effect of Human RBC on Edema Formation in Isolated Rat Lungs Perfused with Hypoxanthine (HX) and Xanthine Oxidase (XO)

Test Conditions (Substances Added to Perfusates)	Lung Weight Gains (g)	Lung Lavage Albumin Concentrations (mg/dL)
None	0.3 ± 0.1 (12)*†	220 ± 15 (12)†
HX + XO	17.0 ± 1.0 (10)	2090 ± 260 (10)
HX + XO + RBC (0.25%)	16.0 ± 0.2 (5)‡	2110 ± 250 (5)‡
HX + XO + RBC (0.5%)	6.2 ± 0.7 (5)†	485 ± 60 (5)†
HX + XO + RBC (1%)	0.8 ± 0.6 (10)†	205 ± 50 (10)†
HX + XO + RBC (5%)	0.4 ± 0.1 (5)†	250 ± 60 (5)†
HX	0.3 (2)†	220 (2)†
XO	0.3 (2)†	220 (2)†

*Mean ± SE (number of determinations).
†Value significantly different ($P<.05$) from value obtained with HX + XO alone.
‡Value not significantly different ($P>.05$) from value obtained with HX + XO alone.

134

Table 10-2
Effect of Human RBC on Lactate Dehydrogenase (LDH) Concentrations in Supernatants from Cultured Bovine Pulmonary Artery Endothelial Cells Treated with H_2O_2

Test Conditions (Substances Added to Cultures)	LDH Concentrations (% Total)
None	13 ± 0.1 (22)*†
H_2O_2 (3 mmol/L)	19 ± 1.5 (4)†
H_2O_2 (10 mmol/L)	23 ± 1.2 (4)†
H_2O_2 (30 mmol/L)	41 ± 4.0 (14)
H_2O_2 (30 mmol/L) + RBC (0.1%)	38 ± 2.5 (4)‡
H_2O_2 (30 mmol/L) + RBC (0.5%)	20 ± 1.8 (4)†
H_2O_2 (30 mmol/L) + RBC (1.0%)	17 ± 0.1 (8)†
H_2O_2 (30 mmol/L) + RBC (5.0%)	7 ± 4.0 (4)†

*Mean ± SE (number of determinations).
†Value significantly different ($P < .05$) from value obtained with H_2O_2 (30 mmol/L) alone.
‡Value not significantly different ($P > .05$) from value obtained with H_2O_2 (30 mmol/L) alone.

Table 10-3
Effect of Human RBC on Oxidation of Reduced Cytochrome c by H_2O_2 in vitro

Test Conditions (Substances Added in vitro)	Oxidation of Reduced Cytochrome c (nm Oxidation/20 min)
None	0 (20)*†
H_2O_2 (1 μmol/L)	3 ± 0.2 (5)†
H_2O_2 (10 μmol/L)	7 ± 0.3 (6)†
H_2O_2 (20 μmol/L)	15 ± 0.3 (30)
H_2O_2 (20 μmol/L) + RBC (0.001%)	15 ± 0.2 (5)‡
H_2O_2 (20 μmol/L) + RBC (0.01%)	8 ± 0.3 (6)†
H_2O_2 (20 μmol/L) + RBC (0.05%)	0.5 ± 0.1 (15)†

*Mean ± SE (number of determinations).
†Value significantly different ($P < .05$) from value obtained with H_2O_2 (20 μmol/L) alone.
‡Value not significantly different ($P > .05$) from value obtained with H_2O_2 (20 μmol/L) alone.

Finally, we have most recently found that RBC from cigarette smokers contain more catalase and glutathione and protect endothelial cells against H_2O_2-mediated injury better than RBC from nonsmokers.[26] Perhaps more importantly, wide individual variations exist in the antioxidant enzyme activities of RBC from various subjects.

These observations on RBC antioxidants raise a number of speculations. First, we suggest that RBC could be effective circulating scavengers of O_2 metabolites. This concept is supported by the present observations, as well as studies showing that H_2O_2 dissipation is critical to tissue protection.[24,25] Although RBC can scavenge H_2O_2 in cell-free[24] and/or stimulated neutrophil systems,[25,27] whether H_2O_2 exists long enough in biological systems to react with RBC or if RBC can penetrate tight neutrophil-endothelial junctions where oxidant injury may be occurring, remains to be determined. At any rate, it is interesting that hemorrhage—a common feature of many pathologic processes—may bring needed, protecting antioxidant enzymes to normally unprotected areas, such as lung alveolar spaces. Likewise, the provocative possibility exists that transfusion of RBC, especially RBC with high antioxidant enzyme contents, may be beneficial in combating oxidant injury.

An additional possibility is that RBC antioxidant enzymes serve as a marker of oxidant stress and/or a predictor of susceptibility to lung or other vascular injury. This hypothesis is based on our observation that RBC from cigarette smokers have more antioxidant enzymes than RBC from nonsmokers. The latter suggests that exposure to oxidants may stimulate synthesis of increased RBC enzymes or glutathione—ostensibly to protect against the increased oxidant load. In addition, wide individual variations were seen in antioxidant enzyme activities of RBC from individual cigarette smokers. Because only a relatively small percentage of cigarette smokers develop lung injury, heart disease, or cancer (all of which have been postulated to be associated with oxidant-induced injury), it suggests that RBC antioxidant enzymes might also serve as a marker of risk for these diseases. For example, with a comparable oxidant load, those individuals with the ability to increase their antioxidant enzymes would have fewer "net" O_2 metabolites and susceptibility to oxidant-induced pathology. In contrast, individuals with lower RBC antioxidant enzyme activities would have a greater net O_2 metabolite load and a greater susceptibility to oxidants. While the aforementioned is based on the theory that RBC antioxidant enzymes are scavengers, the speculations could also be true if antioxidant levels in RBC are indicators of other cell antioxidant capabilities. Specifically, do individuals with higher RBC antioxidant enzyme levels have higher antioxidant enzyme levels in their lung or other cells? Conversely, do individuals with lower RBC antioxidant enzyme levels have lung cells with less antioxidant activities and accordingly a greater susceptibility to oxidant injury?

SUMMARY

Recent knowledge implicating oxidants as contributors to many diseases has prompted intensified examination of potential antioxidant defense mechanisms. This report suggests that antioxidant enzymes in RBC may be an important part of our antioxidant defenses. It will be interesting to assess this possibility as investigators probe the significance of RBC antioxidant enzymes in biological processes and oxidant-induced diseases.

ACKNOWLEDGMENTS

Support for this work was provided by the National Institutes of Health, American Heart Association, American Lung Association, Procter & Gamble Co, Tambrands, and the Council for Tobacco Research.

REFERENCES

1. Johnson KJ, Fantone JC, Kaplan J, et al: *In vivo* damage of rat lungs by oxygen metabolites. *J Clin Invest* 1981;67:983–993.
2. Shasby DM, VanBenthuysen KM, Tate RM, et al: Granulocytes mediate acute edematous lung injury in rabbits and isolated rabbit lungs perfused with phorbol myristate acetate: Role of oxygen radicals. *Am Rev Respir Dis* 1982; 125:443–447.
3. Henderson WR, Klebanoff SJ: Leukotriene B_4, C_4, D_4 and E_4 inactivation by hydroxyl radicals. *Biochem Biophys Res Commun* 1983;110:266–272.
4. Tate RM, Morris HG, Schroeder WR, et al: Oxygen metabolites stimulate thromboxane production and vasoconstriction in isolated saline perfused rabbit lungs. *J Clin Invest* 1984;74:608–613.
5. Harada RN, Vatter AE, Repine JE: Oxygen radical scavengers protect alveolar macrophages from hyperoxic injury *in vitro*. *Am Rev Respir Dis* 1983; 128:761–762.
6. Cochrane CG, Spragg RG, Revak SO, et al: The presence of neutrophil elastase and evidence of oxidation activity in the bronchoalveolar lavage fluid of patients with adult respiratory distress syndrome. *Am Rev Respir Dis* 1983;127:290–300.
7. Klebanoff SJ: Oxygen metabolites and the toxic properties of phagocytes. *Ann Intern Med* 1980;93:480–489.
8. Bowman CM, Toth KM, Vatter AE, et al: Mechanisms of lung injury from hyperoxia: Pulmonary artery endothelial cells but not lung fibroblasts make superoxide anion (O_2^-). *Clin Res* 1983;31:414A.
9. Rosen GM, Freeman BA: Detection of superoxide generated by endothelial cells. *Proc Natl Acad Sci USA* 1985;81:7269–7273.
10. McCord JM: Oxygen-derived free radicals in postischemic tissue injury. *N Engl J Med* 1985;312:159–163.
11. White CW, Repine JE: Pulmonary host defense mechanisms. *Exp Lung Res*, 1985;8:81–96.
12. Lauterberg BH, Smith CV, Hughes H, et al: Biliary excretion of glutathione and glutathione disulfide in the rat. Regulation and response to oxidative stress. *J Clin Invest* 1984;73:124–133.
13. Frank L, Yam J, Roberts R: The role of endotoxin in protection of adult rats from oxygen induced lung toxicity. *J Clin Invest* 1978;61:269–275.
14. Turrens JF, Crapo JD, Freeman BA: Protection against oxygen toxicity by intravenous injection of liposome entrapped catalase and superoxide dismutase. *J Clin Invest* 1984;73:879–885.
15. White CW, Jackson JH, Abuchowski A, et al: Intravenous treatment with polyethylene glycol (PEG)-conjugated superoxide dismutase (SOD) and catalase (CAT) prolongs survival of rats exposed to hyperoxia. *Clin Res* 1984;32:60A.

16. McDonald RJ, Berger EM, White CW, et al: Effect of superoxide dismutase encapsulated in liposomes or conjugated with polyethylene glycol on neutrophil bactericidal activity *in vitro* and bacterial clearance *in vivo*. *Am Rev Respir Dis* 1985;131:633–637.

17. Gilbreath MJ, Swartz GM Jr, Alving CR, et al: Differential inhibition of macrophage microbicidal activity by liposomes. *Infect Immun* 1985; 47:567–569.

18. Tate RM, VanBenthuysen KM, Shasby DM, et al: Oxygen radical-mediated permeability edema and vasoconstriction in isolated perfused rabbit lungs. *Am Rev Respir Dis* 1982;126:802–806.

19. Jackson JH, White CW, Clifford DP, et al: Dimethylthiourea (DMTU), a scavenger of toxic oxygen metabolites, prevents acute edematous lung injury in rabbits following injection of phorbol myristate acetate (PMA). *Am Rev Respir Dis* 1983;127:286.

20. Fox RB: Prevention of granulocyte-mediated oxidant lung injury in rats by a hydroxyl radical scavenger, dimethylthiourea. *J Clin Invest* 1984;74: 456–1464.

21. Ward PA, Till GO, Kunkel R, et al: Evidence for role of hydroxyl radical in complement and neutrophil dependent tissue injury. *J Clin Invest* 1983;72:789–801.

22. Bernard GR, Lucht WD, Nidermeyer ME, et al: Effect of N-acetylcysteine on the pulmonary response to endotoxin in the awake sheep and upon *in vitro* granulocyte function. *J Clin Invest* 1984;73:1772–1774.

23. Tierney D, Ayers L, Herzog S, et al: Pentose pathway and production of re-uced nicotinamide adenine dinucleotide phosphate. A mechanism that may protect lungs from oxidants. *Am Rev Respir Dis* 1973;108:1348–1353.

24. Toth KM, Clifford DP, Berger EM, et al: Intact human erythrocytes prevent hydrogen peroxide-mediated damage to isolated perfused rat lungs and cultured bovine pulmonary artery endothelial cells. *J Clin Invest* 1984;74:292–295.

25. van Asbeck BS, Hoidal JR, Vercellotti GM, et al: Protection against lethal hyperoxia by tracheal insufflation of erythrocytes: Role of red cell glutathione. *Science* 1985;227:756–758.

26. Toth KM, Berger EM, Beehler CJ, et al: Erythrocytes (RBC) from cigarette smokers contain more catalase and glutathione (GSH) and protect endothelial cells (EC) against H_2O_2 better than RBC from non-smokers. *Clin Res* 1985;33:82A.

27. Test ST, Weiss SJ: Quantitative and temporal characterization of the extracellular H_2O_2 pool generated by human neutrophils. *J Biol Chem* 1984; 259:399–405.

11 Interactions of Neutrophils in the Pulmonary Vascular Bed in the Adult Respiratory Distress Syndrome (ARDS)

Kenneth L. Brigham

Inflammation, defined as accumulation of polymorphonuclear neutrophils, is a common finding in the lungs of humans with the adult respiratory distress syndrome (ARDS) and in several animal models of the syndrome. In some animal models, including pulmonary embolism, endotoxemia, and possibly pulmonary oxygen toxicity, injury to the lung microcirculation has been shown to be neutrophil-dependent, that is, when animals are depleted of neutrophils, the magnitude of the injury is decreased.

We have concentrated on the effects of gram-negative bacterial endotoxin on the lung circulation because gram-negative sepsis is a common clinical setting in which ARDS occurs and because, in whole animals, endotoxemia causes pathophysiologic changes in the lungs similar in many respects to those of ARDS in humans.

Data will be presented relevant to the mechanism of endotoxin-induced pulmonary vascular injury from three preparations: (1) chronically instrumented unanesthetized sheep, (2) bovine pulmonary artery intima explants, and (3) cultured bovine pulmonary vascular endothelial cells.

ENDOTOXIN CAUSES NEUTROPHIL-DEPENDENT LUNG VASCULAR INJURY

When *Escherichia coli* endotoxin is infused intravenously (IV) into sheep in doses too small to cause marked alterations in systemic hemodynamics, it causes lung injury.[1] Alterations in lung function include an early phase, reaching a zenith at about one hour following endotoxin infusion, which is characterized by marked decreases in lung compliance, increases in resistance to airflow across the lungs, and dramatic pulmonary hypertension.[2] This constrictor phase of the reaction is followed at two to three hours after endotoxin infusion by a period of sustained increases in the flow of protein-rich lymph from the lungs indicating increased lung vascular permeability.[1,2-4] If sufficient doses of endotoxin are given, severe pulmonary edema and death from respiratory failure results several hours after administering endotoxin.[5]

Structural studies of the lungs over the course of the endotoxin reaction in sheep show accumulation of neutrophils in the lungs.[6] Neutrophils begin to accumulate as early as 30 minutes after endotoxin is infused and large numbers of neutrophils persist in the lung periphery for many hours. In addition, neutrophils undergo an interesting series of interactions with lung microvessels, demonstrated by electron microscopy.[6,7] Both neutrophils and lymphocytes sequester in microvessels early in the endotoxin reaction. This sequestration is followed by degranulation of neutrophils and migration of neutrophils between microvascular endothelial cells into the interstitium. Ultrastructural evidence of pulmonary microvascular endothelial injury is seen as early as one hour after endotoxin and by four hours there is severe endothelial injury with gaps in the endothelial layer.[6-8]

When sheep are depleted of circulating granulocytes by treatment with hydroxyurea, the response to endotoxin is altered. The early changes in lung mechanics are attenuated and the later increase in vascular permeability is much less.[9,10] Thus, in the sense that neutrophils seem necessary for the full expression of the endotoxin effect, endotoxin produces neutrophil-dependent lung vascular injury.

At least one class of drugs, corticosteroids, which prevents accumulation of neutrophils in the lungs following endotoxin infusion, also moderates the lung injury.[11] When sheep are treated with high doses of methylprednisolone prior to infusing endotoxin, the initial pulmonary hypertension is less severe and the late phase of increased lung vascular permeability is markedly attentuated. Structural studies show that methylprednisolone also prevents accumulation of granulocytes in peripheral lung.[12]

IS THE INITIAL ENDOTHELIAL ALTERATION CAUSED BY ENDOTOXIN NEUTROPHIL-DEPENDENT?

If activated neutrophils are responsible for initiating endothelial injury following endotoxemia, then other interventions which activate circulating neutrophils should mimic the endotoxin effect. This may not be the case.

When zymosan-activated plasma (ZAP) is infused IV into sheep in doses sufficient to cause marked pulmonary sequestration of neutrophils, the response is at least quantitatively different from the response to endotoxin. Zymosan-activated plasma infusion causes transient pulmonary hypertension and peripheral leukopenia and a modest increase in lung lymph flow.[13] Although similar numbers of neutrophils sequester in the lung periphery after ZAP infusion as with endotoxin, and although increased numbers of neutrophils persist in the lungs for several hours, severe persistent injury of lung microvascular endothelium does not occur with ZAP.[13] There are transient modest ultrastructural changes in pulmonary endothelial cells, but by four hours following ZAP infusion, endothelium appears normal.[13]

It can be shown in in vitro preparations that neutrophils can migrate across pulmonary endothelium in response to ZAP without causing any detectable injury to the endothelial layer. In bovine pulmonary artery intima explants mounted in Boyden chambers with ZAP in the lower well and a suspension of purified granulocytes in the upper well, granulocytes migrate between endothelial cells, in close contact with the endothelium throughout the migration progress, but there is no ultrastructural evidence of injury.[14] Endothelial cells cultured on micropore filters show similar results. Thus, activation of neutrophils with complement fragments, even when the neutrophils are in close contact with endothelium, is not a sufficient explanation of the severe and persistent endothelial injury caused by endotoxin infusion.[7,8]

Also, endotoxin, in the absence of any inflammatory cells, can injure pulmonary endothelium. In the bovine pulmonary artery intima explant preparation described above, incubation of the explant with endotoxin causes endothelial cell retraction and, after a few hours, endothelial cell death.[15] In cultured bovine pulmonary vascular endothelial monolayers, endotoxin, even in concentrations as low as $0.001~\mu g/mL$ causes cytotoxicity, evidenced by pyknosis of endothelial cells and release of lactic dehydrogenase into the culture medium. After as little as one hour of endotoxin exposure, increased permeability and increased hydraulic conductance of cultured endothelial monolayers can be demonstrated.[15]

CONCLUSIONS

Interactions of neutrophils with the lung microcirculation seem to be important events in the evolution of diffuse lung injury. It is not clear, however, that interaction of activated neutrophils with normal vascular endothelium can initiate endothelial injury. It is possible that diffuse lung injury begins with alterations in the structure, surface properties, or metabolism of endothelium, unrelated to neutrophils, and that activated neutrophils then exaggerate and perpetuate the endothelial injury.

142

ACKNOWLEDGMENTS

This work was supported by grant No. HL 19153 (SCOR in Pulmonary Vascular Diseases) from the National Heart, Lung, and Blood Institute and grants from the John W. Cooke, Jr., and Laura W. Cooke Fund for Lung Research, the Hugh J. Morgan Fund for Cardiology donated by the Martha Washington Straus–Harry H. Straus Foundation, Inc., the Upjohn Company, Kalamazoo, Mich., the Kroc Foundation and the Bernard Werthan, Sr. Pulmonary Research Fund.

Several investigators contributed to this work. Those who assumed primary responsibility for the studies include Drs Barbara O. Meyrick, James R. Snapper, and John H. Newman. Dr Una S. Ryan of the University of Miami collaborated in the studies of cultured endothelial cells.

REFERENCES

1. Brigham KL, Bowers RE, Haynes J: Increased sheep vascular permeability caused by *E. coli* endotoxin. *Circ Res* 1979;45:292-297.
2. Snapper JR, Hutchison AA, Ogletree ML, et al: Effects of cyclooxygenase inhibitors on the alterations in lung mechanics caused by endotoxemia in the unanesthetized sheep. *J Clin Invest* 1983;72:63-76.
3. Brigham KL, Harris TR, Bowers RE, et al: Lung vascular permeability: Inferences from measurement of plasma to lung lymph protein transport. *Lymphology* 1979;12:177-190.
4. Brigham KL, Begley CJ, Bernard GR, et al: Septicemia and lung injury. *Clin Lab Med* 1983;3:719-744.
5. Esbenshade AM, Newman JH, Lams PM, et al: Respiratory failure after endotoxin infusion in sheep: Lung mechanics and lung fluid balance. *J Appl Physiol* 1982;53:967-976.
6. Meyrick B, Brigham KL: Acute effects of *Escherichia coli* endotoxin on the pulmonary microcirculation of anesthetized sheep: Structure:function relationships. *Lab Invest* 1983;48:458-470.
7. Brigham KL, Meyrick B: Granulocyte dependent injury of pulmonary endothelium: A case of miscommunication? *Tissue Cell* 1984;16:137-155.
8. Brigham KL, Meyrick B: Interactions of granulocytes with the lungs. *Circ Res* 1984;54:623-635.
9. Heflin AC, Brigham KL: Prevention by granulocyte depletion of increased lung vascular permeability of sheep lung following endotoxemia. *J Clin Invest* 1981;68:1253-1260.
10. Hinson JM, Hutchison AA, Ogletree ML, et al: Effect of granulocyte depletion on altered lung mechanics after endotoxemia in sheep. *J Appl Physiol* 1983;55:92-99.
11. Brigham KL, Bowers RE, McKeen CR: Methylprednisolone prevention of increased lung vascular permeability following endotoxemia in sheep. *J Clin Invest* 1981;67:1103-1110.
12. Begley CJ, Ogletree ML, Meyrick BO, et al: Modification of pulmonary responses to endotoxemia in awake sheep by steroidal and nonsteroidal anti-inflammatory agents. *Am Rev Respir Dis*, in press.

143

13. Meyrick B, Brigham KL: The effect of a single infusion of zymosan-activated plasma on the pulmonary microcirculation of sheep: Structure-function relationships. *Am J Pathol* 1984;114:32–45.
14. Meyrick B, Hoffman LH, Brigham KL: Chemotaxis of granulocytes across bovine pulmonary artery intimal explants without endothelial cell injury. *Tissue Cell* 1984;16:1–16.
15. Meyrick B: Endotoxin-mediated pulmonary endothelial damage. *Fed Proc*, in press.

12 Mechanisms of Lung Vascular Injury After Thrombin-Induced Pulmonary Microembolism

Asrar B. Malik
Joseph G. Garcia
Siu K. Lo
Jeffrey A. Cooper
Marc B. Perlman
Arnold Johnson

Pulmonary vascular thrombosis is a common pathologic finding in acute lung injury.[1,2] The thrombosis may result from a variety of causes, such as septicemia,[1,3] endothelial damage with exposure of the subendothelial matrix,[4] acute hemorrhagic pancreatitis,[5] and release of thromboplastin into the circulation after head injury and bone fractures. [2,6,7] All these insults are associated with morphologic evidence of intravascular thrombi.[1,8,9]

THROMBIN: ENZYME SPECIFICITY AND INDUCTION OF PULMONARY VASCULAR THROMBOSIS

We have examined the consequences of intravascular coagulation induced in the pulmonary circulation by an intravenous (IV) infusion of thrombin. Electron microscopic examination indicates that fibrin microthrombi and an abundance of platelets are clustered in close proximity to the fibrin "plugs." Neutrophils are seen sequestered in the small pulmonary vessels. Platelets and neutrophils are seen in different stages of degranulation.

We have examined some of the postulated mechanisms by which thrombin leads to neutrophil and platelet sequestration in the pulmonary

146

vessels and the relationship of fibrin to the sequestration of these blood-formed elements. We have also assessed the role of these factors in mediating the pulmonary edema associated with pulmonary intravascular coagulation. This review will concentrate on these experiments.

The thrombin molecule possesses a configuration that separates its protein-binding site or its fibrinogen recognition site from its catalytic and enzymatic sites that cleave proteolytically the fibrinopeptides A and B from the fibrinogen molecule and induce the formation of fibrin[10] (Figure 12-1). In addition, there are specific regions on the molecule which are responsible for leukocyte chemotaxis and platelet aggregatory properties of thrombin.[11] The thrombin molecule also possesses the ability to induce formation of clottable fibrin monomers and to activate factor XIII (fibrin-stabilizing factor) which stabilizes the fibrin clot.

The fibrin microthrombi become entrapped in the pulmonary circulation following IV thrombin infusion. Thrombin also leads to in vivo platelet aggregation and leukocyte sequestration by activating secondary processes such as generation of complement-derived peptides and arachidonate metabolites.[11,12]

The IV infusion of thrombin in experimental animals has been used as a model of inducing pulmonary vascular thrombosis. Thrombin resulted in increases in the pulmonary artery pressure, left atrial pressure and pulmonary vascular resistance, while the pulmonary blood flow decreased (Figure 12-2). The increase in pulmonary vascular pressures is the result of three factors: (1) a direct pulmonary vasoconstrictor action of thrombin[13]; (2) secondary vasoconstriction mediated by release of substances such as thromboxane A$_2$ (TxA$_2$) by the action of thrombin on

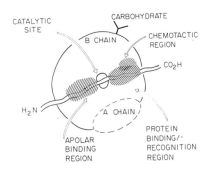

Figure 12-1 Representation of the thrombin molecule showing the specific regions of the molecule. Note that the catalytic (protease) site is distinct from the protein-binding-fibrinogen recognition region. The chemotactic region is also a separate domain. (Figure courtesy of Dr John Fenton, New York State Health Laboratories, Albany, NY.)

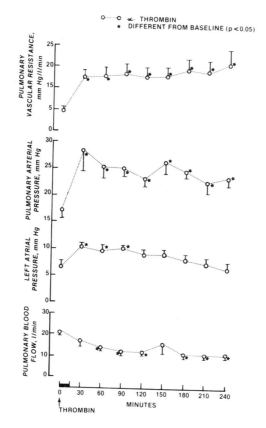

Figure 12-2 Changes in pulmonary blood flow, left atrial pressure, pulmonary arterial pressure, and pulmonary vascular resistance after α-thrombin challenge in anesthetized sheep. Note the increases in pulmonary arterial pressure and pulmonary vascular resistance following thrombin challenge.

the blood-formed elements[14,15]; and (3) pulmonary microvascular obstruction and the resultant decrease in vascular cross-sectional area.[16,17] The role of arachidonic acid metabolites in mediation of the hemodynamic response has been assessed by inhibiting the cyclo-oxygenase or thromboxane synthetase enzymes. In these experiments, the initial pulmonary pressor and resistance responses to thrombin were attenuated.[18] Studies in the isolated-perfused lung indicate that thrombin itself exerts a slow modest pressor effect independent of the cyclo-oxygenase pathway,[19] supporting a direct pressor action of thrombin. This effect may be mediated by thrombin receptors on the pulmonary vascular smooth muscle.

Thrombin infused IV produced rapid decreases in the circulating leukocyte and platelet counts (Figure 12-3). Since decreases in the counts occurred immediately after the infusion of thrombin, the likely site of

148

deposition of these elements is in the pulmonary circulation. This was confirmed by studies in which indium–111 (^{111}In) oxine-labelled neutrophils were shown to accumulate in the lung subsequent to the thrombin infusion (Figure 12-4)).[11] The uptake of the cells was marked but transient. However, it is interesting to note that the decrease in the peripheral leukocyte count was sustained (Figure 12-3); it may be that unlabelled neutrophils released from peripheral sites continue to sequester in the lungs after the initial uptake and release of the labelled cells.

INCREASE IN LUNG VASCULAR PERMEABILITY INDUCED BY THROMBIN

We have examined the alterations in lung transvascular fluid and protein exchange in the sheep lung lymph fistula preparation.[20] This preparation has the unique advantage that studies can be made in the un-

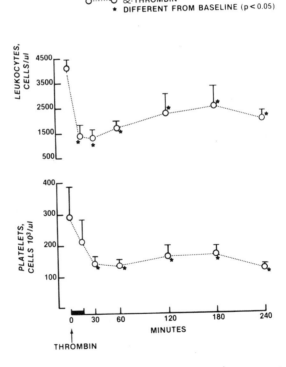

Figure 12-3 Changes in arterial leukocyte and platelet counts in anesthetized sheep challenged with α-thrombin. Note the rapid decrease in leukocyte count which occurred at a more rapid rate than the decrease in the platelet count.

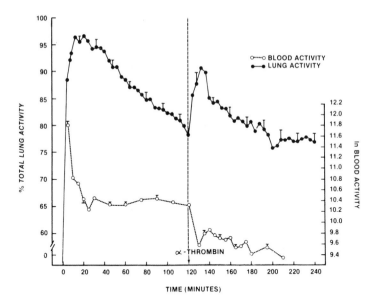

Figure 12-4 Time-dependent change in total lung activity of indium 111 (^{111}In) oxine–labelled neutrophils. The cells were injected at 0 time and α-thrombin was injected at the 120-minute point. There was a large increase in the ^{111}In activity over the lungs. The bottom curve shows the changes in blood ^{111}In activity.

anesthetized animal. Measurement of pulmonary lymph flow provides an assessment of the net transvascular fluid filtration rate and thus it is possible to make inferences about alterations occurring at the level of pulmonary exchange microvessels.

Intravenous infusion of α-thrombin (the native enzyme) resulted in increases in pulmonary lymph flow and the lymph protein clearance (ie, the product of lymph flow and lymph-to-plasma protein concentration ratio).[21] The lymph protein clearance increased markedly (Figure 12-5) suggesting that there is a large increase in the plasma-to-lymph protein transport. This could be due to an increase in the vascular permeability to proteins (ie, resulting from endothelial injury) and to convective transport (ie, the solvent drag associated with increased fluid filtration after a rise in the pulmonary capillary hydrostatic pressure).[22] It is unlikely that increased vascular surface area is a valid explanation of these data because microvascular obstruction with thrombin reduces the surface area.

To address the issue that the rise in lymph protein clearance was indeed the result of increased permeability, we have measured alterations in the pulmonary lymph response to thrombin when the fluid filtration is maximized by raising the pulmonary capillary pressure (with inflation of a left

150

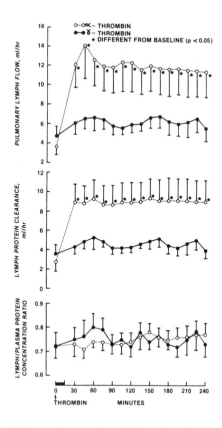

Figure 12-5 Changes in pulmonary lymph flow, lymph-to-plasma protein concentration ratio, and lymph protein clearance following intravenous infusion of α-thrombin or γ-thrombin. Note the large increases in pulmonary lymph flow and lymph protein clearance following the α-thrombin infusion as compared to γ-thrombin. These studies were carried out in the acutely prepared anesthetized sheep lung lymph fistula preparation.

atrial balloon catheter). As shown in Figure 12-6, left atrial hypertension increases the lymph flow and decreases the lymph-to-plasma protein concentration ratio indicating increased filtration of fluid and dilution of the interstitial protein concentration. Infusion of α-thrombin resulted in further increments in pulmonary artery pressure and pulmonary lymph flow, but the lymph-to-plasma protein concentration ratio increased. This finding indicates increased transvascular protein flux as a result of thrombin at very high lymph flows. From this type of experiment, it is possible to calculate the protein reflection coefficient (a measure of vascular permeability to proteins)[1]; a protein reflection coefficient (σ_d) of zero indicates that the membrane is fully permeable to proteins and a σ_d of one

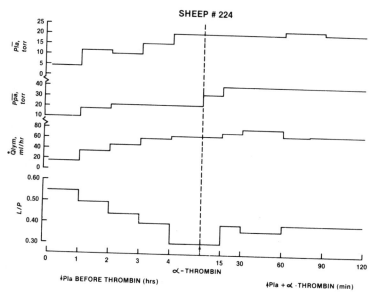

Figure 12-6 Changes in mean left atrial pressure ($P_{\bar{l}a}$), mean pulmonary arterial pressure ($P_{\bar{p}a}$), pulmonary lymph flow (Q_{lym}), and lymph-to-plasma protein concentration ratio (L/P) following the step increases in left atrial pressure. Note the step increases in pulmonary lymph flow as left atrial pressure increased, and the decrease in lymph-to-plasma protein concentration ratio. At five hours into the rise in left atrial pressure, α-thrombin was infused intravenously. This results in a further rise in pulmonary arterial pressure and a small increase in pulmonary lymph flow. The increase in pulmonary lymph flow is associated with an increase in L/P protein concentration ratio indicating increased vascular permeability to protein.

indicates the membrane is impermeable to proteins. We have determined that the σ_d decreases from the value 0.70 to 0.59 after thrombin-induced intravascular coagulation in sheep and to 0.49 in dogs which received a higher concentration of α-thrombin. These studies indicate that thrombin induces an increase in lung vascular permeability to proteins. The σ_d measurements made in our laboratory with various challenges are shown in Table 12-1.

α-Thrombin also causes an increased permeability of the airway epithelium. Technetium 99c-labelled diethylenetriamine pentaacetate (DPTA) was aerosolized into the lungs and this was followed by thrombin infusion. The rate of clearance of DPTA increased markedly during the thrombin infusion and then returned to normal values. There was a rapid tenfold increase in clearance indicating an increase in the permeability of the airway epithelium to the tracer DPTA (molecular weight ~800). The mechanism of the transient increase in epithelial permeability

Table 12-1
**Protein Reflection Coefficient (δd) Measurements
in Sheep and Dogs Following Various Interventions**

Experiment	Species	σ_d
Control	Sheep	0.70
α-Thrombin (80 U/kg)	Sheep	0.59
Platelet-activating factor (PAF)(4 μg/kg/h)	Sheep	0.43
Platelet-depleted (antiplatelet serum)	Sheep	0.40
Control	Dog	0.73
α-Thrombin (300 U/kg)	Dog	0.49

is unclear; it may not be related to the increase in endothelial permeability because the response was transient.

The effects of thrombin on endothelial permeability can be also demonstrated using in vitro systems. Transport of iodine–125 (^{125}I)–labelled albumin across an endothelial monolayer was studied using bovine pulmonary artery endothelial cells grown to confluency on a membrane consisting of a gelatinized micropore filter.[23] The addition of α-thrombin and γ-thrombin to the monolayer caused similar increases in the leakage of albumin across the endothelial membrane (Figure 12-7). Increased permeability was demonstrated at thrombin concentrations of 10^{-6} mol/L which are 100 times greater than those used in the intact animal. Therefore, thrombin in high concentrations exerts a direct permeability-increasing effect in vitro on the endothelium, possibly by inducing endothelial gap formations. The finding that both α- and γ-thrombin (which lacks the fibrinogen recognition site of α-thrombin) were equally effective in increasing endothelial permeability suggests that the catalytic or protease sites or some other site of the molecule mediates the response. Thrombin in low concentration induces a permeability increase in vivo by its action on blood components, ie, fibrinogen and the blood-formed elements; however, thrombin in higher concentrations may have a direct permeability-increasing effect.

ROLE OF BLOOD COMPONENTS
IN MEDIATING INCREASE IN LUNG
VASCULAR PERMEABILITY

Fibrin

To study the role of intravascular coagulation and resulting entrapment of fibrin in the pulmonary vessels, studies have utilized a modified form of thrombin (γ-thrombin) which lacks the fibrinogen recognition site but retains the catalytic and proteolytic sites,[10] ie, it possesses the same esterase and amidolytic activities as α-thrombin. γ-Thrombin is produced by proteolytic conversion of α-thrombin using a limited tryptic digestion method.[10] Figure 12-8 compares the lymph responses of α- and γ-thrombins. The increases in pulmonary lymph flow and lymph protein clearance were marked in the α-thrombin group but absent in the γ-thrombin group. Therefore, the fibrinogen recognition site and formation of fibrin are necessary for the increased vascular permeability response that results from thrombin-induced intravascular coagulation in vivo.

The fibrin hypothesis was also further tested in animals depleted of circulating fibrinogen by pretreatment of purified faction of the Malayan pit viper venom, ancrod.[24] This resulted in markedly reduced concentra-

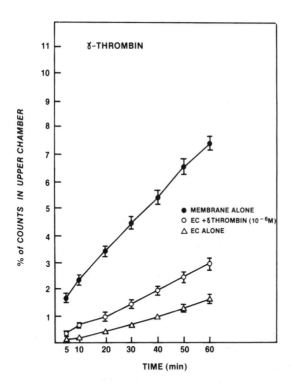

Figure 12-7 Alterations in iodine 125 albumin flux across the endothelial monolayer induced by γ-thrombin. The y-axis indicates counts present in the lower chamber as a percent of the counts in the upper chamber. Note that the endothelium (EC) restricted albumin flux as compared to the membrane alone. The addition of γ-thrombin to the endothelium increased the albumin flux. Results obtained with γ-thrombin are quantitatively similar to those obtained with α-thrombin.

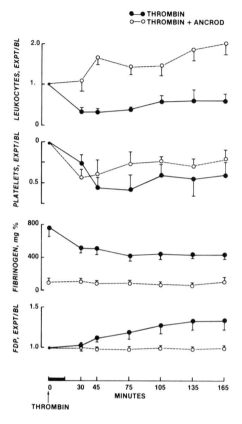

Figure 12-8 The effects of infusion of fibrin degradation products in the control sheep and sheep challenged with thrombin. Infusion of fibrin degradation products enhanced the lymph flow response after thrombin from 10 mL/h to a maximum of 17 mL/h. The effect was associated with a decrease in L/P protein concentration indicating that the increase in lymph flow response was due to a rise in pulmonary capillary hydrostatic pressure. This is also indicated by the finding that fibrin degradation products increase the pulmonary arterial pressure.

tions of fibrinogen. The increases in pulmonary lymph flow were small compared to the control group challenged with thrombin, as were increases in pulmonary arterial pressure. Increasing the left atrial pressure in this group resulted in a decrease in the lymph-to-plasma protein concentration ratio, indicating that defibrinogenation prevented the increase in lung vascular permeability.[13]

It is important to note that the peripheral leukocyte count did not decrease after thrombin infusion in the defibrinogenated group (Figure 12-9). This may explain the protective effect observed after defibrinogenation since our previous studies have indicated that the increases in

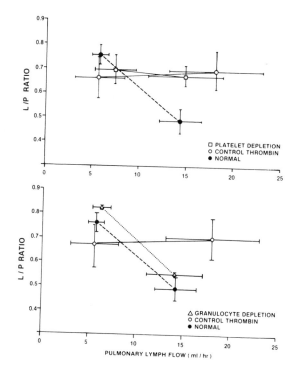

Figure 12-9 Changes in the leukocyte count, platelet counts, fibrinogen concentration, and concentration of fibrin degradation products in control thrombin-challenged sheep and in sheep pretreated with ancrod prior to thrombin challenge. Note the marked reduction in fibrinogen concentration in the ancrod-pretreated animals. The leukocyte count did not decrease in the defibrinogenated animals following thrombin challenge.

lung vascular permeability seen after thrombin-induced pulmonary microembolism are prevented by prior granulocytopenia induced by hydroxyurea.[25,26]

Granulocytes and Platelets

We examined the role of granulocytes in mediating thrombin-induced lung vascular injury by granulocyte depletion using either hydroxyurea or antineutrophil serum. The results were comparable for both agents. Thrombin infusion in both groups resulted in an increase in lymph flow and a decrease in lymph-to-plasma protein concentration ratio. The increase in lymph protein clearance was small compared to the control thrombin-challenged animals. These results indicate an important role of granulocytes in the mediation of the response. When the data from granulocyte and platelet depletion groups (the latter induced by anti-sheep platelet serum) are compared, the results indicate that granulocyte depletion is more protective (Figure 12-10). The increase in lymph flow that occurred after raising the pulmonary capillary hydrostatic pressure with the left atrial balloon in the control thrombin-challenged group was associated with a decrease in the lymph-to-plasma protein concentration ratio. Granulocytopenia prevented the increased permeability response, whereas platelet depletion did not (Figure 12-10). Therefore, the thrombin-induced lung vascular injury depends on the interaction between fibrin and granulocytes.

Plasminogen Activation

An important aspect of the thrombin-induced lung vascular permeability increase may closely relate to the fibrinolytic activity. Thrombin induces fibrin microemboli and entrapment in the pulmonary circulation.[1,9] Subsequent activation of plasminogen conversion to plasmin (an active proteolytic enzyme) occurs on fibrin surface and plasminogen activation requires the presence of fibrin.[27] Plasmin acts as an endopeptidase and is capable of digesting and lysing fibrin microemboli. Plasmin remains bound to fibrin polymer until dissolution of the clot.[27] The circulating α_2-antiplasmin rapidly binds and inactivates the plasmin. However, the plasmin that is in immediate contact with fibrin may reach a high concentration if it is not immediately inactivated by inhibitors as may be the case in the obstructed and poorly perfused vessels. The presence of the free plasmin may have a direct action on neutrophils and cause neutrophils to release injurious substances,[28] although this has not been examined. The generation of plasmin may also lead to complement activation which results in leukostasis and neutrophil activation in the pulmonary circulation.[12] The role of complement in the thrombin model has been evaluated by decomplementing sheep prior to thrombin; decomplementation prevented the increase in lung vascular permeability suggesting complement system is necessary for the response. However, the exact role of complement remains unclear. The generation and release of fibrin degradation products (FDP) subsequent to the clot lysis may also contribute to the lung vascular injury. Saldeen[1] has proposed that FDPs directly induce an increase in lung vascular permeability. An in vitro study showed that FDP injures endothelial cells.[30] The infusion of FDP in dogs and sheep, however, resulted in only slight increases in lymph flow with no increase in lung permeability[30,31]; thus the role of FDP remains controversial. The results of infusion of FDP in sheep are shown in Figure 12-8. Pulmonary lymph flow was increased only in the presence of thrombin and the increase in lymph flow was associated with a decrease in lymph-to-plasma protein concentration ratio, indicating a hydrostatic effect of FDP.

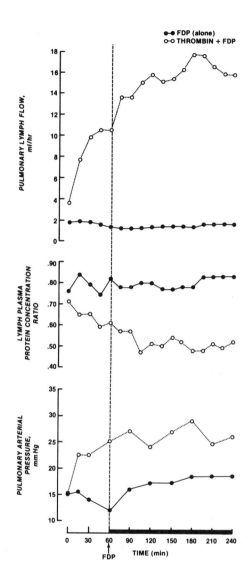

Figure 12-10 Changes in pulmonary lymph flow as a function of lymph/plasma protein concentration ratio (L/P ratio). The upper graph indicates the effects of platelet depletion induced by antiplatelet serum. The lower graph indicates the effects of granulocyte depletion induced by hydroxyurea treatment. Note that increased lymph flow response in the granulocyte-depleted group was a result of hydrostatic pressure increase, whereas the permeability increase persisted in platelet-depleted animals.

We have examined the response of thrombin-induced injury in awake sheep models with and without fibrinolytic depression. Fibrinolysis was depressed by IV tranexamic acid (100 mg) pretreatment (Figure 12-11).

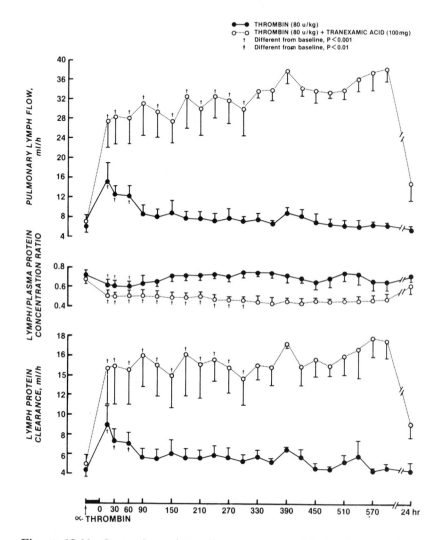

Figure 12-11 Comparison of the effect of thrombin infusion in awake sheep challenged with 80 U/kg of thrombin. There are two groups: animals receiving thrombin alone (solid dots) and animals receiving thrombin plus tranexamic acid (open dots) to depress fibrinolytic system. Note the sustained increases in pulmonary lymph flow and the lymph protein clearance for up to 570 minutes in the latter group. Both lymph flow and lymph protein clearance were elevated at 24 hours after thrombin challenge, although they are much lower than their maximum levels.

Tranexamic acid competes for the lysine binding site of plasminogen on fibrin.[27] The increases in lymph flow and lymph protein clearance were greater in the fibrinolytic-depressed animals and these effects were sustained (Figure 12-8). Therefore, the duration of microthrombi in the pulmonary circulation appears to be a crucial determinant of the increase in lung vascular permeability.

MEDIATORS OF LUNG VASCULAR INJURY AFTER THROMBIN

We have examined the lymph obtained from thrombin-challenged animals with respect to its ability to induce alterations in neutrophil function. The idea behind these studies was that thrombin-induced intravascular coagulation generated humoral factors causing alterations in neutrophil function, which we have shown to be the final effectors of lung vascular injury after thrombin. We observed that lymph contained such substances which resulted in neutrophil chemotaxis and aggregation (Figure 12-12) as well as superoxide anion generation by the neutrophils. The substance was not thrombin because thrombin inactivation using hirudin did not prevent the generation of these substances. An important aspect of response was that it was transient and rapid (with 15 to 30 minutes after thrombin) and that it paralleled uptake of labelled neutrophils after the thrombin infusion (Figure 12-4). These substances have not been characterized; eicosanoids derived from the arachidonic acid cascade (eg, leukotriene B_4) are potent chemotactic and neutrophil-activating agents.[32,33] These substances may also be the complement-derived peptides, such as C3a and C5a, which also induce neutrophil chemotaxis, aggregation, and activation.[34,35]

Thrombin is directly involved in neutrophil chemotaxis and aggregation. Thrombin (10^{-8} mol/L) induces chemotaxis which is comparable to that for zymosan-treated serum and f Met-Leu-Phe (FLMP). Hirudin also has a minor chemotactic effect. The chemotactic effects of both thrombin and hirudin are blocked when thrombin and hirudin are complexed. This suggests that the direct chemotactic activity of the thrombin molecule resides in the site at which hirudin complexes with the thrombin molecule. In addition, thrombin (10^{-8} mol/L) induces neutrophil aggregation, suggesting that thrombin also has a direct effect in inducing pulmonary leukostasis. We observed thrombin-induced neutrophil aggregation comparable to that seen with zymosan-treated serum which contains complement-derived peptides[36] (Figure 12-13). The effect of thrombin in inducing neutrophil chemotaxis and aggregation is blocked by hirudin, suggesting that the aggregation and chemotaxis are mediated by the same site on the thrombin molecule. Therefore, the thrombin molecule is capable of inducing direct alterations in neutrophil function.

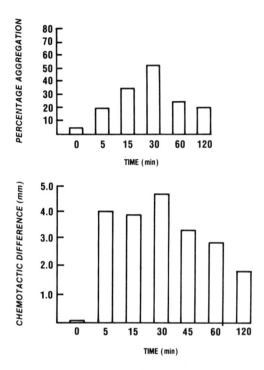

Figure 12-12 Effects of lymph obtained from thrombin-challenged animals on the chemotaxis of sheep neutrophils. Note that the lymph obtained at 30 minutes after thrombin challenge has the most activity in aggregating neutrophils and inducing chemotaxis.

The thrombin molecule may also act on blood components and release secondary mediators which may be present in pulmonary lymph and which also alter neutrophil function (eg, C5a and leukotriene B_4 (LTB$_4$). This was demonstrated by a study in which α-thrombin was incubated with citrated blood. The supernatant resulted in neutrophil aggregation, which could not be inhibited with hirudin (Figure 12-14), indicating that thrombin caused the generation of a neutrophil-aggregatory substance(s) in the blood.

MECHANISMS OF THE NEUTROPHIL-DEPENDENT LUNG VASCULAR INJURY AFTER THROMBIN

The processes involved in mediating the neutrophil-dependent increase in permeability may be related to the generation of oxygen radicals and proteolytic enzymes secondary to neutrophil activation.[23,37,38] The role of oxygen radicals was examined by pretreating sheep with superoxide

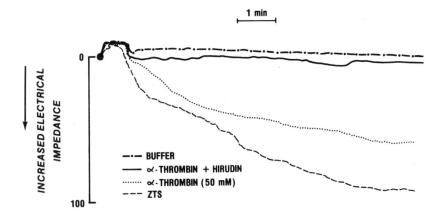

Figure 12-13 This figure shows the thrombin-induced aggregation of sheep neutrophils. The x-axis shows the increased electrical impedance measured on the aggregometer. ZTS indicates zymosan-treated serum. Note that the response to α-thrombin and ZTS were comparable.

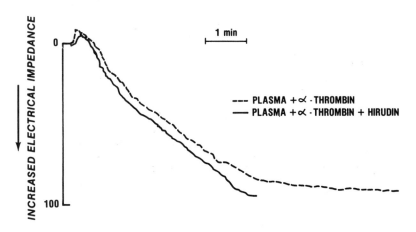

Figure 12-14 The effects of supernatant obtained from incubation of α-thrombin with citrated plasma on sheep neutrophil aggregation as measured by an increase in electrical impedance on the aggregometer meter. Note that supernatant induces full aggregation and that it is not inhibited by adding hirudin (an antithrombin substance), indicating that the response is not due to the effects of thrombin alone. The response may be due to the generation of plasma-derived substances.

162

dismutase (SOD) to scavenge the superoxide anion and to drive the reaction towards hydrogen peroxide (H_2O_2). We showed that pretreatment with the Ficoll-bound SOD blunted the increase in lung vascular permeability after thrombin (Figure 12-15). Therefore, a part of the increase in lung vascular permeability is mediated by the generation of superoxide anions. Perhaps a reason why the response was not completely inhibited may be related to an increase in the H_2O_2 that may be generated by pretreatment with SOD.

CONCLUSIONS

Figure 12-16 summarizes our understanding of the pathophysiology of pulmonary edema after thrombin-induced intravascular coagulation. The activation of thrombin leads to fibrin sequestration in the pulmonary circulation. Fibrin activates neutrophils and this likely involves activation of the complement system and generation of arachidonic acid metabolites such as leukotriene B_4. In addition, thrombin in high concentrations has direct effects on neutrophil chemotaxis and aggregation. Therefore, we believe that pulmonary sequestration of neutrophils after thrombin occurs by direct and indirect mechanisms.

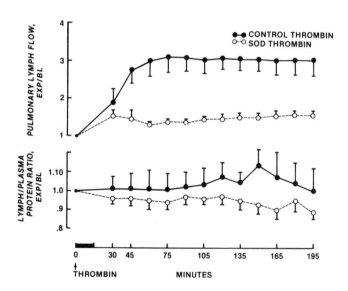

Figure 12-15 Effects of pretreatment of superoxide dismutase (SOD) on the response to thrombin. The response of thrombin is markedly reduced in the SOD-pretreated anesthetized sheep challenged with thrombin.

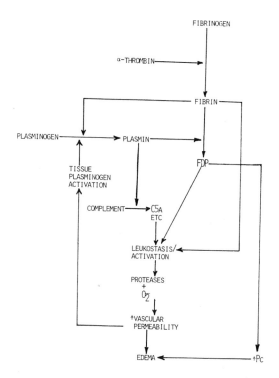

Figure 12-16 Summary of the mechanisms mediating increased lung vascular permeability and pulmonary edema after thrombin-induced intravascular coagulation.

ACKNOWLEDGMENT

The research presented in this review was supported by grant HL-32418 and HL-26551 from the National Institutes of Health.

REFERENCES

1. Saldeen T: The microembolism syndrome: A review, in Saldeen T (ed): *The Microembolism Syndrome*. Stockholm, Almqvist & Wiksell International, 1979, pp 7–44.
2. Schnells G, Voigt WH, Redl H, et al: Electron microscopic investigation of lung biopsies in patients with post-traumatic respiratory insufficiency. *Acta Chir Scand Suppl* 1980;449:9–20.
3. Bachofen M, Weibel ER: Alterations of the gas exchange apparatus in adult respiratory insufficiency associated with septicemia. *Am Rev Respir Dis* 1977;116:589–615.

4. Mason RG, Sharp D, Chuang HYK, et al: The endothelium: roles in thrombosis and hemostasis. *Arch Pathol Lab Med* 1977;101:61–64.
5. Garcia-Szabo RR, Malik AB: Pancreatitis-induced increase in lung vascular permeability. *Am Rev Respir Dis* 1984;129:580–583.
6. Malik AB: Neurogenic mechanisms of pulmonary edema. *Circ Res*, in press.
7. Saldeen T: Fat embolism and signs of intravascular coagulation in a post-traumatic autopsy material. *J Trauma* 1970;10:273–286.
8. Bone RC, Francis PB, Pierce AK: Intravascular coagulation associated with the adult respiratory distress syndrome. *Am J Med* 1976;61:585–589.
9. Minnear FL, Martin D, Taylor AE, et al: Large increase in pulmonary lymph flow after thrombin-induced intravascular coagulation. *Fed Proc* 1983;42:1274.
10. Fenton JW: Thrombin specificity. *Ann NY Acad Sci* 1981;370:468–495.
11. Cooper JA, Solano SJ, Bizios R, et al: Pulmonary neutrophil kinetics after thrombin-induced intravascular coagulation. *J Appl Physiol* 1984;57:826–832.
12. Zimmerman TS, Frero J, Rothberge H: Blood coagulation and the inflammatory response. *Semin Hematol* 1977;14:391–404.
13. Johnson A, Tahamont MV, Malik AB: Thrombin-induced lung vascular injury. Role of fibrinogen and fibrinolysis. *Am Rev Respir Dis* 1983;128:38–44.
14. Garcia-Szabo RR, Minnear FL, Bizios R, et al: Role of thromboxane in the pulmonary response to pulmonary micro-embolization. *Chest* 1983;83S:76S–78S.
15. Hyman AL, Spannhake EW, Kadowitz PJ: Prostaglandins and the lung. *Am Rev Respir Dis* 1978;117:111–136.
16. Malik AB, van der Zee H: Lung vascular permeability following progressive embolization. *J Appl Physiol* 1978;45:590–597.
17. Ohkuda K, Nakahara K, Weidner J, et al: Lung fluid exchange after uneven pulmonary artery obstruction in sheep. *Circ Res* 1978;43:152–161.
18. Bizios R, Minnear FL, van der Zee H, et al: Effect of cyclo-oxygenase and cyclo-oxygenase inhibition on lung fluid after thrombin. *J Appl Physiol* 1983;55:462–471.
19. Kern DF, Kivlen CM, Neumann P, et al: Effects of thrombin in the isolated-perfused lung. *Fed Proc* 1984;43:1029.
20. Staub N, Bland R, Brigham K, et al: Preparation of chronic lung lymph fistulas in sheep. *J Surg Res* 1975;19:315–320.
21. Garcia-Szabo RR, Kern DF, Bizios R, et al: Comparison of α- and γ-thrombin on lung fluid balance in anesthetized sheep. *J Appl Physiol* 1984;57:1375–1383.
22. Staub NC: The forces regulating fluid filtration in the lung. *Microvasc Res* 1978;15:45–55.
23. Shasby DM, Van Benthuysen KM, Tate RM, et al: Granulocytes mediate acute edematous lung injury in rabbits and isolated rabbit lungs perfused with phorbol myristate acetate: Role of oxygen radicals. *Am Rev Respir Dis* 1982;125:443–447.
24. Bell WR, Shapiro SS, Martinez J, et al: The effects of ancrod, the coagulating enzyme from the venom of Malayan pit venom (*A. rhodostoma*) on prothrombin and fibrinogen metabolism and fibrino-peptide A release in man. *J Lab Clin Med* 1978;91:592–604.
25. Barie PS, Malik AB: Role of intravascular coagulation and granulocytes in lung vascular injury after bone marrow embolism. *Circ Res* 1982;50:830–838.
26. Johnson A, Malik AB: Pulmonary edema after glass bead microembolization: protective effect of granulocytopenia. *J Appl Physiol* 1982;52:155–161.
27. Stormophen H: Interrelations between the coagulation, fibrinolytic and the kallidrein-kinin system. *Scand J Haematol Suppl* 1979;34:24–27.

28. Ryan GB: Inflammation and localization of infection. *Surg Clin North Am* 1976;56:831–846.
29. Sueishi K, Nanno S, Tanaka K: Permeability enhancing and chemotactic activities of lower molecular weight degradation products of human fibrinogen. *Thromb Haemost* 1981;45:90–94.
30. Johnson A, Garcia-Szabo RR, Kaplan JE, et al: Effects of fibrin degradation products on lung transvascular fluid and protein exchange. *Thromb Res* 1985;37:543–554.
31. Taylor AE, Parker JC, Ryan J, et al: Effects of fibrinogen degradation products (FDP) on pulmonary vascular permeability to macromolecules, abstracted. *Physiologist* 1983;26(4):A8.
32. Ford-Hutchinson AW, Bray MA, Doig MV, et al: Leukotriene B, a potent chemokinetic and aggregating substance released from polymorphonuclear leukocytes. *Nature* 1980;286:264–265.
33. Goetz EJ, Pickett WC: The human PMN leukocyte chemotactic activity of complex hydroxy-eicosatetronoic acids (HETES). *J Immunol* 1980;125: 1789–1791.
34. Craddock PR, Hammerschmidt DE, Dalmasso AP, et al: Complement (C5a)-induced granulocyte aggregation *in vitro*: a possible mechanism of complement-mediated leukostasis and leukopenia. *J Clin Invest* 1977;60: 260–264.
35. Jacob HS, Craddock PR, Hammerschmidt DE, et al: Complement-induced granulocyte aggregation. *N Engl J Med* 1980;302:789–794.
36. Mueller-Eberhard HJ, Schneber RD: Molecular biology and chemistry of the alternate pathway of complement. *Adv Immunol* 1980;29:1–53.
37. Hammerschmidt DE: Leukocyte in lung injury. *Chest* 1983;83:165–205.
38. Harlan JM, Killen PD, Harker LA, et al: Neutrophil-mediated endothelial injury *in vitro*. Mechanisms of cell detachment. *J Clin Invest* 1981;68: 1394–1405.

13 A Model of Immunologic Lung Injury

Peter R.B. Caldwell

Angiotensin-converting enzyme is membrane-bound in the endothelium of the vasculature.[1-4] We have studied a rabbit model of immunologic lung injury induced by intravenous (IV) administration of heterologous antibodies to converting enzyme.[5,6] In this model, the interaction of goat IgG, (Fab')$_2$ and Fab to converting enzyme produces endothelial injury, platelet and leukocyte aggregation, and fibrin deposition in the pulmonary vascular bed with development of rapidly fatal pulmonary edema.

In recent studies,[7] we have measured platelet-activating factor (PAF) release in this model and found a dose-dependent response to administered IgG to converting enzyme. The release was diminished but still present in animals depleted of polymorphonuclear leukocytes (PMN) by prior administration of nitrogen mustard (Figure 13-1). Studies in isolated lungs also showed release of PAF after administration of IgG to converting enzyme. The same observations were made in isolated aorta strips with intact endothelium and in isolated endothelium containing angiotensin-converting enzyme. Camussi et al[8] next showed that release of PAF could be induced in cultured human endothelial cells reacted with calcium ionophore, angiotensin II, vasopressin, thrombin, or antibody to Factor VIII. Prescott et al[9] subsequently also showed that cultured human endothelial cells produce PAF when stimulated with thrombin. Thus, a variety of stimuli and injury to endothelium may result in release of PAF which mediates pathophysiologic sequelae. Whether this mediator of anaphylaxis accounts for the injury induced by monovalent Fab to converting enzyme remains to be determined.

Antigenic modulation of pulmonary endothelial angiotensin-converting enzyme has been shown in this model using a protocol in which serial administration of heterologous IgG to converting enzyme was given over a four-day period.[10] By immunofluorescence microscopy deposits of

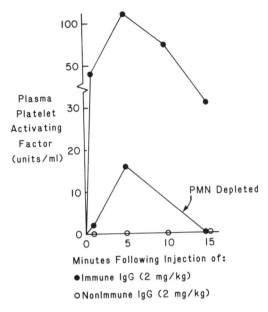

Figure 13-1 Platelet activating factor release following intravenous administration of immune IgG to angiotensin converting enzyme. PMN = polymorphonuclear neutrophil. (Data from Camussi et al.[7])

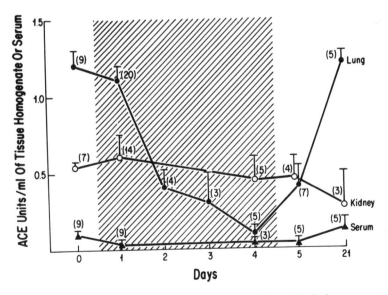

Figure 13-2 Angiotensin-converting enzyme (ACE) activity in homogenates of lung and kidney and serum following serial administration of goat antirabbit ACE indicated by the shaded area. (Reproduced with permission from Barba et al.[10])

IgG were present on the endothelium of all rabbits on day 1, in 57% on day 2, in 33% on day 3, and in none on day 4. Biochemical assay of converting enzyme activity in lung homogenates correlated with the reduction of demonstrable binding of IgG as shown in Figure 13-2.

Whereas in vitro binding of anticonverting enzyme IgG reveals a linear pattern by immunofluorescence, in vivo binding shows redistribution in a granular pattern with fixation of C3 (Figure 13-3). Fab fragments of goat IgG to converting enzyme localized in a linear pattern in vivo without fixation of C3. When the administration of Fab was followed by administration of rabbit antigoat serum, antigenic redistribution occurred giving a granular pattern with deposits of C3. These results show that divalent antibodies to an endothelial membrane antigen promote a rapid redistribution of antigen with fixation of complement. Surviving rabbits lose membrane antigen and are tolerant of antigen-specific antibodies. In this model, since the antigen is an enzyme, immunologic enzymectomy resulted from serial administration of heterologous IgG to angiotensin-converting enzyme. This model may have relevance to antigenic modulation of converting enzyme in other organs as well.

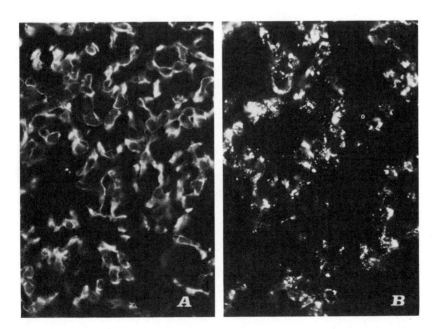

Figure 13-3 Immunofluorescence photomicrographs showing in vitro binding of goat antirabbit ACE IgG (**A**) giving a linear pattern and in vivo binding (**B**) giving a granular pattern (× 600). (Reproduced with permission from Barba et al.[10])

ACKNOWLEDGMENT

This study was supported by USPHS grants HL 33707, AI 10334, The Joe and Emily Lowe Foundation, The Dana Foundation, and a grant from the American Heart Association.

REFERENCES

1. Ryan JW, Ryan US, Schultz DR, et al: A subcellular localization of pulmonary angiotensin converting enzyme (Kininase II). *Biochem J* 1975;146:497–499.
2. Ryan US, Ryan JW, Whitaker C, et al: Localization of angiotensin converting enzyme (Kininase II). II. Immunocytochemistry and immunofluorescence. *Tissue Cell* 1976;8:125–145.
3. Caldwell PRB, Seegal BC, Hsu K, et al: Angiotensin converting enzyme: Vascular endothelial localization. *Science* 1976;191:1050–1051.
4. Takada Y, Unno M, Hiwada K, et al: Immunologic and immunofluorescent studies of human angiotensin converting enzyme. *Clin Sci* 1981;61:253s–256s.
5. Caldwell PRB, Wigger HJ, Das M, et al: Angiotensin converting enzyme: Effects of antienzyme antibody. *FEBS Lett* 1976;63:82–84.
6. Caldwell PRB, Wigger HJ, Fernandez LT, et al: Lung injury induced by antibody fragments to angiotensin converting enzyme. *Am J Pathol* 1981; 105:54–63.
7. Camussi G, Pawlowski I, Bussolino F, et al: Release of platelet activating factor in rabbits with antibody mediated injury of the lung: The role of polymorphonuclear neutrophils and of pulmonary endothelium. *J Immunol* 1983;131:1802–1807.
8. Camussi G, Aglietta M, Malawasi F, et al: The release of platelet activating factor from human endothelial cells in culture. *J Immunol* 1983;131:2397–2403.
9. Prescott SM, Zimmerman GA, McIntyre TM: Human endothelial cells in culture produce platelet-activating factor (1-alkyl-2-acetyl-sn-glycero-3-phosphocholine) when stimulated with thrombin. *Proc Natl Acad Sci* 1984;81:3534–3538.
10. Barba LM, Caldwell PRB, Downie GH, et al: Lung injury mediated by antibodies to endothelium. I. In the rabbit a repeated interaction of heterologous anti-angiotensin converting enzyme antibodies with alveolar endothelium results in resistance to immune injury through antigenic modulation. *J Exp Med* 1983;158:2141–2158.

14 Autonomic Mechanisms in the Pulmonary Vascular Bed

Albert L. Hyman
H. L. Lippton
Louis J. Ignarro
Dennis B. McNamara
K. S. Wood
Philip J. Kadowitz

The autonomic innervation of the pulmonary vascular bed has been studied extensively in recent years.[1-5] Studies in the cat and dog from this laboratory using 6-hydroxydopamine to differentiate adrenergic and cholinergic terminals indicate that the pulmonary vascular bed is innervated by both the sympathetic and parasympathetic systems.[3,4] A periarterial plexus of nerves in the walls of pulmonary arteries extends into the lung to innervate small arteries possessing even a single layer of smooth muscle cells. Adrenergic nerves appear to surround all pulmonary arteries and extend into the tunica media of the large arteries, whereas cholinergic nerves are present in medium- and small-sized pulmonary arteries only.[4] However, the function of adrenergic and cholinergic nerve terminals in the pulmonary vascular bed is not well understood. Adrenergic nerve stimulation increases pulmonary vascular resistance and decreases pulmonary vascular compliance.[6-9] Since these responses are inhibited by α-receptor and neuronal blocking agents, it appears the response to adrenergic nerve stimulation is the result of activation of α-adrenergic receptors by neuronally released norepinephrine.[3,8,10] The existence of postsynaptic α_1- and α_2-adrenergic receptor subtypes that, when stimulated, produce a pressor response in the systemic circulation has been reported recently.[11-13] However, the relative contribution of α-receptor subtype(s) mediating the adrenergic vasoconstrictor response to the lung of the intact animal remains unclear.

Although adrenergic nerve stimulation increases pulmonary vascular resistance, isoproterenol has been shown to decrease pulmonary vascular resistance suggesting that β-adrenergic receptors are present in the pulmonary vascular bed.[14-16] β-Adrenergically mediated vasodilation can be elicited by administration of isoproterenol or epinephrine as well as by norepinephrine when pulmonary vascular tone is elevated by hypoxia and acidemia; however, the actions of neuronally released norepinephrine on β-receptors in the pulmonary circulation are uncertain.[14-16] It has been reported that sympathetic nerve stimulation elicits vasodilation in skeletal muscle, liver, spleen, adipose tissue, and in isolated facial vein of the rabbit.[17-21] The concepts that β-adrenergic receptors in blood vessels are innervated and that neuronally released norepinephrine can elicit vasodilation by stimulating β_2-receptors have been challenged recently.[22,23] Vasodilator responses in the pulmonary circulation may be mediated by the parasympathetic system since decreases in pulmonary arterial pressure, although small and inconsistent, have been observed in response to vagosympathetic nerve stimulation in the dog.[24] In addition to the uncertainty of responses to vagal stimulation, there is disagreement on responses to acetylcholine chloride in the pulmonary vascular bed. Both pressor and depressor responses to acetylcholine chloride have been reported. Moreover, the relaxation of isolated arterial smooth muscle by muscarinic receptor agonists including the cholinergic transmitter is dependent on the presence of undamaged endothelium whereas contraction is the major response with damaged endothelium.[25] In addition to muscarinic receptor agonists, vascular smooth muscle relaxation elicited by bradykinin, divalent cation ionophores such as A23187, and a variety of vasodepressor substances appears to be dependent on an intact endothelial cell layer.[25-28] Furthermore, it has been proposed that acetylcholine-elicited relaxation of vascular smooth muscle is attributed to the release of an endothelium-derived lipoxygenase product of arachidonic acid metabolism which interacts with smooth muscle to increase cGMP formation.[25,29] Moreover, these data are consistent with the hypothesis that activation of guanylate cyclase and subsequent accumulation of cGMP are associated with relaxation of vascular smooth muscle by muscarinic agonists, including acetylcholine chloride, as well as a variety of nitrogen oxide–containing vasodilators such as nitroglycerin and sodium nitroprusside.[30,31] It has also been suggested that the pulmonary vasodilator response to acetylcholine chloride is secondary to its actions on the systemic vascular bed.[32] The variability in response to acetylcholine may depend on species, experimental preparation, dose of acetylcholine, and on the initial level of tone in the pulmonary vascular bed.[14,32-34] Thus, there appears to be a paucity of data describing pulmonary vascular responses to sympathetic and parasympathetic nerve stimulation and an understanding as to the physiologic or pathophysiologic role for the presence of these autonomic neurons remains unclear. The mechanism by which both the cholinergic and adrenergic transmitters produce a vascular response is uncertain. In addition, the contribution of endothelium in pulmonary vascular responses is currently an enigmatic one and the involvement of cyclic nucleotides as mediators in these vascular responses has recently been scrutinized.

The present chapter summarizes the actions of catecholamines and acetylcholine as well as vagal and sympathetic nerve stimulation on the pulmonary vascular bed of the intact-chest cat. The actions of acetylcholine on isolated bovine intrapulmonary arterial rings with and without endothelium were investigated and the association of these effects on isolated smooth muscle to changes in cyclic nucleotide levels was determined as well.

RESULTS

Effects of Norepinephrine

Pulmonary vascular responses to norepinephrine were investigated in the intact-chest cat under conditions of controlled blood flow. In these experiments, the effects of norepinephrine infusions and adrenergic receptor blocking agents were studied under basal conditions and when pulmonary vascular tone had been elevated by infusion of a prostaglandin endoperoxide analog or 15-methyl $PGF_{2\alpha}$. Under resting conditions, intralobar infusions of norepinephrine at rates of 0.5, 1.0, 2.0, and 10.0 μg/kg/min increased lobar arterial pressure in a dose-dependent fashion while lobar venous outflow pressure was maintained constant. In 11 of the animals the effects of propranolol hydrochloride, a β-receptor blocking agent, on the pressor response to norepinephrine in the pulmonary vascular bed were investigated and show that after administration of propranolol, 2 mg/kg intravenously (IV), the increases in lobar arterial pressure in response to norepinephrine infusions at 0.5–10.0 μg/kg/min were greatly enhanced ($P < .01$ at each infusion rate when compared to corresponding control). The dose-response curve for norepinephrine was shifted to the left and the threshold dose was decreased after administration of the β-receptor blocking agent. In eight of the animals, the effects of phenoxybenzamine hydrochloride, an α-receptor blocking agent, were studied and, in these experiments, the increases in lobar arterial pressure in response to norepinephrine infusions at 0.5 and 10.0 μg/kg/min were blocked completely after administration of phenoxybenzamine hydrochloride, 5 mg/kg IV.

The effects of norepinephrine infusions on the pulmonary vascular bed were also investigated in this group of cats when pulmonary vascular tone was elevated by infusion of the endoperoxide analog. In 13 animals, lobar arterial pressure was increased from 13 ± 1 to 39 ± 2 mmHg by infusion of the endoperoxide analog; however, increases in lobar arterial pressure in response to norepinephrine infusions, 0.5 to 10 μg/kg/min, were not significantly different when pulmonary vascular tone was at resting levels or when tone had been enhanced by infusion of the endoperoxide analog. However, when lobar arterial pressure was increased from 13 ± 1 to 42 ± 2 mmHg in eight cats treated with phenoxybenzamine hydrochloride, 5 mg/kg IV, the pressor response to norepinephrine was reversed and infusions of norepinephrine at 0.25 to 10.0 μg/kg IV caused significant dose-dependent decreases in lobar arterial pressure. The reductions in lobar arterial pressure in response to norepinephrine in animals treated with phenoxybenzamine hydrochloride were similar when lobar vascular resistance was enhanced by the endoperoxide analog or by 15-methyl $PGF_{2\alpha}$. In four of the eight animals in which phenoxybenzamine hydrochloride was administered and lobar vascular tone was enhanced, the effect of propranolol on the depressor responses to norepinephrine was investigated. In these four animals treated with phenoxybenzamine hydrochloride, 5 mg/kg IV, and propranolol hydrochloride, 2 mg/kg IV, lobar arterial pressure was increased by the endoperoxide analog, but infusion of norepinephrine, 10 μg/kg/min, had little if any effect in that lobar arterial pressure decreased from 40 ± 2 to 39 ± 3 mmHg ($P < .05$).

Influence of Propranolol

The enhanced response to norepinephrine after administration of propranolol could result from blockade of β-adrenergic receptors or other actions of the drug. To examine these possibilities, the effects of propranolol on responses to phenylephrine hydrochloride and tyramine were investigated. Intralobar infusions of phenylephrine hydrochloride, an agent which acts on α-receptors at 1 to 3 μg/kg/min, increased lobar arterial pressure in a dose-dependent manner. The increases in lobar arterial pressure in response to phenylephrine were not changed after administration of propranolol hydrochloride, 2 mg/kg IV, but were blocked after injection of phenoxybenzamine hydrochloride, 5 mg/kg IV. In another group of animals, the effects of propranolol on pressor responses to tyramine, an indirectly acting agent, were investigated and these experiments show that increases in lobar arterial pressure in response to tyramine were enhanced after administration of propranolol hydrochloride, 2 mg/kg IV, but were blocked after administration of cocaine, 5 mg/kg IV. This dose of cocaine also enhanced the pressor response to intrapulmonary injections of norepinephrine.

Effects of Epinephrine

The effects of epinephrine on the pulmonary vascular bed were also investigated in another group of cats using a similar experimental protocol. Under resting conditions, intralobar infusion of epinephrine at 1 μg/kg/min had no significant effect on lobar arterial pressure. However, when the infusion rate was increased to 2 μg/kg/min there was a small (3.5 ± 0.8 mmHg) but statistically significant ($P < .05$) reduction in lobar arterial pressure. After administration of propranolol hydrochloride, 2 mg/kg IV, in four animals, intralobar infusions of epinephrine at 1 to 10 μg/kg/min caused significant dose-related increases in lobar arterial pressure. When lobar arterial pressure was increased from 14 ± 1 to 45 ± 3 mmHg by infusion of the endoperoxide analog, intralobar infusions of epinephrine at rates of 0.125 to 2.0 μg/kg/min caused significant dose-dependent decreases in lobar arterial pressure. When lobar vascular tone was enhanced in the presence of phenoxybenzamine hydrochloride, intralobar infusions of epinephrine at rates of 0.03 to 0.125 μg/kg/min produced marked dose-dependent decreases in lobar arterial pressure that were not different from responses to isoproterenol when tone was enhanced.

Effects of Isoproterenol

In a fourth series of experiments, intralobar infusions of isoproterenol, a β-agonist, at 62 and 125 ng/kg/min caused small but statistically significant reductions in lobar arterial pressure when lobar vascular resistance was at basal levels. When lobar arterial pressure was increased from 14 ± 1 to 46 ± 2 mmHg by infusion of the endoperoxide analog, intralobar infusions of isoproterenol at rates of 12 to 125 ng/kg/min caused marked dose-dependent decreases in lobar arterial pressure. In addition, when lobar vascular resistance was elevated by the endoperoxide analog, decreases in lobar arterial pressure in response to intrapulmonary infusions of isoproterenol at 62 and 125 ng/kg/min were almost completely blocked after administration of propranolol hydrochloride, 2 mg/kg IV. In contrast, when lobar vascular tone was enhanced by the endoperoxide analog, the decreases in lobar arterial pressure in response to isoproterenol infusions at 25 to 125 ng/kg/min were decreased significantly but not blocked after metoprolol, 2 mg/kg IV (n = 4), or practolol, 4 mg/kg IV (n = 4). The extent of β_1 H blockade was evaluated by comparing the increase in heart rate in response to isoproterenol before and after administration of metoprolol or practolol. In the control period, injection of isoproterenol, 3 μg IV, increased heart rate from 172 ± 6 to 205 ± 5 beats/min. After administration of metoprolol, 2 mg/kg IV (n = 4), or practolol, 4 mg/kg IV (n = 4), injection of isoproterenol, 3 μg/kg IV, increased the heart rate from 142 ± 6 to 147 ± 6 beats/min. The increase in heart rate in response to isoproterenol was decreased significantly after administration of metoprolol or practolol ($P < .05$, paired comparison).

Effects of Sympathetic Nerve Stimulation

In the last series of experiments, the effects of neuronally released norepinephrine and adrenergic blocking agents were investigated in the feline pulmonary vascular bed. Under resting conditions, stimulation of the sympathetic nerves at 3, 10, and 30 c/s caused significant frequency-related increases in lobar arterial pressure while lobar venous outflow pressure was held constant. In 13 of the cats, the effects of phenoxybenzamine on responses to nerve stimulation and bolus injections of norepinephrine were investigated. Under resting conditions, responses to the 1-μg dose of norepinephrine and nerve stimulation at 3 and 10 c/s were completely blocked after phenoxybenzamine hydrochloride, 5 mg/kg IV, whereas responses to nerve stimulation at 30 c/s and norepinephrine at 3 μg were reversed. In additional experiments under resting conditions, responses to norepinephrine were enhanced after administration of β-receptor blocking agents, whereas the β-blocking agents had no significant effect on the response to sympathetic nerve stimulation. In these experiments both propranolol hydrochloride, 2 mg/kg IV (n = 1), and sotalol hydrochloride 4 mg/kg IV (n = 4), an agent which may have fewer membrane effects than propranolol, were used. In 16 of the animals the effects of nerve stimulation and norepinephrine were investigated when lobar vascular tone was enhanced after administration of phenoxybenzamine hydrochloride, 5 mg/kg IV. When lobar arterial pressure was increased from 15 ± 2 to 39 ± 2 mmHg by intrapulmonary infusion of the endoperoxide analog or 15-methyl PGF$_{2\alpha}$ in animals treated with this α-blocking agent, stimulation of the sympathetic nerves at 3, 10, and 30 c/s and intralobar injections of norepinephrine at 1 and 3 μg caused significant frequency- and dose-dependent decreases in lobar arterial pressure. In four of the 16 cats, the decrease in lobar arterial pressure in response to nerve stimulation at 30 c/s was blocked after administration of propranolol hydrochloride, 2 mg/kg IV (control −9 ± 2 mmHg, after propranolol −1 ± 1 mmHg, $P < .05$). In four other cats with enhanced tone and α-receptor blockade, the decrease in lobar arterial pressure in response to nerve stimulation at 30 c/s was not modified after administration of atropine, 1 mg/kg IV (control −8 ± 1 mmHg, after atropine −8 ± 1 mmHg). In four other experiments, the effects of phentolamine and atropine on responses to nerve stimulation were investigated. Responses to nerve stimulation at 3, 10, and 30 c/s were reversed after administration of phentolamine, 2.5 mg/kg IV, when tone was enhanced by intrapulmonary infusion of the endoperoxide analog. The vasodilator responses to nerve stimulation were not modified after administration of atropine, 1 mg/kg IV.

The specificity of the blocking effects of phentolamine and propranolol were investigated in four other animals, and in these experiments phentolamine, 2.5 mg/kg IV, was without significant effect on increases in lobar arterial pressure in response to angiotensin II or PGF$_{2\alpha}$. In addition, phentolamine was without significant effect on decreases in lobar arterial pressure in response to PGE$_1$ or nitroglycerin when lobar vascular resistance was elevated by the endoperoxide analog. In these same experiments, propranolol hydrochloride, 2 mg/kg IV, was without significant effect on decreases in lobar arterial pressure in response to PGE_1 or nitroglycerin when lobar vascular resistance was elevated by the endoperoxide analog.

The effects of bolus injections of phenylephrine hydrochloride, an α-receptor agonist, and UK-14304, an α_2-receptor agonist, were investigated in the pulmonary vascular bed and under base-line conditions intralobar administration of phenylephrine hydrochloride, 1 to 30 μg, or UK-14304, 30 to 300 μg, increased lobar arterial pressure in a dose-related fashion, whereas left atrial pressure remained unchanged. Although UK-14304 and phenylephrine possessed vasoconstrictor activity in the lobar vascular bed, prolonged and marked systemic hypotension was observed only following the intralobar injections of UK-14304.

Pulmonary Vascular Responses to Vagal Stimulation and Acetylcholine

Pulmonary vascular responses to vagal stimulation and acetylcholine chloride were investigated in the intact-chest cat under conditions of controlled pulmonary blood flow. Under base-line (resting tone) conditions in nine cats, stimulation of the left midcervical vagus at stimulus frequencies of 4, 8, and 16 Hz caused small (1 ± 0, 2 ± 1, 3 ± 1 mmHg, respectively) but statistically significant increases in lobar arterial pressure when left atrial pressure was maintained constant. In three of these animals, the effects of α-receptor blockade on the pressor response to vagal stimulation under base-line conditions was investigated. Vagal stimulation increased lobar arterial pressure 1 ± 0, 2 ± 1, and 3 ± 1 mmHg at 4, 8, and 16 Hz, respectively, under base-line conditions, whereas no measurable rise was observed at these stimulus frequencies after administration of phenoxybenzamine hydrochloride, 5 mg/kg IV. In contrast to the effects of vagal stimulation, intralobar injections of acetylcholine chloride in eight of the cats in doses of 0.5 and 1.0 μg caused small (1 ± 0 mmHg) but statistically significant decreases in lobar arterial pressure under base-line conditions.

Since the magnitude of vasodilator responses in the lung is dependent on the existing level of vasoconstrictor tone which is minimal under base-line conditions (forced inspiratory oxygen $[FI_{O_2}]$ = 0.21),[35,36] responses to vagal stimulation and acetylcholine were also investigated when lobar vascular tone was elevated. Intralobar infusion of U-46619, a stable prostaglandin endoperoxide analog (n = 9), or 15-methyl $PGF_{2\alpha}$ (n = 3), increased lobar arterial pressure from 12 ± 1 to 36 ± 2 mmHg in the 12 animals. The increases in lobar arterial pressure in response to the prostaglandin analogs were well maintained during the infusion period. Under conditions of enhanced tone in the group of 12 animals, vagal stimulation at 4, 8, and 16 Hz caused small (1 ± 0, 2 ± 1, 4 ± 1 mmHg, respectively) but statistically significant decreases in lobar arterial pressure. In four of these animals, the effects of β-receptor blockade on the decrease in lobar arterial pressure in response to vagal stimulation were also investigated. Decreases in lobar arterial pressure at stimulus frequencies of 8 and 16 Hz were -2 ± 1 and -4 ± 1 mmHg before and -2 ± 1 and -4 ± 1 mmHg after administration of propranolol hydrochloride, 1 mg/kg IV. However, in eight of the animals, atropine, 1 mg/kg IV, significantly attenuated the decreases in lobar arterial pressure in response to vagal stimulation at 8 and 16 Hz which were -1 ± 0 and -4 ± 1 mmHg before and 0 and -2 ± 0 mmHg after atropine.

Under conditions of enhanced vascular tone, intralobar injections of acetylcholine chloride, 0.05 to 1.0 μg, in eight animals caused significant dose-related decreases in lobar arterial pressure. Pressure decreased 19%, 27%, 45%, and 48% at doses of 0.05, 0.1, 0.5, and 1.0 μg, respectively. Responses to acetylcholine were rapid in onset and lobar arterial pressure returned to control values one to three minutes after the injection. Lobar arterial pressure decreased -6 ± 1, -8 ± 1, -11 ± 1, and -13 ± 2 mmHg at 0.05 to 1.0 μg doses of acetylcholine chloride under enhanced tone conditions, and these decreases in pressure were reduced to a similar extent as observed in 6-hydroxydopamine-treated animals after administration of atropine.

Influence of Adrenergic Neuronal Blockade and Hexamethonium

It has been reported that the vagus is a mixed nerve containing efferent fibers from both the parasympathetic and the sympathetic divisions of the autonomic nervous system.[37] Therefore, responses to vagal stimulation were investigated in animals treated with 6-hydroxydopamine, an agent which interferes with the capacity of adrenergic nerves to store catecholamines.[38] For these experiments, the animals were treated with 6-hydroxydopamine, 100 mg/kg intraperitoneally (IP), for three days and were catheterized on days 4 to 6. In six animals treated with 6-hydroxydopamine, vagal stimulation at 4, 8, and 16 Hz elicited small but statistically significant decreases in lobar arterial pressure of 1 ± 0, 2 ± 1, 2 ± 0 mmHg, respectively. In these animals, as in control animals, intralobar injections of acetylcholine chloride caused small (1 ± 0, 2 ± 0 mmHg, respectively) but significant decreases in lobar arterial pressure at the 0.5- and 1.0-μg doses. However, when lobar arterial pressure was increased from 13 ± 1 to 34 ± 2 mmHg in 12 animals by intralobar infusion of U-46619 (n = 9), or 15-methyl PGF$_{2\alpha}$ (n = 3), vagal stimulation at 2 to 16 Hz caused marked frequency-dependent decreases in lobar arterial pressure. The responses were slow in onset, reaching a steady state 30 to 60 seconds after onset of stimulation, and the decreases in lobar arterial pressure were well maintained during nerve stimulation for periods of up to 90 seconds. Lobar arterial pressure decreased 12%, 18%, 25%, and 38% at frequencies of 2, 4, 8, and 16 Hz, respectively, and pressure returned to control level over a one- to three-minute period after vagal stimulation was terminated. When lobar vascular resistance was elevated by infusion of U-46619 (n = 5) or 15-methyl PGF$_{2\alpha}$ (n = 3), intralobar injections of acetylcholine chloride (0.05, 0.1, 0.5, and 1.0 μg) caused significant dose-related reductions in lobar arterial pressure of 7 ± 1, 9 ± 1, 12 ± 1, 13 ± 1 mmHg, respectively. These responses were not significantly different from those observed in eight control animals when lobar vascular resistance was elevated to comparable levels by infusion of U-46619.

In three of the 6-hydroxydopamine-treated animals, the effects of β-receptor blockade on the decreases in lobar arterial pressure in response to vagal stimulation were studied. The decreases in lobar arterial pressure at 8 and 16 Hz (-8 ± 1 and -11 ± 1 mmHg, respectively) in 6-hydroxydopamine-treated animals under enhanced tone conditions were not significantly different (-7 ± 1 and -11 ± 2 mmHg) after administration of propranolol hydrochloride, 1 mg/kg IV. However, the decreases in lobar arterial pressure in response to vagal stimulation and to acetylcholine chloride in 6-hydroxydopamine-treated animals were blocked after administration of atropine, 1 mg/kg IV. In other experiments, the effect of ganglionic blockade on responses to vagal stimulation and acetylcholine chloride were investigated in 6-hydroxydopamine-treated animals. In experimental animals (n = 5), when lobar vascular resistance was elevated by infusion of U-46619, the reductions in lobar arterial pressure in response to vagal stimulation were blocked after administration of hexamethonium bromide, 5 mg/kg IV. However, decreases in lobar arterial pressure in response to acetylcholine chloride injections were not modified by the ganglionic blocking agent.

The functional extent of depletion of catecholamines from adrenergic nerves was assessed by comparing responses to tyramine, an indirectly acting sympathomimetic agent, in control animals and in animals treated with 6-hydroxydopamine. In control animals (n = 5), intralobar injections of tyramine, 200 μg, increased lobar arterial and systemic arterial pressures 5 ± 1 and 24 ± 4 mmHg, respectively. In 6-hydroxydopamine-treated animals (n = 4), this dose of tyramine increased lobar arterial and systemic arterial pressure 1 ± 0 and 4 ± 1 mmHg, respectively. The increases in lobar arterial and systemic arterial pressures were significantly less in 6-hydroxydopamine-treated animals, compared with controls. The effect of treatment with 6-hydroxydopamine was further investigated by comparing responses to norepinephrine in control animals (n = 6) and in cats treated with the adrenergic neuronal blocking agent, 100 mg/kg IP, for three days and studied on days 4 to 6. In control animals, intralobar infusion of norepinephrine, 0.25 μg/kg/min for two to three minutes, increased lobar arterial pressure from 12 ± 1 to 16 ± 1 mmHg. In animals treated with 6-hydroxydopamine (n = 4), a similar increase in lobar arterial pressure (10 ± 1 to 13 ± 1 mmHg) was observed at a norepinephrine infusion rate of 0.025 μg/kg/min which was one tenth the control rate.

In addition to experiments with 6-hydroxydopamine, the effects of a second adrenergic neuronal blocking agent were investigated in another group of five cats. These animals were treated with reserpine, 1 mg/kg intramuscularly (IM), and the animals were catheterized on day 2 or 3. In these animals, vagal stimulation at 8 and 16 Hz and acetylcholine chloride injections at the 1-μg dose caused small but significant decreases in lobar arterial pressure. However, when lobar vascular resistance was increased by infusion of U-46619, vagal stimulation at 4 to 16 Hz and acetylcholine chloride injections, 0.1 to 1.0 μg, caused significant frequency- and dose-dependent decreases in lobar arterial pressure. Although decreases in lobar arterial pressure in response to intralobar injections of acetylcholine were similar in animals treated with 6-hydroxydopamine or reserpine, responses to vagal stimulation were significantly smaller at 4, 8, and 16 Hz in reserpine-treated animals.

Effect of Physostigmine

If responses to vagal stimulation are the result of release of acetylcholine chloride from cholinergic terminals, then these responses should be enhanced by physostigmine, a cholinesterase inhibitor. In another group of cats treated with 6-hydroxydopamine, decreases in lobar arterial pressure in response to vagal stimulation at 1 and 2 Hz (n = 5), and to acetylcholine chloride at 0.5 and 1.0 μg (n = 5), were enhanced significantly to 2 ± 0, 3 ± 1 mmHg and 2 ± 0, 3 ± 1 mmHg, respectively, after administration of physostigmine, 1 mg/kg IV. Furthermore, when lobar vascular resistance was elevated by infusion of U-46619, the frequency-response curve for vagal stimulation was shifted to the left by physostigmine and the threshold frequency for stimulation was decreased from 2.0 Hz to 0.25 Hz. The dose-response curve for acetylcholine was also shifted to the left by the cholinesterase inhibitor and the threshold dose was reduced.

Influence of Systemic Hypotension
and Bronchial Obstruction

Although bradycardia and systemic hypotension in response to vagal stimulation were minimized by ventricular pacing, using an electrode catheter in the right ventricle, aortic pressure was decreased from 130 ± 5 to 115 ± 6 mmHg in control animals and from 105 ± 4 to 95 ± 5 mmHg in 6-hydroxydopamine-treated animals. Moreover, a decrease in systemic arterial pressure could change lobar arterial pressure by altering bronchopulmonary shunt flow.[39] Therefore, the effects of vagal stimulation were compared when aortic pressure was at normal levels and when pressure was reduced during a period of ventricular fibrillation. In four animals treated with 6-hydroxydopamine, a short period of high-frequency stimulation of the right ventricular free wall by way of an electrode catheter induced ventricular fibrillation, during which time aortic pressure decreased from 110 ± 6 to 50 ± 7 mmHg. The reduction in aortic pressure had no significant effect on lobar arterial pressure (control 35 ± 2 and 34 ± 2 during fibrillation) or on the response to vagal stimulation at 16 Hz (control -10 ± 1, during fibrillation -9 ± 2 mmHg). The period of ventricular fibrillation was two to three minutes, and normal sinus rhythm was reestablished by direct current defibrillation.

Vagal stimulation increases bronchomotor tone.[39] Therefore, the contribution of changes in bronchomotor tone to the response to vagal stimulation was investigated in four cats treated with 6-hydroxydopamine in which the left lower lobe bronchus was obstructed by inflation of a 5 F balloon catheter. The decreases in lobar arterial pressure in response to vagal stimulation at 4 and 8 Hz and to acetylcholine chloride at 0.5 and 1.0 μg were not significantly different during normal ventilation, or when the left lower lobe bronchus was obstructed, blocking airflow.

Responses During Alveolar Hypoxia

The effects of vagal stimulation were also investigated in another group of cats treated with 6-hydroxydopamine when lobar arterial pressure was increased by ventilatory hypoxia. Ventilation with 10% O_2 in N_2 caused a significant increase in lobar arterial pressure without altering left atrial pressure. When lobar arterial pressure was increased by ventilation with 10% O_2, vagal stimulation caused a significant reduction in lobar arterial pressure without altering left atrial pressure.

Results from Studies in Isolated Intrapulmonary Vessels

Relaxant responses to acetylcholine chloride Isolated rings rather than the more conventional helical strip preparations were used in these experiments because rings were more consistently isolated with an intact or functioning endothelium, as assessed by reproducible relaxations in response to acetylcholine chloride. The most consistent submaximal contractions to phenylephrine and relaxations to acetylcholine chloride were obtained when arterial rings were first depolarized with potassium and then submaximally contracted with phenylephrine. Acetylcholine chloride produced a concentration-dependent relaxation of phenylephrine-precontracted arterial rings and this response was antagonized by atropine. Although acetylcholine chloride also relaxed rings that were precontracted with 30 mol/L KCl, acetylcholine chloride was tenfold more potent when phenylephrine was used to precontract the rings. A 10-μmol/L concentration of quinacrine hydrochloride partially antagonized acetylcholine-elicited relaxation without affecting the contractile response to phenylephrine. Higher concentrations (20 to 50 μmol/L) of quinacrine hydrochloride, however, markedly depressed or abolished contractions to phenylephrine and were not employed in this study. Methylene blue enhanced contractile responses to phenylephrine and markedly antagonized relaxant responses to acetylcholine chloride.

Contractile responses to acetylcholine   Isolated rings prepared with a damaged endothelium contracted in response to acetylcholine chloride. Acetylcholine chloride further contracted arterial rings that had been submaximally precontracted by phenylephrine. Contractile responses to acetylcholine were antagonized by atropine and enhanced by methylene blue. Quinacrine hydrochloride, at a concentration (10 μmol/L) which depressed relaxant responses to acetylcholine also depressed contractile responses to acetylcholine.

Effects of acetylcholine on arterial accumulation of cGMP and cAMP   In all of the present experiments, cyclic nucleotide determinations were made in arterial ring preparations that had been previously equilibrated under 6 g of tension, depolarized with potassium, and submaximally precontracted with phenylephrine. In addition, changes in isometric force were recorded until the time of freeze-clamping. The reason for this is that a considerable number of initial experiments in which arterial rings were incubated in the absence of tension, whether or not depolarization or contraction was induced, yielded inconsistent and highly variable values for cyclic nucleotide levels.

Acetylcholine elicited a time-dependent increase in arterial cGMP accumulation which correlated well with the development of relaxation. The onset of cGMP accumulation (5 seconds) preceded the onset of relaxation (15 seconds). Furthermore, peak levels of cGMP which occurred at 30 seconds preceded peak relaxant responses to acetylcholine. At 60 seconds after addition of 10^{-6} mol/L acetylcholine chloride, cGMP levels were elevated 15-fold to 331 ± 21 pmol/g of tissue. At this time point (60 seconds), acetylcholine elicited 75% to 80% relaxation, which is less than that for maximal relaxation by 10^{-6} mol/L acetylcholine chloride, because maximal responses take about 120 seconds to develop. Concentration-dependent responses to acetylcholine appear to be relatively flat, which suggests that multiple endothelial-dependent mechanisms are involved in the regulation of the contractile state mediated by muscarinic receptors. Atropine and methylene blue markedly inhibited both relaxation and cGMP accumulation caused by acetylcholine. Quinacrine hydrochloride caused a highly significant antagonism of relaxation without altering cGMP accumulation in response to acetylcholine. Quinacrine hydrochloride at concentrations of 50 to 100 μmol/L markedly inhibited cGMP accumulation elicited by acetylcholine, but the effects on relaxation could not be assessed because such high concentrations of quinacrine markedly depressed phenylephrine-induced precontractions.

Resting levels of cAMP in arterial rings were 331 ± 16 pmol/g of tissue or about 15-fold greater than those of cGMP. Cyclic levels remained relatively constant at times when both cGMP levels and relaxation were increasing in response to acetylcholine.

Cyclic guanosine monophosphate levels were determined also in intrapulmonary arterial rings that had been prepared with a damaged endothelium. Resting cGMP levels were 26 ± 1 pmol/g of tissue and were unaltered by phenylephrine. Acetylcholine elevated cGMP after 60 seconds by approximately sixfold to 153 ± 12 pmol/g of tissue, and also elicited a contractile response. Atropine abolished both responses to acetylcholine, whereas methylene blue markedly inhibited cGMP accumulation and enhanced the contractile response to acetylcholine. Quinacrine depressed contractions to acetylcholine and failed to alter arterial cGMP accumulation. Methylene blue (10^{-5} mol/L) by itself lowered resting levels of cGMP from 26 ± 1 to 14 ± 1 pmol/g of tissue. Similarly, in arterial rings possessing a functional endothelium, methylene blue (10^{-5} mol/L) lowered the resting levels of cGMP from 25 ± 3 to 11 ± 2 pmol/g of tissue.

DISCUSSION

Results of the present study show that stimulation of the sympathetic nerves to the lung and norepinephrine administration increase lobar arterial pressure in the cat. Inasmuch as lobar blood flow and lobar venous outflow pressure were maintained constant, the increases in lobar arterial pressure indicate that nerve stimulation and norepinephrine increase pulmonary lobar vascular resistance. The increases in lobar arterial pressure in response to norepinephrine and nerve stimulation were dose- and frequency-dependent and these responses were blocked after administration of α-receptor blocking agents. These data indicate that the feline pulmonary vascular bed is functionally innervated by the sympathetic nervous system and that under basal conditions both exogenously administered and neuronally released norepinephrine cause vasoconstriction by stimulating α-receptors. These results are similar to those of previous studies on the canine pulmonary vascular bed.[3,6,10] However, the present experiments extend the work of previous studies by showing that, when pulmonary vascular tone was elevated in animals treated with α-receptor blocking agents, adrenergic nerve stimulation caused frequency-dependent decreases in lobar arterial pressure that were not blocked by atropine. The atropine-resistant neurogenically induced vasodilator responses were well maintained during the period of stimulaton, and these responses were of greater magnitude than were the increases in lobar arterial pressure observed under basal conditions.

Norepinephrine also caused dose-dependent decreases in lobar arterial pressure after α-receptor blockade when pulmonary vascular tone was elevated. The vasodilator responses to norepinephrine and nerve stimulation were blocked by propranolol, a β-receptor blocking agent. These data indicate that the adrenergic transmitter acts on both α- and β-adrenergic receptors and when pulmonary vascular tone is elevated and α-receptors are masked, norepinephrine causes vasodilation in the pulmonary vascular bed. The present data for the pulmonary vascular bed are in agreement with previous studies in skeletal muscle, liver, spleen, and adipose tissue and in isolated facial vein of the rabbit and support the hypothesis that norepinephrine liberated from sympathetic nerves can act on β_2-receptors in blood vessels.[17-19,21,40,41] However, other investigators have not been able to elicit vasodilator responses to adrenergic stimulation in a variety of organ systems.[23,37,42,43]

The hypotheses that vascular β (β_2)-receptors are innervated and that neuronally released norepinephrine elicits vasodilation have been challenged recently.[23] These investigators were unable to confirm the classic studies in which nerve stimulation caused atropine-insensitive vasodilation in skeletal muscle.[21] In these studies, responses to adrenergic stimulation were reversed after intra-arterial administration of dibozane, a substance which is poorly soluble at neutral pH, whereas responses to nerve stimulation were not reversed by phentolamine. However, when dibozane was administered IV at a dose of 10 mg/kg, vasodilator responses to nerve stimulation were blocked by atropine.[23] Moreover, results of the present study show that neuronally released norepinephrine can cause vasodilation and indicate that β_2-receptors in the pulmonary vascular bed are innervated. In the present study, responses to nerve stimulation were reversed by phenoxybenzamine or phentolamine in doses that did not significantly alter responses to $PGF_{2\alpha}$, angiotensin II, PGE_1, or nitroglycerin in the pulmonary vascular bed. In addition, vasodilator responses to nerve stimulation were not modified by doses of atropine that reduced responses to acetylcholine in the feline pulmonary vascular bed. These data suggest that reversal of the response to nerve stimulation was not dependent on the type of α-blocker employed and did not involve a cholinergic mechanism. The reasons for the difference in results in the present study and in those of other investigators[23] are uncertain but may suggest differences in nerve terminal–adrenergic receptor relationships in the skeletal muscle and the pulmonary vascular beds. The hypothesis that the feline pulmonary vascular bed is well supplied with β-receptors is suggested by the observation that isoproterenol, a potent β-agonist, had marked vasodilator activity when pulmonary vascular tone was elevated. Moreover, the observation that vasodilator responses to isoproterenol were only partially decreased by metoprolol or practolol but were almost completely blocked by propranolol suggests that the vascular β-receptors in the lung are of the β_2 type, as previously suggested.[44] Although metoprolol or practolol had only a small effect on the pulmonary vasodilator response to isoproterenol, these agents almost completely blocked the increases in heart rate in response to isoproterenol, confirming the cardioselective nature of these antagonists.[45,46]

It has been reported that vasoconstrictor tone in the feline pulmonary vascular bed is minimal under resting conditions and that vasodilator responses to prostaglandins and nitroglycerin are dependent on the existing level of tone in the bed.[35] Vasodilation in response to β-receptor activation is caused by relaxation of basal tone, and variations in response to β-agonists may result from variations in the level of existing tone.[18] The present studies with isoproterenol are consistent with the results of studies in the hepatic bed and support the concept that responses to β-agonists are dependent on the existing level of vasoconstrictor tone.[18,47]

Epinephrine stimulates both α- and β-receptors, and its potency on β-receptors is between that of norepinephrine and isoproterenol.[25] Reports in the literature on the pulmonary vascular effects of epinephrine vary with the study.[15,48] Results of the present study show in the cat with an intact chest that epinephrine infusions produced modest decreases in pulmonary vascular resistance. Moreover, these decreases were greatly enhanced when pulmonary vascular tone was elevated. In addition, when tone was elevated and α-receptors were blocked, epinephrine had potent vasodilator activity. Moreover, vasodilator responses to epinephrine after α-blockade were nearly equal to vasodilator responses to isoproterenol when vasoconstrictor tone was elevated. These results indicate that epinephrine has good β-receptor-stimulating activity in the feline pulmonary vascular bed but suggests that this activity is dependent on the existing level of tone in the bed. These data support our hypothesis that the feline pulmonary vascular bed is well supplied with β-receptors. The present data are in agreement with results of a recent study in skeletal muscle in regard to the relative potency of isoproterenol, epinephrine, and norepinephrine in stimulating vascular β-receptors.[23] Although epinephrine had no apparent vasoconstrictor activity when infused at rates of 1 or 2 μg/kg/min, these concentrations caused significant vasoconstriction when β-receptors were blocked with propranolol. In addition, vasoconstrictor responses to norepinephrine were increased greatly after β-adrenergic blockade. These data suggest that in the feline pulmonary vascular bed, epinephrine and norepinephrine act on both α- and β-receptors and that the resulting response is the algebraic summation of these two opposing actions. Therefore, when β-receptors are blocked, both catecholamines have potent α-receptor-stimulating activity.

The possibility that propranolol was enhancing pressor responses to norepinephrine and epinephrine by a mechanism other than β-receptor blockade was investigated by evaluating the effects of the antagonist on responses to phenylephrine, tyramine, PGF$_{2\alpha}$, and antiotensin II. Since phenylephrine is a selective α-receptor agonist, propranolol would not be expected to enhance the response to this agent.[49] The present studies show that propranolol in doses that blocked vasodilator responses to isoproterenol and enhanced vasoconstrictor responses to norepinephrine was without significant effect on the pressor response to phenylephrine infusion. Tyramine is an indirectly acting amine which must be taken up by the adrenergic nerves in order to displace norepinephrine.[50] However, propranolol, in doses that blocked β-receptors in the feline pulmonary vascular bed, enhanced the pressor response to tyramine. In addition, propranolol did not modify pressor responses to PGF$_{2\alpha}$ and angiotensin II which are nonadrenergic agonists. These data suggest that propranolol does not enhance pressor responses to norepinephrine or epinephrine by blocking uptake of these substances into adrenergic nerves or by a nonspecific effect on vascular smooth muscle. Although propranolol did not block responses to tyramine, the effects of this indirectly acting substance are inhibited by cocaine, an agent which blocks neuronal uptake.[51] The doses of cocaine that blocked responses to tyramine-enhanced responses to norepinephrine suggests that neuronal uptake may be an important mechanism for terminating the actions of catecholamines in the pulmonary vascular bed. In addition, the observation that tyramine causes an indirectly mediated pressor response supports our hypothesis that the feline pulmonary vascular bed is innervated by the adrenergic nervous system. The enhanced pressor response to norepinephrine and the significant vasoconstrictor response to epinephrine after propranolol provide further support for the hypothesis that these catecholamines act on both α- and β-receptors in the feline pulmonary vascular bed.

Although responses to sympathetic nerve stimulation were reversed after α-receptors were blocked and tone was elevated, these responses were not enhanced after administration of β-blocking agents. Thus, in the same group of cats in which pressor responses to exogenously administered norepinephrine were augmented, responses to nerve stimulation were not modified. The explanation for the inability to enhance neurogenic responses is uncertain; however, it is possible that the β-blocking agents may have a depressant action on the processes by which norepinephrine is liberated by stimulation of the sympathetic nerves. Neither sotalol nor propranolol enhanced the response to nerve stimulation, and since sotalol has little, if any, "membrane stabilizing activity," the depressant action is probably not nonspecific.[45] The inability of the β-blockers to enhance responses to nerve stimulation, whereas these agents enhanced responses to tyramine and norepinephrine in the present study, suggests a very specific action on the neurogenic release process for norepinephrine in the adrenergic terminal. It has been reported that activation of presynaptic β-receptors enhances neuronal release of norepinephrine and that β-blocking agents such as sotalol decrease the release of the adrenergic transmitter.[52,53] It is, therefore, possible that the β-blocking agents may block presynaptic receptors and decrease the release of norepinephrine in response to nerve stimulation. This action would oppose the effects of blockade of vascular β_2-receptors.

Results of the present study indicate that the feline pulmonary vascular bed is innervated by the sympathetic nervous system and that α- and β_2-adrenergic receptors are present. In addition, these results suggest that neuronally released and blood-borne norepinephrine can act on β-receptors, but vasodilator responses are dependent on the existing level of vasoconstrictor tone in the bed.

Recent studies have indicated that in addition to postsynaptic α_1-adrenoceptors, postsynaptic α_2-receptors, which produce a pressor response when activated, exist as well.[11-13] Results from previous experiments have demonstrated the presence of both α-receptor subtypes at the effector sites of vascular smooth muscle of the systemic circulation. Results from the present study demonstrate that in the intact animal, selective α_1- and α_2-receptor agonists produce a pressor response in the pulmonary vascular bed. Phenylephrine as an α_1-receptor agonist, when compared to UK-14304, an α_2-agonist, has 20 to 30 times greater pressor activity in the feline pulmonary vascular bed. It has been shown in isolated rabbit pulmonary arterial strips that postsynaptic α_1-adrenoceptors, which mediate a contractile response, and not α_2-receptors are present in vascular smooth muscle from the lung.[54] In contrast, results from the present study demonstrate that in the intact animal, substances which selectively activate α_1- or α_2-adrenoceptors may produce a pressor response in the pulmonary vascular bed of the cat. Additional experiments are necessary to fully characterize the nature of responses due to activation of α-receptor subtypes and to determine which population of α-receptor subtypes has an intra- and/or extrasynaptic location in the feline pulmonary vascular bed.

Results of the present investigation in the intact-chest cat also show that, under normal resting conditions, electrical stimulation of the peripheral segment of the vagus nerve in the midcervical region increases lobar arterial pressure. However, when vasoconstrictor tone in the pulmonary vascular bed was increased by several mechanisms, the pressor response was reversed and a depressor response was unmasked. The pressor response under base-line conditions was blocked by phenoxybenzamine, whereas the depressor response under enhanced tone conditions was blocked by atropine. These data suggest that in the cat, in the cervical region, the vagus is composed of efferent fibers from both sympathetic and parasympathetic divisions of the autonomic nervous system, as has been reported previously in the dog.[24] Since efferent fibers from both sympathetic and parasympathetic systems are represented in the cervical vagus, the effects of 6-hydroxydopamine, an agent which destroys the integrity of adrenergic terminals, on responses to vagal stimulation were investigated.[38] Treatment with 6-hydroxydopamine markedly inhibited pressor responses to tyramine and enhanced pressor responses to norepinephrine in the systemic and lobar vascular beds, suggesting that the neuronal blocking agent depleted adrenergic terminals of norepinephrine and inhibited uptake of adrenergic transmitter.[3,55,56]

After treatment with 6-hydroxydopamine, stimulation of efferent vagal fibers decreased lobar arterial pressure, and responses to vagal stimulation were greatly enhanced when vasoconstrictor tone was increased to a high steady level during infusion of 15-methyl $PGF_{2\alpha}$ or U-46619, a stable prostaglandin endoperoxide analog whose actions may mimic those of thromboxane A_2 (TxA_2).[57] Since lobar blood flow and left atrial pressure were maintained constant, the reductions in lobar arterial pressure in response to vagal stimulation suggest that pulmonary lobar vascular resistance is decreased. The reductions in lobar arterial pressure in response to vagal stimulation were not modified by propranolol, suggesting that the vasodilator response is not mediated in part through activation of β-receptors by neuronally released norepinephrine.[36] When vasoconstrictor tone was enhanced during infusion of U-46619 or 15-methyl $PGF_{2\alpha}$, intralobar infusions of acetylcholine decreased lobar arterial pressure and the response was not altered by treatment with 6-hydroxydopamine. However, decreases in lobar arterial pressure in response to vagal stimulation and acetylcholine in 6-hydroxydopamine-treated animals with enhanced tone were blocked by atropine, a muscarinic receptor-blocking agent. In contrast to experiments with atropine, responses to vagal stimulation and to acetylcholine in 6-hydroxydopamine-treated animals with enhanced tone were greatly increased by physostigmine, a cholinesterase inhibitor. These data suggest that vagal stimulation decreases lobar arterial pressure by releasing acetylcholine, which acts on muscarinic receptors in the pulmonary vascular bed. Vasodilator responses to vagal stimulation were blocked after treatment with hexamethonium, a ganglionic blocking agent, whereas responses to acetylcholine were not affected after ganglionic blockade. These data indicate that the decreases in lobar arterial pressure in response to vagal stimulation are due to activation of preganglionic cholinergic neurons.

In a recently published study, it has been shown that small- and medium-sized intrapulmonary arteries in the cat have cholinergic terminals.[4] However, the effects of cholinergic (vagosympathetic) nerve stimulation are uncertain, since reports in the literature show modest increases, modest decreases, a biphasic response, or no change in pulmonary vascular resistance.[24,39] It has been shown in a perfused dog lung preparation that stimulation of the cervical vagosympathetic trunk increased pulmonary arterial pressure in two animals, decreased pulmonary arterial pressure in six, and elicited a biphasic response in two animals.[24] The decreases in pressure in response to vagal stimulation were small (1 to 4 mmHg) and were blocked by atropine.[24] However, these investigators concluded from their results that a final decision as to the existence of atropine-sensitive pulmonary vasodilator fibers must await further studies, including experiments designed to ensure that the pulmonary arterial pressure changes are not secondary to alterations in the transfer of blood from the bronchial (systemic) to the pulmonary circulation.[24] Results of the present investigation extend the work of these investigators by demonstrating that efferent vagal stimulation caused larger-than-previously-recognized, consistent, stimulus-related decreases in lobar vascular resistance in intact–chest animals after treatment with 6-hydroxydopamine when vasoconstrictor tone was increased. The dilator responses were blocked by atropine and enhanced by physostigmine, and similar responses were elicited by intralobar injections of acetylcholine, suggesting that they were cholinergic in nature.

The contribution of the bronchial circulation to the response to vagal stimulation was minimal in these experiments, since transfer of blood from the lobar vascular bed to the systemic vascular bed woud not occur when systemic arterial pressure was maintained at normal levels by cardiac pacing. In addition, experiments showing that responses to vagal stimulation and to acetylcholine were similar when systemic arterial pressure was decreased to levels approximately equal to or lower than lobar arterial pressure during a period of ventricular fibrillation suggests that alterations in bronchial blood flow contribute little, if anything, to the lobar vascular response to vagal stimulation or acetylcholine. In addition, a marked reduction in systemic arterial pressure had no significant effect on lobar arterial pressure, suggesting that changes in bronchial flow, which is less than 5% of pulmonary flow, had no measurable effect on lobar hemodynamics in the cat. Similar observations have been made in the intact-chest dog.[8,58]

It has been reported that vagal stimulation can increase bronchomotor tone, and it is possible that changes in bronchomotor tone could influence the vascular response to vagal stimulation.[6,24,39,50] To assess the contribution of changes in bronchomotor tone and lung volume on responses to vagal stimulation and acetylcholine, we compared responses during normal ventilation and when airflow to the left lower lobe was interrupted by inflation of a balloon catheter positioned in the left lower lobe bronchus. Since responses to vagal stimulation and to acetylcholine were not altered during the period of bronchial occlusion, these experiments suggest that changes in bronchomotor tone and lung volume contribute little, if anything, to the response of the pulmonary lobar vascular bed to vagal stimulation or acetylcholine. The data showing that responses to vagal stimulation occur independent of changes in bronchopulmonary shunt flow, bronchomotor tone, or lung volume, along with the recent demonstration of the presence of numerous cholinergic terminals in intrapulmonary arteries, suggest that vagal stimulation dilates the pulmonary vascular bed by releasing acetylcholine from postganglionic cholinergic terminals. The transmitter then acts on muscarinic receptors in pulmonary vessels.[4]

The results of the present study indicate that the vagus in the mid-cervical region in the cat carries efferent fibers innervating lung vessels which have adrenergic and cholinergic terminals, and that, in order to demonstrate a vasodilator response to vagal stimulation, it is necessary to interfere with the integrity of the adrenergic nerves and to enhance vasoconstrictor tone, since the pulmonary vascular bed has little, if any, vasoconstrictor tone under resting conditions.[35,36,60] The physiological significance of the cholinergic dilator system is uncertain at resting tone ($FI_{O_2} = 0.21$) conditions. However, when vasoconstrictor tone is elevated by ventilatory hypoxia ($FI_{O_2} = 0.10$), the present data show that this neurogenic system could produce significant vasodilation. In addition to hypoxic vasoconstriction, pulmonary vascular resistance is increased by prostaglandins and TxA_2 in a number of pulmonary disorders, including endotoxin shock and embolism.[61-63] The present data suggest that, in pathophysiologic states in which tone is elevated by $PGF_{2\alpha}$ or TxA_2, the neurogenic cholinergic vasodilator system could produce marked unloading of the right ventricle, since the actions of U-46619 closely mimic those of TxA_2.[57]

In all previously discussed experiments in which a vasodilator response to vagal stimulation was described, 6-hydroxydopamine was used to destroy the integrity of adrenergic terminals. To determine whether the vasodilator response to vagal stimulation could be demonstrated when adrenergic neuronal activity is inhibited with another neuronal blocking agent, the effects of reserpine were investigated. Reserpine also impairs adrenergic transmission by depleting nerve terminal stores of norepinephrine.[21,64] In animals pretreated with reserpine, vagal stimulation and intralobar acetylcholine injections caused significant decreases in lobar arterial pressure, and these responses were greatly enhanced when lobar vascular resistance was increased to a high steady-state level with U-46619. When lobar vascular resistance was increased by the thromboxane analog, U-46619, decreases in lobar arterial pressure in response to vagal stimulation and acetylcholine became frequency- and dose-dependent. However, in reserpine-pretreated animals, decreases in lobar arterial pressure in response to vagal stimulation were significantly smaller than in

6-hydroxydopamine-treated animals when lobar vascular resistance was increased to comparable levels during infusion of U-46619. The explanation for the difference in magnitude of response to vagal stimulation in 6-hydroxydopamine and reserpine-pretreated animals is uncertain. However, responses to acetylcholine were similar in both groups of animals, suggesting that the difference may be related to the extent of adrenergic neuronal blockage achieved with the two agents in these experiments.

Results of the present study demonstrate that efferent vagal stimulation can elicit both vasoconstrictor and vasodilator responses in the feline pulmonary vascular bed. Moreover, when the integrity of the adrenergic nerves to the lung was destroyed and vasoconstrictor tone was elevated, vagal stimulation caused marked frequency-dependent decreases in pulmonary vascular resistance. Injections of acetylcholine also dilated the pulmonary vascular bed, and responses to vagal stimulation and acetylcholine were blocked by atropine and enhanced by physostigmine. Vasodilator responses to vagal stimulation were not dependent on changes in bronchomotor tone and lung volume, or changes in aortic pressure and bronchopulmonary shunt flow. The present studies indicate that stimulation of cholinergic fibers in the vagus releases acetylcholine which acts on muscarinic receptors to dilate the pulmonary vascular bed. Studies with hexamethonium, a ganglionic blocking agent, suggest that the feline pulmonary vascular bed is well supplied with functional cholinergic terminals whose preganglionic fibers travel in the cervical vagus. The ability of acetylcholine to dilate pulmonary vessels may be dependent on the integrity of the endothelial cell layer and changes in the concentration of intracellular cGMP.[65]

The observations in this study indicate clearly that acetylcholine-elicited relaxation of phenylephrine-precontracted rings of bovine intrapulmonary artery possessing an unrubbed intimal surface is accompanied by increases in arterial cGMP but not cAMP levels. Acetylcholine produced a time- and concentration-dependent accumulation of arterial cGMP which correlated well with relaxation. Moreover, the findings that both atropine and methylene blue inhibited not only relaxation but also arterial cGMP accumulation are consistent with the close association of elevated cGMP levels and intrapulmonary arterial relaxation.

The inhibition by atropine of the increase in cGMP levels in response to acetylcholine provides evidence in support of a link between muscarinic receptors and cGMP accumulation. We have previously demonstrated that methylene blue inhibits (1) the activity of soluble guanylate cyclase prepared from vascular smooth muscle,[66-68] (2) vascular cGMP accumulation elicited by nitrogen oxide–containing vasodilators,[31,69] and (3) vascular smooth muscle relaxation caused by the above vasodilators.[31,66,67,70] Similarly, in the present study the inhibitory effect of methylene blue on acetylcholine-stimulated cGMP accumulation is likely the result of the inhibition of guanylate cyclase activity. These observations point to a muscarinic receptor-mediated increase in arterial cGMP formation by acetylcholine.

Acetylcholine elevates cGMP levels in a variety of tissues, including smooth muscle, in a calcium-dependent manner.[65,71,72] The inability of many investigators to demonstrate significant activation of soluble or particulate guanylate cyclase by acetylcholine and related agents indicates that the stimulation of tissue cGMP formation occurs by an indirect mechanism. Elevated intracellular concentrations of calcium probably do not directly stimulate cGMP formation because micromolar concentrations of calcium markedly inhibit soluble guanylate cyclase activity.[70] Furchgott et al[29] have forwarded the hypothesis that acetylcholine-mediated arterial relaxation is caused indirectly by the formation of a lipoxygenase metabolite or arachidonic acid in endothelial cells, which interacts with the adjacent smooth muscle to cause relaxation. The latter view was based on the observations that atropine, quinacrine (a phospholipase A_2 inhibitor) and ETYA (an inhibitor of both cyclo-oxygenase and lipoxygenase) antagonized the relaxant effect of acetylcholine, whereas indomethacin (a cyclo-oxygenase inhibitor) did not.

Several observations, however, appear to be inconsistent with a mediator effect of an endothelium-derived lipoxygenase metabolite of arachidonic acid on intrapulmonary arterial cGMP accumulation caused by acetylcholine. At concentrations that antagonized relaxation by acetylcholine, quinacrine failed to inhibit arterial cGMP accumulation. In addition, endothelium-damaged intrapulmonary arterial rings that contracted to acetylcholine also displayed a marked accumulation of cGMP and the latter response was unaltered by quinacrine, whereas contraction was partially inhibited. Quinacrine is a nonspecific agent and possesses multiple actions. For example, quinacrine has been reported to inhibit guanylate cyclase activity and interfere with certain direct effects of added cGMP on specific cellular functions.[73] Moreover, a recent study showed that quinacrine was less effective than indomethacin or meclofenamate sodium in inhibiting phospholipase A_2 activity in rat aorta.[54] Nonspecific effects were evident also in the present study. Concentrations of quinacrine (20 to 50 μmol/L) just in excess of those (5 to 10 μmol/L) which inhibited relaxation by acetylcholine also markedly inhibited arterial contractions to phenylephrine and KCl. Even low concentrations (2 to 10 μmol/L) of quinacrine inhibited arterial contraction elicited by acetylcholine. The observations that atropine and methylene blue nearly abolished relaxation and cGMP accumulation whereas quinacrine partially inhibited only relaxation in response to acetylcholine suggests that the latter is a nonspecific effect of quinacrine.

Definitive conclusions cannot be drawn until selective inhibitors of lipoxygenase and phospholipase A_2 become available for study. In addition, a lipoxygenase metabolite must be identified and demonstrated to stimulate cGMP accumulation and cause relaxation of endothelium-damaged vessels. It may not be as important to show that such a metabolite directly activates guanylate cyclase because this activation, if it occurs, may be an indirect effect. In view of our findings that concentrations of quinacrine which inhibited acetylcholine-elicited relaxation failed to influence cGMP accumulation, it is conceivable also that an endothelium-derived factor other than an arachidonic acid metabolite could be responsible for the stimulation of arterial cGMP accumulation in bovine intrapulmonary artery. Moreover, an endothelium-derived factor is not obligatory for acetylcholine-mediated increases in cGMP formation because acetylcholine markedly increased cGMP levels in endothelium-damaged arteries which contracted in response to acetylcholine.

The observations that both arterial cGMP accumulation and relaxation elicited by acetylcholine were antagonized by atropine are consistent with the possibility that cGMP mediates muscarinic receptor-linked relaxation of intrapulmonary arterial smooth muscle. Additional evidence for this view derives from the findings that methylene blue, an inhibitor of vascular soluble guanylate cyclase,[66-68] inhibited both cGMP accumulation and relaxation caused by acetylcholine. More definitive conclusions regarding a "mediator" role of cGMP in acetylcholine-elicited vascular smooth muscle relaxation, however, awaits further experimentation.

Acetylcholine is well known to contract certain endothelium-damaged arterial segments. Earlier reports indicated that vascular cGMP accumulation accompanied arterial contraction caused by acetylcholine.[62,72,74,75] Similarly, in the present study acetylcholine contracted endothelium-damaged rings of intrapulmonary artery and stimulated the arterial accumulation of cGMP. Atropine nearly abolished both responses suggesting that muscarinic receptors in vascular smooth muscle are linked to cGMP formation. On the other hand, methylene blue abolished the increase in cGMP levels but potentiated the contractions elicited by acetylcholine. The latter observations are similar to those recently reported by Kukovetz et al.[65,76] These findings indicate clearly that methylene blue is not a muscarinic receptor antagonist because this agent enhanced contractions to acetylcholine while abolishing cGMP accumulation. Methylene blue also enhanced contractile responses to phenylephrine. Moreover, methylene blue significantly lowered resting arterial levels of cGMP. These observations suggest that maintaining low arterial concentrations of intracellular cGMP, a known vascular smooth muscle relaxant,[77,78] could result in enhanced contractile responses.

The findings that acetylcholine increases cGMP levels in both endothelium-intact and endothelium-damaged intrapulmonary artery, whereas the former undergoes relaxation and the latter undergoes contraction, could be taken as evidence to dissociate arterial relaxation from cGMP accumulation. However, several explanations of these seemingly divergent observations are possible. In the absence of a functioning endothelium, muscarinic receptor activation may elicit a more pronounced increase in calcium ion concentration in vascular smooth muscle, resulting in a contractile response which overrides any potential relaxant response attributable to the concomitant accumulation of cGMP. In addition, although acetylcholine-mediated increases in tissue cGMP levels are a calcium-independent process,[65,71,72] this calcium effect is most likely indirect because elevated concentrations of calcium directly inhibit guanylate cyclase activity.[70]

In the presence of an intact endothelium, the mechanism by which acetylcholine causes relaxation instead of contraction may be attributed to the generation of an unknown endothelium-derived relaxing factor which stimulates cGMP formation without appreciably elevating intracellular calcium ion concentrations. Indeed, it is more reasonable to suspect that calcium concentrations would be lowered. In this regard, it is noteworthy that nitrogen oxide–containing vasodilators stimulate cGMP formation by a calcium-independent mechanism,[79,80] and these vasodilators as well as cGMP appear to relax vascular smooth muscle in a calcium-independent manner.[81] In a recent report, Lincoln[81] showed that reducing the concentration of calcium in vascular smooth muscle results in the enhancement of relaxation by sodium nitroprusside and 8-bromo-cGMP. Alternative explanations are not ruled out, including the possibility that the apparently close association between acetylcholine-elicited cGMP accumulation and relaxation is merely fortuitous. Clearly, additional experiments are essential to directly establish that cGMP mediates relaxation. Attention should now be focused, perhaps, on biochemical events linking cGMP to relaxation, assuming that such a link exists.

In summary, responses to vagal stimulation, acetylcholine, catecholamines, and sympathetic nerve stimulation were investigated in the feline pulmonary vascular bed under conditions of controlled pulmonary blood flow and constant left atrial pressure. Under base-line conditions, electrical stimulation of vagal efferent fibers, sympathetic nerve stimulation, and norepinephrine increased lobar arterial pressure in a frequency- and dose-related fashion, whereas acetylcholine produced modest decreases in lobar arterial pressure. When pulmonary tone was enhanced, vagal stimulation produced a depressor response. The pressor response to vagal stimulation under base-line conditions and the depressor response under enhanced tone conditions were blocked by phenoxybenzamine and atropine. When pulmonary vascular tone is enhanced and α-receptors blocked, norepinephrine and sympathetic nerve stimulation caused dose- and frequency-dependent decreases in pulmonary vascular resistance. The decreases in pulmonary vascular resistance in response to norepinephrine and sympathetic nerve stimulation were not altered by atropine but were blocked with propranolol. Under conditions of enhanced tone, selective β_1-receptor antagonists had little effect on vasodilator responses to isoproterenol, whereas responses to this substance were blocked by propranolol. These data suggest that, in the cat, the vagus is composed of efferent fibers from both the sympathetic and parasympathetic systems. Furthermore, these results suggest the presence of α- and β_2-adrenoreceptors in the feline pulmonary vascular bed and that both types of adrenergic receptors are innervated by the sympathetic nervous system.[82] Selective α_1- and α_2-receptor agonists produced dose-related increases in lobar arterial pressure under base-line conditions suggesting the presence of both α_1- and α_2-receptor subtypes, which when activated, may produce a vasoconstrictor response in the pulmonary vascular bed.

After chemical sympathectomy with 6-hydroxydopamine, vagal stimulation and acetylcholine caused frequency- and dose-related decreases in lobar arterial pressure when pulmonary vascular resistance was actively enhanced. Depressor responses to vagal stimulation and acetylcholine in 6-hydroxydopamine-treated animals were blocked by atropine and enhanced by physostigmine. Decreases in lobar arterial pressure in response to vagal stimulation in 6-hydroxydopamine-treated animals with enhanced tone were blocked by hexamethonium, whereas responses to injected acetylcholine were not altered by the ganglionic blocking agent. Decreases in lobar arterial pressure in response to vagal stimulation and acetylcholine were similar when the lung was ventilated and when the left lower lobe bronchus was obstructed. The present data also suggest that the feline pulmonary vascular bed is functionally innervated by cholinergic nerves and that vagal stimulation has the potential to dilate the pulmonary vascular bed when vasomotor tone is enhanced.

The present study also provides some evidence that muscarinic receptor stimulation is linked to both arterial cGMP accumulation and relaxation. In contrast, vascular smooth muscle contraction is readily dissociated from acetylcholine-stimulated cGMP accumulation. Consistent with the observations of others, muscarinic receptor-mediated relaxation of arterial smooth muscle is dependent on the presence of a functioning endothelium.[25-27,29] Moreover, the good correlation between cGMP accumulation and relaxation elicited by either acetylcholine or nitrogen oxide–containing vasodilators is consistent with the hypothesis that cGMP mediates vascular smooth muscle relaxation.[30,31,66,69,76,80] Muscarinic receptor–mediated stimulation of cGMP formation and relaxation of bovine intrapulmonary artery appear to be dependent on an endothelium-derived factor, as originally proposed for other arterial beds by Furchgott and coworkers.[25,29] However, the nature of this endothelium-derived factor remains unknown. Resolution of this problem necessitates the isolation and unequivocal identification of this factor.

196

SUMMARY

Responses to sympathetic nerve stimulation, catecholamines, vagal stimulation, and acetylcholine were analyzed in the feline pulmonary vascular bed under conditions of controlled pulmonary blood flow and constant left atrial pressure. Results of these studies indicate that, in the cat, α- and β_2-adrenoreceptors appear to be present in the feline pulmonary vascular bed and both types of adrenergic receptors are innervated by the sympathetic nervous system. Selective α_1- and α_2-receptor agonists produce pulmonary vasoconstrictor responses suggesting the presence of both α_1- and α_2-receptor subtypes in the feline pulmonary vascular bed. The vagus is composed of efferent fibers from both the sympathetic and parasympathetic systems. The present data also suggest that the feline pulmonary vascular bed is functionally innervated by cholinergic nerves and that vagal stimulation dilates the pulmonary vascular bed by releasing acetylcholine which acts on muscarinic receptors in pulmonary vessels. Moreover, the present data suggest that the effects of acetylcholine in the pulmonary vascular bed may be endothelial-dependent in nature. Relaxation of bovine intrapulmonary artery with an intact endothelium by acetylcholine is closely associated with the accumulation of cGMP. Although nitrogen oxide–containing vasodilators, including nitroglycerin, have similar actions in intrapulmonary artery with a damaged endothelium, there appears to be a clear dissociation between contraction and cGMP accumulation elicited by acetylcholine.

ACKNOWLEDGMENTS

Ms Janice Ignarro provided editorial assistance. Our research was supported in part by NIH grants HL11802, HL15580, HL29456, HL18070, AM17692, and HL27713.

REFERENCES

1. Fillenz M: Innervation of pulmonary and bronchial blood vessels of the dog. *J Anat* 1970;196:449–461.
2. Hebb C: Motor innervation of the pulmonary blood vessels of mammals, in *Pulmonary Circulation and Interstitial Space*. Chicago, University of Chicago Press, 1959, pp 195–222.
3. Kadowitz PJ, Knight DS, Hibbs RG, et al: Influence of 5- and 6-hydroxy-dopamine on adrenergic transmission and nerve terminal morphology in the canine pulmonary vascular bed. *Circ Res* 1976;39:191–199.
4. Knight DS, Ellison PJ, Hibbs GR, et al: A light and electron microscopic study of the innervation of pulmonary arteries in the cat. *Anat Rec* 1981;201:513–521.
5. Verity MA, Bevan JA: Fine structural study of the terminal factor plexus; neuromuscular relationships in the pulmonary artery. *J Anat* 1968;103:49–63.
6. Daly ID, Ramsay DJ, Waaler BA: The site of action of nerves in the pulmonary vascular bed in the dog. *J Physiol* 1970;209:317–339.

7. Ingram RH, Szidon JP, Skalak R, et al: Effects of sympathetic nerve stimulation on the pulmonary arterial tree of the isolated lobe perfused *in situ*. *Circ Res* 1968;22:801–815.

8. Kadowitz PJ, Joiner PD, Hyman AL: Influence of sympathetic stimulation and vasoactive substances on the canine pulmonary veins. *J Clin Invest* 1975;56:354–365.

9. Kadowitz PJ, Hyman AL: Effect of sympathetic nerve stimulation on pulmonary vascular resistance in the dog. *Circ Res* 1973;32;221–227.

10. Kadowitz PJ, Joiner PD, Hyman AL: Differential effects of phentolamine and bretylium on pulmonary vascular responses to norepinephrine and nerve stimulation. *Proc Soc Exp Biol Med* 1973;144:172–176.

11. Doeherty JR, McGrath JC: An examination of factors influencing adrenergic transmission in the pithed rat, with special reference to noradrenaline uptake mechanisms and postjunctional α-adrenoceptors. *Naunyn Schmiedebergs Arch Pharmacol* 1980;313:101–111.

12. Langer SZ, Massingham R, Shepperson NB: Presence of postsynaptic α_2-adrenoceptors of predominantly extrasynaptic location in the vascular smooth muscle of the dog hindlimb. *Clin Sci* 1980;59:225s–228s.

13. Timmermans PBMWM, Van Zwieten PA: Vasoconstriction mediated via postsynaptic α_2-adrenoceptor stimulation. *Naunyn Schmiedebergs Arch Pharmacol* 1980;313:17–20.

14. Hyman AL: The direct effects of vasoactive agents on pulmonary veins. Studies of responses to acetylcholine, serotonin, histamine and isoproterenol in intact dogs. *J Pharmacol Exp Ther* 1969;168:96–105.

15. Porcelli RJ, Bergofsky E: Adrenergic receptors in pulmonary vasoconstrictor responses to gaseous and humoral agents. *J Appl Physiol* 1973;34:483–488.

16. Silvone ED, Inoue T, Grover RF: Comparison of hypoxia, pH and sympathomimetic drugs on bovine pulmonary vasculature. *J Appl Physiol* 1968;24:355–365.

17. Greenway CV, Lawson AE, Stark RD: Vascular responses of the spleen to nerve stimulation during normal and reduced blood flow. *J Physiol* 1968; 194:421–433.

18. Greenway CV, Lawson AE: β-Adrenergic receptors in the hepatic arterial bed of the anesthetized cat. *Can J Physiol Pharmacol* 1969;47:415–419.

19. Ngai SH, Rosell S, Wallenberg LR: Nervous regulation of blood flow in the subcutaneous adipose tissue in dogs. *Acta Physiol Scand* 1966;68:397–403.

20. Pegram BL, Bevan RD, Bevan JA: Facial vein of the rabbit: neurogenic vasodilation mediated by β-adrenergic receptors. *Circ Res* 1976;39:854–860.

21. Viveros OH, Arqueros L, Connet RJ, et al: Mechanism of secretion from the adrenal medulla. IV. The fat of the storage vesicles following insulin and reserpine administration. *Mol Pharmacol* 1969;5:69–82.

22. Hawthorn MH, Broadley KJ: Evidence from use of neuronal uptake inhibition that β_1 adrenoceptors, but not β_2 adrenoceptors, are innervated. *J Pharm Pharmacol* 1982;34:664–666.

23. Russell MP, Moran NC: Evidence for lack of innervation of β-2 adrenoreceptors in the blood vessels of the gracilis muscle of the dog. *Circ Res* 1980; 46:344–352.

24. Daly ID, Hebb CO: Pulmonary vasomotor fibers in the cervical vagosympathetic nerve of the dog. *Q J Exp Physiol* 1952;37:19–43.

25. Furchgott RJ, Zawadzki JV: The obligatory role of endothelial cells in the relaxation of arterial smooth muscle by acetylcholine. *Nature* 1980; 288:373–376.

26. Chand N, Altura BM: Acetylcholine and bradykinin relax intrapulmonary arteries by acting on endothelial cells: role in lung vascular diseases. *Science* 1981;213:1376–1379.

27. De Mey JG, Claeys M, Vanhoutte PM: Endothelium-dependent inhibitory effects of acetylcholine, adenosine triphosphate, thrombin and arachidonic acid in the canine femoral artery. *J Pharmacol Exp Ther* 1982;222:166–173.

28. Regoli D, Mizrahi J, D'Orleans-Juste P, et al: Effects of kinins on isolated blood vessels. Role of endothelium. *Can J Physiol Pharmacol* 1982;60:1580–1583.

29. Furchgott RF, Zawadzki JV, Cherry PD: Role of endothelium in the vasodilator responses to acetylcholine, in *Vasodilatation*. New York, Raven Press, 1981, pp 49–66.

30. Ignarro LJ, Gruetter CA, Hyman AL, et al: Molecular mechanisms of vasodilatation, in *Dopamine Receptor Agonists*. New York, Plenum Press, 1983, pp 259–288.

31. Ignarro LJ, Lippton H, Edwards JC, et al: Mechanism of vascular smooth muscle relaxation by organic nitrates, nitrites, nitroprusside and nitric oxide: evidence for the involvement of S-nitrosothiols as active intermediates. *J Pharmacol Exp Ther* 1981;218:739–749.

32. Lock JE, Hamilton F, Luide H, et al: Direct pulmonary vascular responses in the conscious newborn lamb. *Am J Physiol* 1980;48:188–196.

33. Dawes GS, Mott JC: The vascular tone of the foetal lung. *J Physiol* 1962;146:465–477.

34. Rudolph AM, Scarpelli EM: Drug action on pulmonary circulation of unanesthetized dogs. *Am J Physiol* 1964;206:1201–1206.

35. Hyman AL, Kadowitz PJ: Pulmonary vasodilator activity of prostacyclin (PGI$_2$) in the cat. *Circ Res* 1979;45:404–409.

36. Hyman AL, Nandiwada P, Knight DS, et al: Pulmonary vasodilator responses to catecholamines and sympathetic nerve stimulation in the cat: evidence that vascular beta-2 adrenoreceptors are innervated. *Circ Res* 1981;48:407–415.

37. Glick G, Epstein SE, Wechsler AS, et al: Physiological differences between the effects of neuronally released and blood borne norepinephrine on beta adrenergic receptors in the arterial bed of the dog. *Circ Res* 1967;21:217–227.

38. Kostrzewa RM, Jacobowitz DM: Pharmacological actions of 6-hydroxydopamine. *Pharmacol Rev* 1974;18:619–629.

39. Daly ID, Hebb CO: *Pulmonary and Bronchial Vascular Systems*. London, Edward Arnold Ltd, 1966.

40. Lundvall J, Jarhult J: Beta adrenergic micro-vascular dilation evoked by sympathetic stimulation. *Acta Physiol Scand* 1974;92:572–574.

41. Lundvall J, Jarhult J: Beta adrenergic dilator component of the sympathetic vascular response in skeletal muscle. Influence on the micro-circulation and on transcapillary exchange. *Acta Physiol Scand* 1976;96:180–192.

42. Dawes PM, Faulkner DC: The effect of propranolol on vascular responses to sympathetic nerve stimulation. *Br J Pharmacol* 1975;53:517–524.

43. Rosell S, Belfrage E: Adrenergic receptors in adipose tissue and their relation to adrenergic innervation. *Nature* 1975;253:738–739.

44. Lands EM, Arnold A, McAuliff JP, et al: Differentiation of receptor systems activated by sympathomimetic amines. *Nature* 1967;214:597–598.

45. Fishman W: Clinical pharmacology of the new beta-adrenergic blocking drugs. I. Pharmacodynamics and pharmacokinetic properties. *Am Heart J* 1979;97:663–670.

46. Lertora JJL, Mark AL, Johannsen UJ, et al: Selective beta-1 receptor blockade with oral practolol in man. *J Clin Invest* 1975;56:719-725.

47. Bevan JA: Some bases of differences in vascular responses to sympathetic activity. *Circ Res* 1979;45:161-171.

48. Hauge A, Lunde PKM, Waaler BA: Effect of prostaglandin E₁ and adrenaline on the pulmonary vascular resistance (PVR) in isolated rabbit lungs. *Life Sci* 1967;6:673-680.

49. Eckstein JW, Abboud FM: Circulatory effects of sympathomimetic animals. *Am Heart J* 1962;63:119-135.

50. Trendelenburg U, Muskus A, Fleming WW, et al: Modification by reserpine of the action of sympathomimetic amines. *J Pharmacol Exp Ther* 1962; 138:170-180.

51. Tainter ML, Chang DK: The antagonism of the pressor action of tyramine by cocaine. *J Pharmacol Exp Ther* 1927;30:193-207.

52. Adler-Graschinsky E, Langer SZ: Possible role of a β-adrenoreceptor in the regulation of noradrenaline release by nerve stimulation through a positive feedback mechanism. *Br J Pharmacol* 1975;53:43-50.

53. Yamaguchi N, DeChamplain J, Nadeau RA: Regulation of norepinephrine release from cardiac sympathetic fibers in the dog by presynaptic α- and β-receptors. *Circ Res* 1977;41:108-117.

54. Thakkar JK, Sperelakis N, Pang D, et al: Characterization of phospholipase A₂ activity in rat aorta smooth muscle cells. *Biochim Biophys Acta* 1983; 750:134-140.

55. Shibata S, Kuchii M, Kurahashi K: The supersensitivity of isolated rabbit atria and aortic strips produced by 6-hydroxydopamine. *Eur J Pharmacol* 1972;18:271-280.

56. Tucker A: Pulmonary and systemic vascular responses to vasoactive agents after chemical sympathectomy. *Proc Soc Exp Biol Med* 1980;163:534-539.

57. Coleman RA, Humphrey PPA, Kennedy I, et al: Comparison of the actions of U-46619, a prostaglandin H₂ analog, with those of prostaglandin H₂ and thromboxane A₂ on some isolated smooth muscle preparations. *Br J Pharmacol* 1981;73:773-778.

58. Hyman AL, Knight DS, Joiner PD, et al: Bronchopulmonary arterial shunting without anatomic anastomosis in the dog. *Circ Res* 1975;37:285-298.

59. Daly ID, Hebb CO: Bronchomotor and pulmonary arterial pressure responses to nerve stimulation. *Q J Exp Physiol* 1942;31:211-226.

60. Kadowitz PJ, Nandiwada P, Gruetter CA, et al: Pulmonary vasodilator responses to nitroprusside and nitroglycerin in the dog. *J Clin Invest* 1981;67:893-902.

61. Casey LC, Fletcher JR, Zmudka MI, et al: Prevention of endotoxin-induced pulmonary hypertension in primates by the use of a selective thromboxane synthetase inhibitor, OKY-1581. *J Pharmacol Exp Ther* 1982;222:441-446.

62. Demling R, Gee M, Flynn J: Changes in lung vascular permeability and lung lymph prostaglandins after endotoxin in sheep. *Am Rev Respir Dis* 1980; 121:429-436.

63. Utsunomiya T, Krauz MM, Levine L, et al: Thromboxane mediation of cardiopulmonary effects of embolism. *J Clin Invest* 1982;70:361-368.

64. Iggo A, Vogt M: Preganglionic sympathetic activity in normal and in reserpine-treated cats. *Br J Pharmacol* 1960;150:114-133.

65. Kukovetz WR, Scholz N, Paietta E: Influence of extracellular Ca^{2+} on acetylcholine-induced changes in cyclic nucleotides and tone of smooth muscle. *Naunyn Schmiedebergs Arch Pharmacol* 1976;294(R):13.
66. Gruetter CA, Barry BK, McNamara DB, et al: Relaxation of bovine coronary artery and activation of coronary arterial guanylate cyclase by nitric oxide, nitroprusside and a carcinogenic nitrosoamine. *J Cyclic Nucleotide Res* 1979;5:211-224.
67. Gruetter CA, Barry BK, McNamara DB, et al: Coronary arterial relaxation and guanylate cyclase activation by cigarette smoke, N'-nitrosonornicotine and nitric oxide. *J Pharmacol Exp Ther* 1980;214:9-15.
68. Gruetter CA, Kadowitz PJ, Ignarro LJ: Methylene blue inhibits coronary arterial relaxation and guanylate cyclase activation by nitroglycerin, sodium nitrite and amyl nitrite. *Can J Physiol Pharmacol* 1981;59:150-156.
69. Gruetter CA, Gruetter DY, Lyon JE, et al: Relationship between cyclic GMP formation and relaxation of coronary arterial smooth muscle by glyceryl trinitate, nitroprusside, nitrite and nitric oxide: effects of methylene blue and methemoglobin. *J Pharmacol Exp Ther* 1981;209:181-186.
70. Gruetter DY, Gruetter CA, Barry BK, et al: Activation of coronary arterial guanylate cyclase by nitric oxide, nitroprusside and nitrosoguanidine inhibition by calcium, lanthanum and other cations, enhancement by thiols. *Biochem Pharmacol* 1980;29:2943-2950.
71. Goldberg ND, Haddox MK: Cyclic GMP metabolism and involvement in biological regulation. *Annu Rev Biochem* 1977;46:823-896.
72. Schultz G, Hardman JG, Schultz K, et al: The importance of calcium ions for the regulation of guanosine 3',5'-cyclic monophosphate levels. *Proc Natl Acad Sci USA* 1973;70:3889-3893.
73. Greenberg RN, Guerrant RL, Chang B, et al: Inhibition of *Escherichia coli* heat-stable enterotoxin effects on intestinal guanylate cyclase and fluid secretion by quinacrine. *Biochem Pharmacol* 1982;31:2005-2009.
74. Andersson R, Nilsson K, Wikberg J, et al: Cyclic nucleotides and the contraction of smooth muscle. *Adv Cyclic Nucleotide Res* 1975;5:491-518.
75. Clyman RI, Snadler JA, Manganiello VC, et al: Guanosine 3',5'-monophosphate and adenosine 3',5'-monophosphate content of human umbilical artery. *J Clin Invest* 1975;55:1020-1025.
76. Kukovetz WR, Holzmann S, Wurm A, et al: Evidence for cyclic GMP-mediated relaxant effects of nitro-compounds in coronary smooth muscle. *Naunyn Schmiedebergs Arch Pharmacol* 1979;310:129-138.
77. Napoli SA, Gruetter CA, Ignarro LJ, et al: Relaxation of bovine coronary arterial smooth muscle by cyclic GMP, cyclic AMP and analogs. *J Pharmacol Exp Ther* 1980;212:469-473.
78. Schultz KD, Bohme E, Kreye VAW, et al: Relaxation of hormonally stimulated smooth muscular tissues by the 8-bromo derivative of cyclic GMP. *Naunyn Schmiedebergs Arch Pharmacol* 1979;306:1-9.
79. Katsuki S, Murad F: Regulation of adenosine cyclic 3',5'-monophosphate and guanosine cyclic 3',5'-monophosphate levels and contractility in bovine tracheal smooth muscle. *Mol Pharmacol* 1977;13:330-341.
80. Schultz KD, Schultz K, Schultz G: Sodium nitroprusside and other smooth muscle relaxants increase cyclic GMP levels in rat ductus deferens. *Nature* 1977;265:750-751.
81. Lincoln TM: Effects of nitroprusside and 8-bromo-cyclic GMP on the contractile activity of the rat aorta. *J Pharmacol Exp Ther* 1983;224:100-107.
82. Nandiwada PA, Hyman AL, Kadowitz PJ: Pulmonary vasodilator responses to vagal stimulation and acetylcholine in the cat. *Circ Res* 1983;53:86-95.

15 Eicosanoids and Pulmonary Hypertension

Myron B. Peterson
W. David Watkins

Vasoactive derivatives of arachidonic acid, commonly known as eicosanoids, have been intensively studied in different animal models of acute lung injury and pulmonary hypertension for almost a decade. It is clear that this family of compounds can be involved in different types of lung pathology and that their synthesis can be induced by diverse stimuli such as endotoxin, hypoxia, and oleic acid.[1-3] Specifically, we have been able to establish a causative role for thromboxane, a powerful vasoconstrictor eicosanoid, in the genesis of pulmonary hypertension utilizing different animal model systems of lung injury.[4,5] This was accomplished by direct end-product analysis (thromboxane B_2) in plasma, the use of cyclooxygenase inhibitors (eg, ibuprofen), and specific thromboxane synthetase inhibitors (imidazole or imidazole-like compounds). We demonstrated that endogenous thromboxane production correlated to rises in pulmonary vascular resistance and that the lung was the site of production of this compound. Although no specific intrapulmonary cell type was identified as the source of production we felt this to be an important observation. Prior to this time platelets were considered to be the major source of endogenous thromboxane synthesis. These experiments also strengthened the concept that eicosanoids act as local "hormones" near their sites of synthesis and also indicate that cell-to-cell interactions may play a major role in metabolic regulation of the arachidonic acid cascade. Further, these investigations also showed that synthesis of the pulmonary vasodilator prostacyclin was altered. However, increased prostacyclin synthesis, or at least the appearance of the stable metabolite 6-keto-$PGF_{1\alpha}$, in both lymph from the lung or plasma, was not coincident with rises in thromboxane metabolite and occurred at a later time. Thus, the arachidonic acid cascade appears to be specifically controlled and generalized increases in end products do not occur, at least in the model systems we have studied.

In general, it seems that thromboxane causes or is associated with acute pulmonary vasoconstriction and prostacyclin is synthesized either in response to pulmonary vasoconstriction or thromboxane synthesis and correlates to decreases in pulmonary vascular resistance. The basic mechanisms of this relationship are unknown at present but this concept is consistent with the known vasoactive properties of each compound, ie, vasoconstrictor and vasodilator, respectively. Although we know that specific cells have a propensity to synthesize certain of the eicosanoids, eg, endothelial cells synthesize primarily prostacyclin, the metabolic capacity often is present for production of all the arachidonic acid metabolites. Thus, sophisticated inhibitor mechanisms probably exist for the control of these synthetic pathways that may be (1) negative or positive feedback loops, or (2) substrate-limited steps. Studies addressing these problems are just now being instituted and will probably be quite valuable in actually defining the role these compounds play in the control of pulmonary vascular physiology.

We believe thromboxane and prostacyclin to be important local effectors in the pathogenesis of acute lung injury, including pulmonary hypertension. Other products of arachidonic acid probably are involved as well and can be metabolized through either the cyclo-oxygenase or lipoxygenase enzyme systems. However, these relationships are not as well defined as those of thomboxane and prostacyclin.

Because of the positive correlations obtained in animal models we became interested in examining the role of eicosanoids in pulmonary hypertension in man. We believe this to be an important line of inquiry from both mechanistic and therapeutic points of view, since the approach to treatment of pulmonary hypertension would naturally be simplified if more were understood of the underlying molecular mechanisms. Specifically, we wondered if the eicosanoids are causally involved, and if so, which ones are primary effectors.

The production of prostacyclin and thromboxane is enzymatically catalyzed as shown in Figure 15-1. This is important because one can modify pulmonary vascular resistance or tone, in some instances, by inhibition of the cyclo-oxygenase enzyme. However, this causes a reduction in all end products, including thromboxane and prostacyclin. If one believes that thromboxane is involved in pulmonary vasoconstriction and prostacyclin in vasodilation and that other of the cyclo-oxygenase products are also vasoactive, it is not optimal to inhibit synthesis of all these metabolites. We believe specific inhibition of the enzyme thromboxane synthetase to be the most rational pharmacologic approach, particularly since the prototype drugs are safe and specific in their actions.

A second approach to the treatment of pulmonary hypertension is by direct pharmacologic intervention with vasodilator eicosanoids such

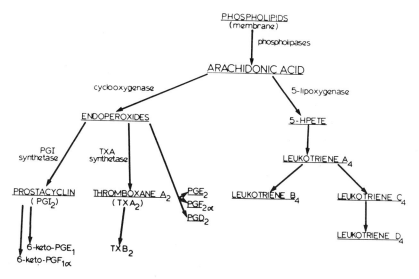

Figure 15-1 The arachidonic acid cascade.

as PGE_1 or prostacyclin. Both have already proved effective in certain types of pulmonary hypertension in man.

We have initiated a number of human studies involving pulmonary hypertension in both normal and sick patients in an attempt to define the role of thromboxane and prostacyclin in this pathology. Since many of our studies are conducted in the face of different unrelated invasive insults we initially made multiple serial determinations of circulating eicosanoids by standard radioimmunoassay in patients without respiratory distress syndrome to assess the effect of these procedures. We were particularly concerned that thromboxane could be easily perturbed by mechanical means. Figure 15-2 is an example of serial prospective analysis of thromboxane and prostacyclin in a patient following left upper lobectomy. Clearly, a variety of common intensive care unit (ICU) events such as chest physical therapy, atelectasis, and movement from supine to upright positions had no effect on either of these compounds. There also appeared to be no diurnal variation. We have found this to be true in over 15 prospectively studied ICU patients and assume that pertubations in these metabolites should be related to underlying pathology or physiology and not artifactual generation. But only if proper sample collection techniques are utilized. A second important point is demonstrated in Figure 15-3. This sequence shows that a specific response in eicosanoid metabolism — thromboxane synthesis — can occur in relation to a pathophysiologic event without pertubations in other products of arachidonic acid. This is important because of the ofttimes opposing biological actions inherent in

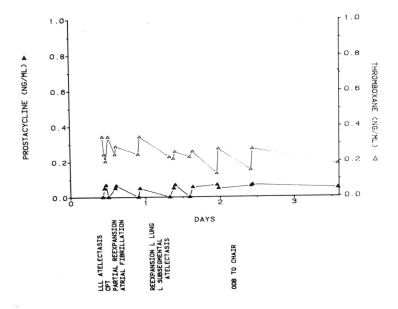

Figure 15-2 Arterial plasma thromboxane B_2 and 6-keto-PGF$_{1\alpha}$ during common intensive care unit events. CPT = chest physical therapy, OOB = out of bed.

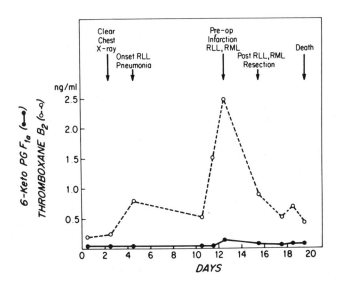

Figure 15-3 Arterial plasma thromboxane B_2 and 6-keto-PGF$_{1\alpha}$ during lobar infarction.

different eicosanoids. Further, synthetic sequencing of this nature strongly suggests that metabolic feedback loops control eicosanoid synthesis. Following these observations we initiated multiple studies in man which are patterned after our animal studies. Specifically, we focused on well-defined insults linked to prospective physiologic and biochemical determinations.

Mild pulmonary hypertension due to hypoxic breathing was studied in normal man in collaboration with Drs Hallemans, Naeije and associates at the Institute of Interdisciplinary Research in Brussels, Belgium, and Dr Michael Rie at Massachusetts General Hospital, Boston. Invasive procedures were done 40 minutes prior to base-line physiologic and biochemical measurements. After 15 minutes breathing 21% oxygen, measurements were repeated and 15 minutes of 12.5% oxygen breathing was conducted. Measurements were taken at the end of this period. Inhibitors, which included ibuprofen or dazoxibin, were administered orally or intravenously (IV) and the above sequences repeated. Table 15-1 shows that mild pulmonary hypertension and hypoxia developed, but no changes in circulating thromboxane or prostacyclin were found. The addition of ibuprofen had no effect on these physiologic parameters or the circulating eicosanoids. We then elected to study specific inhibitor pharmacology because it appeared that (1) tissue sites were not made accessible by ibuprofen and (2) stable circulating thromboxane does not necessarily rule out thromboxane as a mediator. We initially showed that the specific thromboxane synthetase inhibitor dazoxibin, in controls, had no effects on the parameters we were interested in, ie, no change in pulmonary

Table 15-1
Physiologic and Biochemical Determinations in Four Patients Breathing Room Air, 12.5% O_2 and 12.5% O_2 After Ibuprofen

	Control	Control	Ibuprofen
Fi_{O_2}	0.21	0.125	0.125
PAP (mmHg)	13	21	23
PCWP (mmHg)	9	9	7
CI (L/min/m²)	3.8	4.8	4.8
PaO_2 (mmHg)	95	41	38
$PaCO_2$ (mmHg)	40	39	38
6-keto-PGF$_{1\alpha}$ (pg/mL)	40	<40	49
TxB$_2$ (pg/mL)	145	180	118

Fi_{O_2} = fraction of inspired O_2, PAP = mean pulmonary artery pressure, PCWP = pulmonary capillary wedge pressure, CI = cardiac index, PaO_2 = arterial O_2 pressure, $PaCO_2$ = arterial CO_2 pressure, TxB$_2$ = thromboxane B_2.

vascular tone was elicited by the administration of dazoxibin. Further, we found no suppression of circulating thromboxane. We then administered dazoxibin to patients prior to hypoxic breathing. There was neither attenuation of pulmonary hypertension nor of thromboxane (Table 15-2) in these subjects.

Table 15-2
Physiologic and Biochemical Determinations in Five Patients Breathing Room Air, 12.5% O_2 and 12.5% O_2 After Dazoxibin

	Control	Control	Dazoxibin
FiO_2	0.21	0.125	0.125
PAP (mmHg)	14	22	21
PCWP (mmHg)	10	9	9
CI (L/min/m^2)	3.8	4.8	4.5
PaO_2 (mmHg)	94	43	38
$PaCO_2$ (mmHg)	39	38	38
6-keto-PGF$_{1\alpha}$ (pg/mL)	43	<40	45
TxB_2 (pg/mL)	122	181	132

For abbreviations, see footnote to Table 15-1.

We were not sure how to interpret these inhibitor data since we measured plasma ibuprofen concentrations that we know are more than adequate to inhibit cyclo-oxygenase, and dazoxibin, at the doses we utilized, has been shown to specifically inhibit thromboxane synthetase in man. Assay of serum following incubation of arterial blood at 37°C for five minutes proved that significant inhibition of both cyclo-oxygenase and thromboxane synthetase could be easily achieved (Table 15-3). However, this probably involves formed elements of the blood such as the platelet. If one takes into account circulating plasma concentrations in these same patients, it is clear that there are tissue sites that are not being accessed by either inhibitor. This is important to appreciate since it points to the need for end-product analysis as well as plasma determinations of inhibitors. Lack of inhibitor effect on metabolic pathways cannot be ascer-

Table 15-3
Serum and Plasma Thromboxane Concentrations of Nine Patients Before and After Administration of Ibuprofen or Dazoxibin

Serum (ng/mL)		Plasma (pg/mL)	
Control	Drug	Control	Drug
217	17	133	125

tained from a physiologic response alone. Because of this, we also administered inhibitors over a number of days in four subjects in an attempt to improve tissue penetration but our results were the same. Because others have studied prolonged or repetitive hypoxic breathing in animals and suggested that these modes of exposure may have different physiologic expression, we studied prolonged (60 minutes) hypoxic breathing as well as repetitive hypoxic breathing in four volunteers. The results were the same as in our initial group. Thus, we were unable to demonstrate that thromboxane was directly involved in the mild pulmonary hypertension of hypoxia but we could not rule it out. Finally, we wondered if PGE_1, a known pulmonary vasodilator, would reverse the pulmonary hypertension. We designed the experiment so that cyclo-oxygenase inhibition or thromboxane synthetase inhibition, to whatever extent possible, was used in an attempt to remove the influence of other eicosanoids and allow for unopposed vasodilation. In four patients PGE_1, infused at a peak rate of 30 ng/kg/min, was not effective in reducing pulmonary hypertension. This was unexpected since we know PGE_1 to be a very effective pulmonary vasodilator.

Further information concerning pulmonary hypertension was obtained from five patients undergoing mitral valve replacement in collaboration with Dr Mortimer Buckley and associates at Massachusetts General Hospital. Briefly, all these patients had severe preoperative pulmonary hypertension and none could be successfully taken off cardiopulmonary bypass either at the end of the operation or in the immediate perioperative period because of pulmonary hypertension and acute right heart failure. Multiple pharmacologic interventions were unsuccessful in decreasing pulmonary vascular resistance in these patients. Thus, PGE_1 infusions were begun. Within three to five minutes clear effects of PGE_1 were present including increased pulmonary blood flow noted by direct vision in three of the patients. Table 15-4 shows one-hour and 24-hour values obtained on PGE_1. All patients were successfully weaned from PGE_1 within 72 hours and eventually discharged. It should be noted that peak PGE_1 infusions ranged from 30 to 150 ng/kg/min which necessitated systemic blood pressure support via left atrial administration of norepinephrine. Previous investigators have reported similar results in patients with mitral valve pathology when PGE_1 challenge was electively studied. Thus, it appears that different mechanisms operate in hypoxia-induced pulmonary hypertension compared to those associated with mitral valve pathology.

Finally, we studied nine normal and seven diffuse interstitial fibrosis patients during exercise in collaboration with Drs C Risk, M Crigler and associates at Boston University Hospital. These patients' resting hypoxia worsens and they develop pulmonary vasoconstriction at very low levels of exercise. Initially, we studied thromboxane profiles in patients with indwelling arterial lines and were able to identify thromboxane elaboration during exercise in patients with diffuse interstitial fibrosis, but not in normals (Table 15-5). We assumed that hypoxic pulmonary vasoconstriction was present but no direct measurements were made.[6] We have just completed a similar study in which seven of these patients were hospitalized at which time complete hemodynamic monitoring was done during repeat studies. Then dazoxibin was given overnight and the studies were repeated. Preliminary results indicate that in three of seven patients exercise-induced pulmonary vasoconstriction was abolished with dazoxibin. Similar to our study of hypoxic pulmonary vasoconstriction in resting patients, basal plasma concentrations of thromboxane were not altered by dazoxibin. However, in this study it appears that no increases were present in response to exercise. This suggests that thromboxane plays a role in pulmonary hypertension in some of these patients.

Table 15-4
Physiologic Parameters in Five Patients Treated with PGE_1 Infusion Because of Severe Perioperative Pulmonary Hypertension

	Before Operation	After Operation	PGE_1 1 h	PGE_1 24 h
PAP, systolic (mmHg)	81	73	49	51
PAP, diastolic (mmHg)	44	55	26	26
PCWP (mmHg)	33	—	—	—
LAP (mmHg)	—	6	14	16
CI (L/min/m²)	1.6	0.7	2.4	2.4

LAP = left atrial pressure; see also footnote to Table 15-1.

Table 15-5
Physiologic and Biochemical Determinations in Nine Normal Seven Severe Diffuse Interstitial Pulmonary Fibrosis (DPF) Patients at Rest and During Exercise

	Normal	DPF
Rest		
PaO_2 (mmHg)	107	68
TxB_2 (pg/mL)	177	148
Peak aerobic exercise		
Time (min)	7.8	4.7
V_{O_2} (mL/kg/min)	20	9.3
PaO_2 (mmHg)	102	51
TxB_2 (pg/mL)	186	390

V_{O_2} = oxygen uptake; see also footnote to Table 15-1.

In summary, we believe that basic molecular mechanisms of pulmonary hypertension are quite different and are more complex[7] than we had initially anticipated. Thus, before rendering definitive rather than symptomatic treatment of these cardiopulmonary disorders, it is incumbent on us to better define the disease process. To do this we must better define the molecular basis of physiologic events that are monitored clinically. This involves a multifaceted approach to therapeutics. This includes careful prospective monitoring of physiologic end points, concomitant metabolic events, and the pharmacokinetics of drugs used to alter these events.

REFERENCES

1. Hyman AL, Mathe AA, Lippton HL, et al: Prostaglandins and the lung. *Med Clin North Am* 1981;65:789–808.
2. McKeen CR, Brigham KL, Bowers RE, et al: Pulmonary vascular effects of fat emulsion infusion in unanesthetized sheep. Prevention by indomethacin. *J Clin Invest* 1978;61:1291–1297.
3. Parrett JR, Sturgess RM: Evidence that prostaglandin release mediates pulmonary vasoconstriction induced by *E. coli* endotoxin. *J Physiol* 1975;246:79–80.
4. Peterson MB, Huttemeier PC, Zapol WM, et al: Thromboxane mediates acute pulmonary hypertension in sheep extracorporeal perfusion. *Am J Physiol* 1982;243:471–479.
5. Huttemeier PC, Watkins WD, Peterson MB, et al: Acute pulmonary hypertension and lung thromboxane release after endotoxin infusion in normal and leukopenic sheep. *Circ Res* 1982;50:688–694.
6. Risk C, Peterson MB, Woods B, et al: Thromboxane and prostacyclin (epoprostenol) during exercise in diffuse pulmonary fibrosis. *Lancet* 1982;3:1183–1185.
7. Das UN: Prostaglandins in pulmonary hypertension. *Int J Clin Pharmacol Res* 1982;2:171–176.

16 Regulation of Pulmonary Vascular Tone by Autonomic Mediators, Peptides, and Leukotrienes

Sami I. Said

Neurohumoral Control

A variety of neurogenic and humoral factors influence pulmonary vascular tone. These neurohumoral influences include the autonomic innervation of pulmonary vessels and a number of vasoactive compounds that are present or can be released in the vicinity of pulmonary vascular smooth muscle (Table 16-1). Among the humoral agents are peptides, some of which are primarily neuropeptides, ie, they are localized in neurons and released as neurotransmitters by nerve terminals. The influence of these neuropeptides can thus be considered both neurogenic and humoral.

Neurogenic (Autonomic) Control

Adrenergic and cholinergic innervation   The effects of α- and β-adrenergic and cholinergic innervation on pulmonary vessels have been extensively investigated. It is generally accepted that α-adrenergic agonists constrict, and β-agonists and acetylcholine relax pulmonary vascular smooth muscle.[1-3] Until recently the adrenergic and cholinergic systems were thought to constitute the entire autonomic influence on pulmonary vessels.

Investigators of airway, gastrointestinal (GI), and other smooth muscle, however, have long recognized the existence of a component of neurogenic relaxation that cannot be explained by either adrenergic or cholinergic transmission.[4,5] The existence of this nonadrenergic, noncholinergic component, considered the dominant relaxant influence in human airways, has not, to our knowledge, been previously explored in pulmonary vessels.

The nonadrenergic, noncholinergic system   In order to investigate the possible existence and relative importance of a nonadrenergic, noncholinergic relaxant (inhibitory) system in pulmonary vessels, we

Table 16-1
Neurohumoral Regulation of Pulmonary Vascular Tone

	Action
Neurogenic Influences	
Cholinergic	Relaxation
Adrenergic	
α-	Constriction
β-	Relaxation
Noncholinergic, nonadrenergic	Relaxation
Humoral Influences	
Biogenic amines	Mostly constriction (eg, histamine, serotonin)
Peptides	Constriction: substance P, "spasmogenic lung peptide"
	Relaxation-vasoactive intestinal peptide
Lipids	Mostly constriction: leukotrienes, $PGF_{2\alpha}$, PGD_2, thromboxanes
	Relaxation: prostacyclin

examined the responses of isolated strips of cat pulmonary artery to electrical field stimulation and analyzed the modification of these responses by specific pharmacologic blockers. The typical response (Figure 16-1) was an initial, brief contraction, followed by a more sustained relaxation. The relaxation was more evident if the resting tone had been raised by a vasoconstrictor, such as prostaglandin H_2 (PGH_2) analog U-44069. The pharmacologic blockers were added sequentially, and the field stimulation was repeated after each addition. Phenoxybenzamine hydrochloride, producing α-adrenergic blockade, abolished the contraction. Cholinergic muscarinic blockade with atropine, and β-adrenergic blockade with propranolol hydrochloride, each moderately (21% to 25%) reduced the relaxation. Only tetrodotoxin (a neurotoxin) or lidocaine (local anesthetic) abolished or greatly attenuated the relaxation. The findings show that pulmonary arterial relaxation in cats (and probably also in other mammalian species) is mediated in large measure by a system that is neither adrenergic nor cholinergic.[6]

Of the possible transmitters of nonadrenergic, noncholinergic relaxation of pulmonary vessels, the neuropeptide vasoactive intestinal peptide (VIP) appears to be a likely candidate: It is the one neuropeptide present in nerves supplying pulmonary vessels[7] and capable of dilating these vessels[8,9]; it has neurotransmitter/neuromodulator properties; and there is good evidence that it may be a transmitter of the same relaxant system in the airways,[10] lower esophageal sphincter,[11,12] and other sites.[13] Whether VIP is in fact the transmitter of nonadrenergic, noncholinergic relaxation

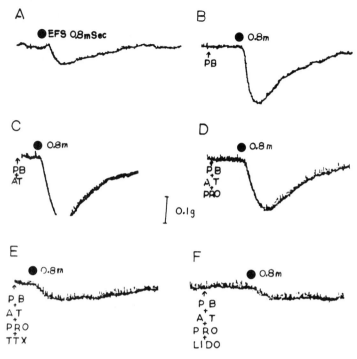

Figure 16-1 Electrical field stimulation (EFS)–induced relaxation of cat pulmonary artery segment. Phenoxybenzamine (PB) abolished the initial contraction and accentuated the subsequent relaxation. Atropine (AT) and propranolol (PRO) had little effect on relaxation, which was markedly reduced by tetrodotoxin (TTX) or lidocaine (LIDO).

in the pulmonary circulation is now under active investigation. Answers are being sought to these questions, among others: Is the pulmonary arterial relaxation that is induced by electrical field stimulation in the presence of adrenergic and cholinergic blockade associated with VIP release? Does the peptide release correlate with the degree of relaxation? Does anti-VIP antiserum inhibit the relaxation?

Humoral Control

Humoral agents that affect, and may regulate, pulmonary vascular tone include biogenic amines, peptides, and lipids (Table 16-1). Most of these, eg, histamine, serotonin, substance P, spasmogenic lung peptide, the leukotrienes, $PGF_{2\alpha}$, PGD_2, and the thromboxanes have a contractile effect. A few, including VIP and prostacyclin (PGI_2), induce relaxation.

Lung peptides At least fourteen biologically active peptides have been identified in the lung[14] (Table 16-2). Most of these peptides, eg, angiotensin II, spasmogenic lung peptide, substance P, and bombesin,

Table 16-2
Biologically Active Peptides in the Lung

1. ACTH	8. Eosinophil-chemotactic peptides
2. Angiotensin II	9. Neurotensin
3. Bombesin-like (GRP)	10. PHI/PHM
4. Bradykinin	11. Somatostatin
5. Calcitonin	12. "Spasmogenic lung peptide"
6. CCK	13. Substance P
7. Enkephalins	14. VIP

ACTH = adrenocorticotrophic hormone, GRP = gastrin-releasing peptide, CCK = cholecystokinin-pancreozymin, PHI = peptide with N-terminal histidine and C-terminal isoleucine, PHM = peptide with N-terminal histidine and C-terminal methionine, VIP = vasoactive intestinal peptide.

contract pulmonary vascular smooth muscle with varying degrees of potency and efficacy.[14-16] Vasoactive intestinal peptide is the only peptide found in the lung that relaxes pulmonary vessels. This relaxant action has been demonstrated in vitro in isolated pulmonary artery segments from several species, including humans. As a relaxant of cat and human pulmonary artery segments, VIP is up to 200 times as potent on a molar basis as prostacyclin[8,9,17] (Figure 16-2). Vasoactive intestinal peptide also exhibits

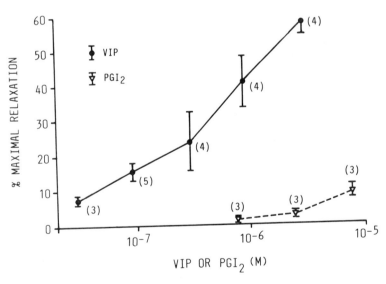

Figure 16-2 Dose-related relaxation (percent of maximal relaxation) of isolated strip of human pulmonary artery (pretreated with 1 µg/mL indomethacin) in response to vasoactive intestinal peptide (VIP) or prostacyclin (PGI$_2$).

pulmonary vasodilator activity in vivo in anesthetized cats, tending to reduce pulmonary arterial pressure while augmenting cardiac output.[18]

There is less information on whether certain peptides have a physiologic regulatory influence on pulmonary vessels. For example, can lung peptides modify pulmonary vascular reactivity? Does one vasoactive lung peptide (eg, angiotensin II) contribute to normal pulmonary vascular tone while another (eg, VIP) provides a relaxant background? The pulmonary vasodilator activity of angiotensin-converting enzyme inhibitors suggests such a role for angiotensin II.[19] The question concerning VIP should be resolved once its relationship to nonadrenergic, noncholinergic relaxation (see above) has been ascertained.

Leukotrienes The leukotrienes (LTs) are peptidolipids generated from arachidonic acid via lipoxygenase-catalyzed pathways.[20] Endogenously occurring LTs include LTB_4, LTC_4, LTD_4, and LTE_4. The latter three are the main constituents of the "slow-reacting substance of anaphylaxis."[20,21] Systemic effects of LTC_4 and LTD_4 include arteriolar constriction, increased peripheral resistance, decreased glomerular filtration, and augmented vascular permeability.[20-23] Acting on the lungs, LTC_4 and LTD_4 induce constriction of airways (peripheral more than central airways), contraction of lung parenchyma, pulmonary vasoconstriction, and increased pulmonary microvascular permeability.[22,23] Leukotriene B_4, a potent chemotactic agent, promotes neutrophil infiltration and increases the adhesion of neutrophils to endothelial cells in small vessels.[24,25] Specific pulmonary receptors for leukotrienes have been identified in the lung, suggesting a physiologic regulatory role for these compounds in the lung.[26]

We have recently examined the effects of LTD_4 on pulmonary vascular dynamics, lung mechanics, and the development of pulmonary edema. In isolated, perfused, and ventilated guinea pig lungs, LTD_4 (1 to 3 μg/kg) dose-dependently increased pulmonary arterial pressure and pulmonary vascular resistance (by > 50%), airway pressure (by up to 400%), and pulmonary resistance (by > 700%). Leukotriene D_4 also reduced pulmonary compliance (by > 60%), and significantly increased the wet/dry lung weight ratio (from 5.3 ± 0.1 to as high as 6.8 ± 0.2) (Figure 16-3).[27] These drastic alterations in lung function were associated with sharp increases in the pulmonary perfusate concentrations of thromboxane B_2 (TxB_2) and other cyclo-oxygenase metabolites, and were markedly attenuated or abolished by UK-37248 (thromboxane synthetase inhibitor), indomethacin (cyclo-oxygenase inhibitor), or FPL-55712 (LT antagonist).[27] These experiments thus show LTD_4 to be a potent constrictor of pulmonary vessels and airways, and capable of inducing pulmonary edema, all due in large part to the release of thromboxanes and other cyclo-oxygenase products.

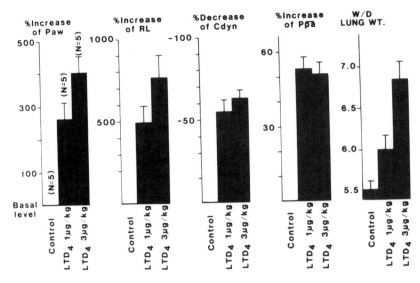

Figure 16-3 Effects of leukotriene D₄ (LTD₄) (1 μg/kg and 3 μg/kg) on mechanics and hemodynamics in isolated, perfused and ventilated guinea pig lungs. Paw = airway pressure; RL = pulmonary resistance; Cdyn = dynamic lung compliance; Ppa = mean pulmonary arterial pressure; W/D Lung Wt. = wet/dry lung weight ratio. Except for last function, all other measurements are expressed as percent changes of basal values.

Summary and Conclusions

Pulmonary vascular tone is influenced, and probably regulated, by multiple neurohumoral factors. These include the autonomic nervous system and a variety of vasoactive peptides and lipids. The autonomic neurogenic influences include the α- and β-adrenergic and cholinergic components, as well as a third, nonadrenergic, noncholinergic component which may be mediated by the neuropeptide VIP. Lung peptides, some present in neuroendocrine cells, have potent actions (relaxation or constriction) on pulmonary vessels and may participate in regulating vascular tone. Leukotrienes and other biologically active lipids generally constrict pulmonary vessels and promote microvascular permeability.

ACKNOWLEDGMENTS

Supported by NIH Research Grants HL-30450 and HL-31039 and by research funds from the Veterans Administration. Ms Teresa Long helped with the preparation of the manuscript.

REFERENCES

1. Cassin S, Dawes GS, Mott JC, et al: The vascular resistance of the foetal and newly ventilated lung of the lamb. *J Physiol* 1964;171:61–79.
2. Cassin S, Dawes GS, Ross BB: Pulmonary blood flow and vascular resistance in immature foetal lambs. *J Physiol* 1964;171:80–89.
3. Barrett CT, Heymann MA, Rudolph AM: Alpha- and beta-adrenergic function in fetal sheep. *Am J Obstet Gynecol* 1972;112:1114–1121.
4. Richardson JB, Beland J: Nonadrenergic inhibitory nervous system in human airways. *J Appl Physiol* 1976;41:764–771.
5. Burnstock G, Hökfelt T, Gershon MD, et al: Non-adrenergic, non-cholinergic autonomic neurotransmission mechanisms. *Neurosci Res Program Bull* 1979;17:379–519.
6. Hamasaki Y, Saga T, Said SI: Autonomic innervation of pulmonary artery: Evidence for nonadrenergic, noncholinergic relaxation. *Am Rev Respir Dis* 1983;127:300A.
7. Dey DA, Shannon WA, Said SI: Localization of VIP-immunoreactive nerves in airways and pulmonary vessels of dogs, cats and human subjects. *Cell Tissue Res* 1981;220:231–238.
8. Mojarad M, Said SI: Vasoactive intestinal peptide (VIP) dilates pulmonary vessels in anesthetized cats. *Am Rev Respir Dis* 1981;122:239A.
9. Hamasaki Y, Mojarad M, Said SI: Relaxant action of VIP on cat pulmonary artery: Comparison with acetylcholine, isoproterenol and PGE_1. *J Appl Physiol* 1983;54:1607–1611.
10. Matsuzaki Y, Hamasaki Y, Said SI: Vasoactive intestinal peptide: A possible transmitter of non-adrenergic relaxation of guinea pig airways. *Science* 1980;210:1252–1253.
11. Goyal RK, Rattan S, Said SI: VIP as a possible neurotransmitter of non-cholinergic non-adrenergic inhibitory neurones. *Nature* 1980;288:378–380.
12. Biancani P, Walsh JH, Behar J: Vasoactive intestinal polypeptide: A neurotransmitter for lower esophageal sphincter relaxation. *J Clin Invest* 1984;73:963–967.
13. Grider JR, Cable MB, Said SI, et al: Vasoactive intestinal peptide: Relaxant neurotransmitter in tenia coli of the guinea pig. *Gastroenterology*, 1985;89:36–42.
14. Dey RD, Said SI: Peptides and the pulmonary circulation, in Said SI (ed): *The Pulmonary Circulation and Acute Lung Injury*. Mount Kisco, NY, Futura Publishing Company, Inc, 1985, pp 101–122.
15. Said SI: Peptide hormones and neurotransmitters of the lung, in Becker KL, Gazdar A (eds): *The Endocrine Lung in Health and Disease*. Philadelphia, WB Saunders Co, 1984, pp 267–275.
16. Said SI, Mutt V, Erdös EG: The lung in relation to vasoactive polypeptides, in *Ciba Found Symp 78: Metabolic Activities of the Lung*. 1980;217–237.
17. Saga T, Said SI: Vasoactive intestinal peptide relaxes isolated strips of human bronchus, pulmonary artery, and lung parenchyma. *Trans Assoc Am Physicians* 1984;97:304–310.
18. Mojarad M, Said SI, Hyman AL: Vasoactive intestinal peptide (VIP) dilates pulmonary vessels in anesthetized cats. *Clin Res* 1980;28:89A.
19. Niarchos AP, Roberts AJ, Laragh JH: Effects of the converting enzyme inhibitor (SQ 20881) on the pulmonary circulation in man. *Am J Med* 1979;67:785–791.

20. Samuelsson B: Leukotrienes: Mediators of immediate hypersensitivity reactions and inflammation. *Science* 1983;220:568–575.
21. Bach MK: The leukotrienes: Their structure, actions and role in diseases, in *Current Concepts*. Kalamazoo, Mich, The Upjohn Co, 1983.
22. Hanna CJ, Bach MK, Pare PD, et al: Slow reacting substances (leukotrienes) contract human airway and pulmonary vascular smooth muscle *in vitro*. *Nature* 1981;290:343–344.
23. Drazen JM, Venugopalan CS, Austen KF, et al: Effects of leukotriene E on pulmonary mechanics in the guinea pig. *Am Rev Respir Dis* 1982;125:290–294.
24. Ford-Hutchinson AW: Neutrophil aggregating properties of PAF-acether and leukotriene B_4. *Int J Immunopharmacol* 1983;5:17–21.
25. Lindbom L, Hedqvist P, Dahlen S-E, et al: Leukotriene B_4 induces extravasation and migration of polymorphonuclear leukocytes *in vivo*. *Acta Physiol Scand* 1982;116:105–108.
26. Lewis RA, Austen KF: The biologically active leukotrienes. Biosynthesis, metabolism, receptors, functions, and pharmacology. *J Clin Invest* 1984; 73:889–897.
27. Saga T, Yoshii K, Said SI: Protection by FPL 55712 or indomethacin of leukotriene D_4-induced pulmonary edema and airway constriction in guinea pig. *Am Rev Respir Dis* 1984;129:A333.

17 The Effects of β-Agonists and Aminophylline on Lung Fluid Balance

Warren Summer
Irving Mizus
Gail Gurtner

Acid aspiration causes damage to air spaces and adjacent capillary endothelium resulting in increased capillary permeability and pulmonary edema.[1-3] In addition, acid lung injury usually produces increases in pulmonary arterial and mean capillary filtration pressure.[4] Recently, it has been clearly demonstrated that when microvascular permeability is increased, small changes in pulmonary vascular pressure have striking effects on the amount of pulmonary edema when compared to normal.[4-6] Thus, it is not surprising that vasodilators or inhibitors of mediators that elevate pulmonary artery pressure have been shown to reduce pulmonary edema in animal models of acute lung injury.[7,8]

Normal function of the endothelium depends upon the cytoskeleton of the individual endothelial cells and the tight junctions that exists between them.[9,10] Ultrastructural studies by Majno and coworkers demonstrate the development of gaps in systemic vascular endothelium with extravasation of colloidal carbon following exposure to bradykinin or histamine.[11,12] Pietra et al found a similar response in bronchial postcapillary venules in response to histamine.[13] Endothelial cells, with their cytoskeleton composed of actomyosin filaments,[14,15] have been found to be contractile.[15,16] This contractile process is known to involve cAMP and cGMP,[17-20] which appeared to act antagonistically, with increased cAMP causing relaxation and increased cGMP allowing for contraction.

Isoproterenol and terbutaline sulfate have been shown to block the macromolecular leakage across the systemic vascular endothelium induced by bradykinin and histamine[21-24] and are known to generate increasing cAMP levels within cells.[25] Evidence for β-agonist modulation of macromolecular leak has been obtained in different tissues involving several species including the guinea pig lung.[26] This suggests the existence of a permeability-reducing β-receptor function. In addition, a recent study

219

using an acid–lung injury model demonstrated that isoproterenol reduced pulmonary edema more than another vasodilator at relatively similar pulmonary artery pressures.[27] Thus, β-adrenergic agonists as well as compounds known to generate cAMP seem to protect against increased vascular permeability at comparable or low vascular pressures.[28-30]

Although it is usually assumed that increased capillary permeability results from direct anatomical insult, there is considerable experimental evidence for early functional injury.[31,32] In addition, a number of clinical conditions of presumed capillary leak syndrome rapidly reverse suggesting a dynamic rather than a destructive etiology. *Postictal* and *heroin*-associated pulmonary edema may reverse in hours and some cases of apparent severe acid aspiration may clear in one to two days.[33]

We sought to determine if isoproterenol and aminophylline significantly influenced lung fluid balance in models of increased capillary permeability pulmonary edema and to distinguish whether the mechanism responsible for such an effect is due solely to a reduction in capillary hydrostatic pressure or some additional attenuation in pulmonary capillary permeability.[34] We examined isolated perfused rabbit and rat lungs following intratracheal acid injury and after pulmonary artery injection of t-butylhydroperoxide. The initial goal was to establish that early lung injury has a functional component that is modulated by isoproterenol. We then tested the hypothesis that the beneficial effect of isoproterenol is related to the β-receptor through blockade by propranolol. We also tried to mimic the effects of isoproterenol on lung fluid balance with terbutaline and other drugs known to increase cAMP as well as analogues of cAMP. In addition, we attempted to quantify the relative contribution of capillary hydrostatic pressure in determining lung fluid balance by examining lung fluid flux at various microvascular filtration pressures generated through increases in pulmonary blood flow or elevated pulmonary venous pressure.[35]

METHODS

Isolated lung preparation Three-kg male New Zealand white rabbits were given 4000 units of heparin and their chests were widely exposed with the heart and lung left in situ. The rabbits were rapidly exsanguinated. The pulmonary artery and left atrial appendage were cannulated with stainless steel cannulae. The ligature around the pulmonary artery was also placed around the aorta, preventing loss of perfusate into the systemic circulation. Eighty milliliters of autologous blood were mixed with 80 mL of Krebs-Henseleit solution and recirculated at 65 mL/min with a Sarns blood pump. The trachea was cannulated and the lungs ventilated with room air plus 5% CO_2 using a Harvard small animal ventilator with a tidal volume of 10 mL/kg and 3 cm of H_2O positive end-expiratory pressure (PEEP).

Experimental measurements Pulmonary artery pressure (PAP) and left atrial pressure (LAP) were zero-referenced to the level of the left atrium and continuously recorded using Statham P23db pressure transducers and a Grass polygraph Model F. Left atrial pressure was maintained at 0 mmHg by adjusting the height of the perfusate reservoir. Lung weight changes were continuously recorded as the inverse of the weight change of the perfusate reservoir which was freely suspended from a force displacement strain gauge transducer (Grass FT 10C). Control uninjured lungs are stable for several hours. The lung weight gain that occurred following acid challenge was expressed as weight gain in grams per 30 minutes. The 30-minute period was chosen because preliminary experiments indicated that, by this time after acid instillation, severe pulmonary edema had developed. Thirty minutes after acid injury the perfusate flow rate was increased in each lung until the PAP was maintained at 25 mmHg. The gain in lung weight was then measured over the next three to five minutes and expressed as grams per minute and as grams per 100 mL per minute rate of perfusion. In a separate group of experiments, after 30 minutes, the pulmonary venous pressure was increased to 10 torr and the rate of edema formation measured. In these experiments pulmonary microvascular pressure was estimated by double occlusion[35] at five minutes and 30 minutes postinjury and during pulmonary venous pressure elevation.

Experimental protocol *Acid-injured rabbits* Five groups of experiments were performed using the following protocol. Measurements were made during three periods: (1) a stable 15-minute control period; (2) a 30-minute period following the intratracheal instillation of 0.1N HCl (2mL/kg followed by a breath that was 150% of the control tidal volume); and (3) a three-minute period after the mean PAP had been increased to 25 mmHg by increasing the perfusion rate. The following groups were studied:

Group 1 (control): This group did not receive hydrochloric acid or treatment.

Group 2 (acid): This group received HCl (2 mL/kg 0.1N HCl) without treatment.

Group 3 (acid plus isoproterenol pretreatment): This group was pretreated with isoproterenol (3 μg/min) which was continuously infused into the perfusion circuit beginning five minutes before HCl instillation and continuing throughout the experiment. Prior to instilling HCl, the perfusate flow rate was increased to return the mean PAP to the preisoproterenol level.

Group 4 (acid plus aminophylline pretreatment): During the control period, a single dose of aminophylline (16 mg/kg body weight) was given into the reservoir. After aminophylline was administered, the perfusion rate was increased in the control period to return the PAP to the preaminophylline level. HCl was then instilled.

Group 5 (acid plus isoproterenol posttreatment): In this group, a continuous infusion of isoproterenol (3 μg/min) was begun three minutes after HCl was instilled and continued throughout the rest of the experiment. In one animal, isoproterenol treatment was begun 33 minutes after acid instillation.

An additional set of experiments was performed to test the hypothesis that β-adrenergic blockade would reverse the protective effect of isoproterenol. A continuous infusion of isoproterenol (3 μg/min) was begun five minutes before and continued for 60 minutes after acid instillation. Thirty minutes after acid instillation, propranolol (3 mg) was added to the reservoir and measurements were made throughout another 30 minutes.

Studies performed by other members of our group included similar experiments using a rat model preinfused with terbutaline and pressure stressed by elevation of the left atrial reservoir,[36] a rabbit model injured with t-butylhydroperoxide pretreated with isoproterenol, aminophylline, and dibutyryl-A 3:5-MP, a cAMP analogue,[37] and a pig model injured with endotoxin and pretreated with isoproterenol.[38]

These later studies will be referred to briefly only to establish the consistency of these effects under various conditions of injury and microvascular manipulation. In addition, reference to the rat model is included because after acid injury this model develops little acute increase in pulmonary vascular pressure and less than a 0.5 mmHg difference in microvascular filtration pressure estimated by double occlusion[35] with or without terbutaline.

Statistics Data were analyzed by analysis of variance or the Student's t-test. Results are presented as the mean ± standard error of the mean (SEM).

RESULTS

Perfusion rate The perfusion rate was 65 mL/min in the no-acid control group, the acid control group, and the acid plus isoproterenol posttreatment group. The perfusion rate was increased from 65 to 150 mL/min in the aminophylline and isoproterenol pretreatment groups in order to maintain a constant pulmonary artery pressure during the control period.

Lung weight gain The change in lung weight throughout the various 30 minute experimental periods is shown in Figure 17-1. Lung weight did not increase in the no-acid control group. In fact, lung weight in this preparation can remain unchanged for at least three hours. Acid instillation, however, increased lung weight in the acid control group by 19.2 ± 5.1 g ($P < .001$). This is more than a doubling of water and was corroborated by a more than doubling of the wet/dry weight ratios. Isoproterenol pretreatment essentially prevented pulmonary edema after instillation ($P < .001$) while aminophylline markedly attenuated weight gain ($P < .01$).

Treatment with isoproterenol beginning three minutes after instilling acid also strikingly reduced the amount of pulmonary edema ($P < .01$). In this isoproterenol postacid treatment group, the gain in lung weight over time was initially similar to that in the acid control group, but after isoproterenol the gain in lung weight markedly decreased. Lung weight gain was significantly less with isoproterenol pretreatment ($P < .01$) than with either aminophylline pretreatment or isoproterenol posttreatment.

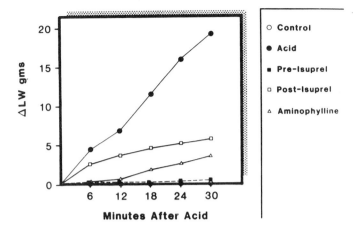

Figure 17-1 The time course of lung weight gain (LW) is shown after intratracheal instillation of acid for four groups: control (○), acid (●), pretreatment with isoproterenol (■) or aminophylline (△), and posttreatment with isoproterenol (□). Treatment with aminophylline or isoproterenol significantly reduced LW after acid instillation.

In a single experiment in which isoproterenol was given 33 minutes after acid instillation, there was an abrupt attenuation in the rate of lung weight gain over the next 30 minutes. When the isoproterenol infusion was discontinued, the gain in lung weight resumed.

Effect of propranolol In a separate group of experiments, 30 minutes after acid injury, the addition of propranolol reversed the beneficial effect of isoproterenol and significantly increased lung fluid flux ($P < .01$) similar to those in the acid control group (Figure 17-2). In additional control experiments, treatment with isoproterenol prevented the development of pulmonary edema for up to 60 minutes after acid instillation.

Pulmonary artery pressure The change in pulmonary artery pressure over time is shown in Figure 17-3. In the no-acid control group mean PAP remained constant throughout the experimental period. Thirty minutes after acid instillation the PAP in the acid control group had increased 67%, from 15 ± 2 to 25 ± 4 mmHg ($P < .01$). Treatment with isoproterenol or aminophylline prevented the increase in PAP following hydrochloric acid.

Flow stress Thirty minutes after acid challenge the perfusion flow was increased in each until the PAP was 25 mmHg and fluid flux was then measured for three minutes. The perfusion rates required to produce a mean PAP of 25 mmHg differed markedly between the groups. The perfusion flow rate was 70 to 80 mL/min in the acid control group and

224

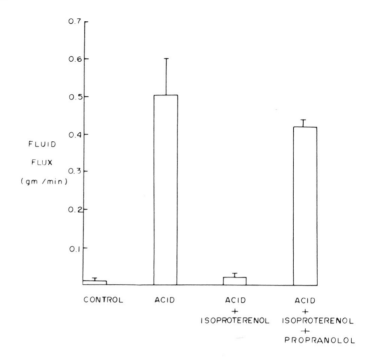

Figure 17-2 The effect of propranolol in isoproterenol-pretreated lungs. The addition of propranolol to lungs treated with isoproterenol reversed the protective effect, increasing fluid flux ($P < .01$) to levels similar to those in the acid control group.

200 to 250 mL/min in the isoproterenol and aminophylline pretreatment groups. Fluid flux was less with isoproterenol ($0.17 \pm .06$ g/min) or aminophylline (0.41 ± 0.04 g/min) compared with $0.96 \pm .30$ g/min in the acid control group (Figure 17-4). When the large disparity between perfusion rates is taken into account by normalizing fluid flux per 100 mL perfusion, the protective effect is even more obvious with isoproterenol ($0.08 \pm .03$ g/100 mL) and aminophylline (0.18 ± 0.2 g/100 mL) compared with $0.86 \pm .18$ g/100 mL in the acid control groups ($P < .01$).

We calculated the relative fluid conductance in the control, acid, acid plus isoproterenol, and acid plus aminophylline groups of experiments by plotting the respective fluid flux and PAP for each group just before and after increasing flow to achieve a PAP of 25 mmHg (Figure 17-5). The resulting slope or conductance was 0.42 mL/min/mmHg in the acid untreated group, decreasing by more than tenfold with aminophylline treatment, to 0.035 mL/min/mmHg, and about 25-fold with isoproterenol treatment, to 0.017 mL/min/mmHg.

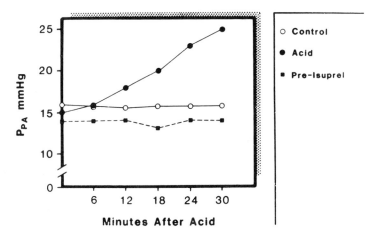

Figure 17-3 The time course of pulmonary artery pressure (P$_{Pa}$) is shown after intratracheal instillation of 2 mL/kg 0.1N HCl for three groups: control (○), acid instillation alone (●), and isoproterenol pretreatment (■). Pulmonary artery pressure (P$_{Pa}$) increased steadily in the acid control group. Treatment with isoproterenol and aminophylline prevented the increase after acid instillation.

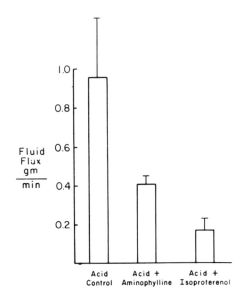

Figure 17-4 The effect of isoproterenol and aminophylline on fluid flux (g/min) after acid injury at a similar pulmonary artery pressure of 25 mmHg. Fluid flux in g/min was significantly reduced by isoproterenol and aminophylline ($P < .01$). Not shown in this figure was fluid flux normalized for perfusion flow rate. Fluid flux in g/100 mL perfusion was reduced by both aminophylline and isoproterenol ($P < .01$).

226

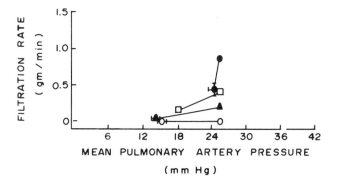

Figure 17-5 Results of the flow stress maneuver. Thirty minutes after acid challenge pulmonary artery pressure (PAP) and the rate of lung weight gain was measured. Flow was then increased sufficiently to increase PAP to 25 mmHg and the rate of lung weight gain was again measured. Measurements were made in control lungs which were not challenged (O), acid-challenged lungs (●), and acid-challenged lungs pretreated with isoproterenol (▲) or aminophylline (□). The slope of the relationship between fluid filtration and PAP for each group has units (g/min/mmHg) and represents the fluid hydraulic conductance. The slopes for the four groups were control 0, acid 0.42, isoproterenol 0.017, and aminophylline 0.035.

Other experiments carried out in our laboratories support the hypothesis that drugs that increase cAMP inhibit edema formation in lung injury by directly reducing vascular permeability.

Gregory et al have tried to distinguish the relative hydrostatic anti-permeability effects of terbutaline, a predominant β_2-agonist, on macromolecular lung fluid flux by estimating microvascular filtration pressure at low or high LAPs in a rat model of acid injury.[36] This preparation was similar in most respects to the rabbit model. However, this model has little if any increase in PAP following acid injury. Elevation of LAP confirmed the well-known predominant effect of microvascular pressure on lung fluid balance. However, double occlusion estimates of microvascular filtration pressure show that terbutaline significantly reduces lung fluid flux at essentially identical hydrostatic pressure between 0 and 10 mmHg by 75% to 35% respectively.

Other studies in our laboratory using a similar rabbit model but injured with four sequential pulmonary artery injections of t-butylhydroperoxide showed comparable attenuations of lung leakage with isoproterenol and aminophylline.[37] In addition, pretreatment with dibutyryl-A 3:5 MP, a cAMP analogue, resulted in quantitatively similar alterations in lung fluid balance.

In a similar isolated blood-perfused pig preparation, Walman et al measured the effect of isoproterenol pretreatment on lung weight gain and

PAP after administration of *Escherichia coli* endotoxin.[38] The effect of changing microvascular pressure was measured by transiently increasing LAP from -5 to $+5$ torr. Lung weight gain was significantly smaller in the isoproterenol pretreated group. The difference in lung weight gain between groups was accentuated by increasing LAP. Similar to acid injury, the beneficial effect of isoproterenol was blocked by propranolol. These results in pigs are consistent with the findings during acid or t-butylhydroperoxide injury in rabbits and rats and suggests a common pathophysiologic mechanism.

DISCUSSION

The major observation of this study is that premedication with isoproterenol and aminophylline strikingly reduce the pulmonary edema that follows acid lung injury. Pulmonary edema was reduced because isoproterenol and aminophylline prevented the increases in pulmonary vascular pressure and permeability that occur after acid instillation. Treatment with isoproterenol at three or 33 minutes after acid instillation also markedly reduced the formation of pulmonary edema. The beneficial effect of isoproterenol involves activation of β-adrenergic receptors; propranolol reverses this effect. Isoproterenol may work by increasing cAMP; treatment with aminophylline, a drug known to increase intracellular cAMP through inhibition of phosphodiesterase, also produces comparable effects on pulmonary vascular pressure and permeability. A cAMP analogue similarly inhibits edema formation in an oxidant injury model.[37]

Gross observation of injured lungs following intratracheal acid show patchy hemorrhage. Similar inhomogeneous injury has been visualized in other models of capillary leak syndrome by computed tomography (CT)[39] and is assumed to be a characteristic of clinical syndromes.[40] It is possible that the reduction in fluid filtration observed with these drugs was due to changes in microvascular pressure alone as reported by others.[8] This explanation would appear less tenable during periods of flow or pressure stress. However, redistribution of blood flow and regional difference in perfusion pressure are also likely in this model and could explain the changes in lung fluid balance following isoproterenol. In fact, Winn et al [41] recently reported pulmonary vasoconstriction in goats after acid aspiration which directs blood flow away from nonventilated alveoli. In our experiments, the pulmonary artery hypertension after acid instillation appeared to develop in vessels upstream to exchanging vessels since little of the increase in pressure over time (Figure 17-3) seemed to be reflected in increasing rates of weight gain (Figure 17-1). In fact, in the acid control group, fluid flux was linear and independent of the PAP ($r = .05$). The high perfusion flow in the treatment groups indicate that the pulmonary arterial bed was dilated. If the vasodilatation was predominantly upstream to the nonexchanging vessels, then it should have little effect on fluid filtration. If the vasodilatation occurred in all vessels, then more of the PAP may have been transmitted to the exchanging vessels. This would make the protective effect of isoproterenol and aminophylline even more striking.

It is qualitatively possible that isoproterenol and aminophylline acted by effecting the distribution of vascular resistance downstream from the site of leak. In studies by Hakim et al[42] and Gregory and Gurtner[43] using inflow and outflow occlusion techniques, a substantial portion of pulmonary vascular resistance lies upstream or in close proximity to the capillary. In our studies, the marked decrease in fluid flux with isoproterenol secondary to vasodilatation Figure 17-2 would require a vascular resistance model with almost all of the vasodilatation downstream from the site of leak.

The reduction in pulmonary vascular permeability following these drugs is well illustrated in Figure 17-4 where fluid flux at 25 mmHg is recorded. In the acid control group this required only a small increase in flow to obtain the increased pressure because the base-line resistance was high and the pressures at 30 minutes were close to 25 mmHg. Despite this minimal elevation in PAP there was a marked increase in fluid flux consistent with transmission of the small amount of additional pressure to a highly permeable membrane.[4,8,10,44] In the treated groups the perfusion flow was three- to fourfold higher indicating a marked decrease in pulmonary resistance and an open vascular bed. In spite of these high flows, at similar pressures fluid filtration was substantially less than acid control. The filtration rate was even greater between the acid-alone and treated groups when normalized for flow at 25 mmHg.

That isoproterenol and aminophylline are capable of markedly attenuating the pulmonary edema developing as a result of acid–lung injury independent of their effect on perfusion pressure is also demonstrated by looking at a plot of fluid flux v PAP (Figure 17-5). The plot reveals a reduction in the fluid flux in the treatment group as compared with the untreated group over a range of similar PAPs. This decreased slope or fluid conductance in each treated group as compared with acid injury alone demonstrates that treatment results in an increased "resistance barrier" or decreased conductance to fluid leak. These results are consistent with measurements of fluid filtration and filtration coefficients obtained by stepwise pressure elevation in isolated normal dog lungs following instillation of oleic acid.[44] Recent studies in our rat model by Gregory[36] have shown similar effects with fluid filtration following terbutaline at low and high LAPs and microvascular pressures measured by double occlusion. The apparent decrease in fluid flux at similar hydrostatic pressures and the reduced membrane conductants and/or filtration coefficient observed with therapy are consistent with closure of endothelial gaps.

An increase in cAMP might prevent the pulmonary vasoconstriction following acid instillation either by preventing the production of vasoconstricting substances or by directly inhibiting vascular smooth muscle contraction. Pulmonary vasoconstriction following acid instillation appears to be due to the production of thromboxane.[45] The effect of isoproterenol on thromboxane production following acid instillation was not studied in these experiments, but we have recently found that isoproterenol does not prevent the production of thromboxane following lipid peroxide infusion in this rabbit preparation.[46] A more likely mechanism for the pulmonary vasodilation with isoproterenol is an increase in cAMP which can prevent smooth muscle contraction by decreasing intracellular calcium or by inhibiting the activation of myosin light chain kinase.[17,18]

An increase in cAMP might reduce vascular permeability following acid injury by preventing mediator release, which results in direct endothelial injury, or by preventing the formation of vascular endothelial gaps. Of course, a host of mediators have been shown to increase endothelial gaps.[47] A number of investigators believe that the development of gaps between vascular endothelial cells increases the permeability of systemic[11,21,24] and bronchial[13] vessels. In systemic vessels isoproterenol and terbutaline prevent the formation of endothelial gaps and the increase in vascular permeability.

Isoproterenol administration appears to have been effective in reducing edema formation even when given 30 minutes after acid injury. This suggests that the alveolar-capillary injury may be reversible and markedly influenced by pharmacologic therapy. Isoproterenol pretreatment was significantly more effective than aminophylline pretreatment in reducing lung weight gain. One possible explanation might be that isoproterenol, which stimulates cAMP production, may be more effective in increasing cAMP levels than is aminophylline, which inhibits cAMP degradation.

The amount of isoproterenol and aminophylline used in this study exceeded the usual dosages used in humans. Other investigators, however, have found that isoproterenol administered in the unusual clinical range reduced pulmonary edema after acid aspiration in isolated dog lungs[27] and after E. coli endotoxin infusion in intact sheep.[8] Final testing of clinical efficacy will, of course, require human studies.

Pulmonary edema has been generally considered the basic abnormality in patients with the adult respiratory distress syndrome (ARDS). However, it is not clear whether this initial injury is an alteration of structure or function. Microscopic examination of animal lungs sacrificed one hour after acid aspiration reveal only mild structural abnormalities. In some ARDS patients interstitial and alveolar exudates seem to be reabsorbed almost as swiftly as the edema fluid in hemodynamic pulmonary edema. Isoproterenol and aminophylline prevent the increase in both pulmonary vascular pressures and permeability following acid lung injury, an accepted model of nonhydrostatic pulmonary edema. The above findings suggest: (1) the edema following hydrochloric acid may be a reversible physiologic leak and not due to direct anatomical destruction; (2) the edema can be initially markedly reduced by agents that increase cAMP. Endothelial cell contraction by mediators is an attractive way of explaining the reversible increased gap formation and increased permeability to macromolecules[26,31,45] The potential anti-inflammatory role of a physiologic antagonist that alters lung fluid balance irrespective of the mediator producing the leak could have practical value in the initial treatment of patients with ARDS.

ACKNOWLEDGMENT

This study was supported in part by a grant from Merrell-Dow Laboratories.

REFERENCES

1. Wynne JW: Aspiration pneumonitis: correlation of experimental models with clinical disease, in *Symposium on Adult Respiratory Distress Syndrome. Clinical Chest Medicine*. Philadelphia, WB Saunders Co, 1982.
2. Jones JG, Berry M, Huland GH, et al: The time course and change of alveolar capillary membrane permeability induced by aspiration of hydrochloric acid and hypotonic saline. *Am Rev Respir Dis* 1978;118:1007–1013.
3. Awe WC, Fletcher WS, Jacab SW: The pathophysiology of aspiration pneumonitis. *Surgery* 1966;60:232–239.
4. Grimbert FA, Parker JC, Taylor AE: Increased pulmonary vascular permeability following acid aspiration. *J Appl Physiol* 1981;51:335–345.
5. Guyton AC, Lindsey AW: Effect of elevated left atrial pressure and decreased plasma protein concentration on the development of pulmonary edema. *Circ Res* 1957;7:649–657.
6. Erdmann AJ III, Vaughan TR Jr, Brigham KL, et al: Effect of increased vascular pressure on lung fluid balance in unanesthetized sheep. *Circ Res* 1975;37:271–284.
7. Utsunomiya T, Krausz MM, Dunham B, et al: Modification of inflammatory response to aspiration with ibuprofen. *Am J Physiol* 1982;243:H903–910.
8. Foy T, Marrion J, Brigham KL, et al: Isoproterenol and aminophylline reduce lung capillary filtration during high permeability. *J Appl Physiol* 1979; 46:146–151.
9. Hurley JV: Types of pulmonary microvascular injury. *Ann NY Acad Sci* 1982;384:269–286.
10. Shasby DM, Shasby SS, Peach MJ: Granulocytes and phorbol myistate acetate increase permeability to albumin of cultured endothelial monolayers and isolated perfused lungs. *Am Rev Respir Dis* 1983;127:72–76.
11. Majno G, Palade GE: Studies on inflammation. The effect of histamine and serotonin on vascular permeability: an electron microscopic study. *J Biophys Biochem Cytol* 1961;11:571–605.
12. Majno G, Gilmore V, Leventhal M: On the mechanism of vascular leakage caused by histamine-type mediators. *Circ Res* 1967;21:833–847.

13. Pietra GG, Szidon JP, Leventhal MM, et al: Histamine and interstitial pulmonary edema in the dog. *Circ Res* 1971;29:323-337.
14. Wong AJ, Pollard TD, Herman IM: Actin filament stress fibers in vascular endothelial cells in vivo. *Science* 1983;219:867-869.
15. Becker CG, Machman RL: Contractile proteins of endothelial cells, platelets and smooth muscle. *Am J Pathol* 1973;71:1-22.
16. DeClerck F, DeBrabender M, Meels H, et al: Direct evidence for the contractile capacity of endothelial cells. *Thromb Res* 1981;23:505-520.
17. Rasmussen H, Goodman DBP: Relationships between calcium and cyclic nucleotides in cell activation. *Physiol Rev* 1977;57:421-509.
18. Conti M, Adelstein RS: Phosphorylation by cyclic adenosine 3',5'-monophosphate-dependent protein kinase regulates myosin light chain kinase. *Fed Proc* 1980;39:1569-1573.
19. Davison PM, Karasek MA: Human dermal microvascular endothelial cells in vitro: effect of cAMP on cellular morphology and proliferation rate. *J Cell Physiol* 1981;106:253-258.
20. Kukovetz WR, et al: Function of cGMP in acetylcholine-induced contraction of coronary smooth muscle. *Naunyn Schmeidebergs Arch Pharmacol* 1982;319:29-33.
21. Grega GJ, Maciejko JJ, Raymond RM, et al: The interrelationship among histamine, various vasoactive substances, and macromolecular permeability in the canine forelimb. *Circ Res* 1980;46:264-275.
22. O'Donnell SR, Persson CGA: Evidence for a β adrenoreceptor mediated inhibition by terbutaline of histamine induced dye leakage in guinea pig skin. *Br J Pharmacol* 1978;62:321-324.
23. Svensjo E: Bradykinin and prostaglandin E_1 E_2,F_2-alpha induced macromolecular leakage in the hamster cheek pouch. *Prostaglandins Med* 1978;1:397-410.
24. Svensjo E, Arfors KE, Raymond RM, et al: Morphological and physiological correlation of bradykinin induced macromolecular efflux. *Am J Physiol* 1979;236:H600-H606.
25. Kuo JF, Kuo WK: Regulation by β adrenergic receptors and cholinergic receptors activation of intracellular cAMP and cGMP levels in rat lung slices. *Biochem Biophys Res Commun* 1973;55:660-665.
26. Persson CGA, Erjefalt I, Grega GJ, et al: The role of β-receptor agonists in the inhibition of pulmonary edema. *Ann NY Acad Sci* 1982;384:544-557.
27. Broe PJ, Toung TJK, Permutt S, et al: Aspiration pneumonia: treatment with pulmonary vasodilators. *Surgery* 1983;94:95-99.
28. Persson CGA, Ekman M, Erjefalt I: Vascular anti-permeability effects of beta receptor agonists and theophylline in the lung. *Acta Pharmacol Toxicol* 1979;44:216-220.
29. Svensjo E, Persson A, Rutillia O: Inhibition of bradykinin induced macromolecular leakage from post capillary vessels by β_2 adrenoreceptor stimulant, terbutaline. *Acta Physiol Scand* 1977;101:504-506.
30. Dobbuis DE, Soika CY, Permen AJ, et al: Blockade of histamine and bradykinin-induced increase in lymph flow and protein transport by terbutaline in vivo. *Microcirc* 1982;2:127-150.
31. Brigham KL: Mechanisms of lung injury. *Clin Chest Med* 1982;3:9-24.
32. Bachofen M, Weibel ER: Structural alterations of lung parenchyma in the adult respiratory distress syndrome. *Clin Chest Med* 1982;3:35-56.
33. Bynum L, Pierce AK Jr: Pulmonary aspiration of gastric contents. *Am Rev Respir Dis* 1976;114:1129.

34. Mizus I, Summer W, Farrukh I, et al: Agents that increase cAMP attenuate pulmonary edema after acid lung injury. *Am Rev Respir Dis* 1985;131:256–259.
35. Dawson CA, Linehan JH, Rickaby DA: Pulmonary microcirculatory hemodynamics. *Ann NY Acad Sci* 1982;384:90–106.
36. Gregory TJ, Weinberg AB, Summer WR: β_2-agonists reduce lung fluid accumulation at low and high microvascular filtration pressures. *Am Rev Respir Dis* 1985(suppl);131:A415.
37. Farrukh IS, Michael JR, Gurtner GH: Agents that increase cAMP prevent pulmonary vasoconstriction and edema in oxidant lung damage. *Fed Proc* 1984;43:884.
38. Walman AT, Parker SD, Traystman RY, et al: Isoproterenol protects against pulmonary edema in endotoxin lung injury. *Anesthesiology* 1984;61:A113.
39. Hedlung L, Effmann E, Bates W, et al: Pulmonary edema: A CT study of regional changes in lung density following oleic acid injury. *J Comput Assist Tomogr* 1982;6:939–946.
40. Rutili G, Parker JC, Taylor AE: Fluid balance in ANTU-injured lungs during crystalloid and colloid infusions. *J Appl Physiol* 1984;56:993–998.
41. Winn R, Stothert J, Nadir B, et al: Lung fluid balance, vascular permeability, and gas exchange after acid aspiration in awake goats. *J Appl Physiol* 1984;56:979–985.
42. Hakim T, Michael R, Chong H: Partitioning of pulmonary vascular resistance by arterial and venous occlusion. *J Appl Physiol* 1982;52:710–715.
43. Gregory TJ, Gurtner GH: The longitudinal distribution of pulmonary vascular resistance in oxidant induced vasoconstriction, abstracted. *Am Rev Respir Dis* 1983;127:310.
44. Earhart IC, Granger WM, Hofman WF: Filtration coefficient obtained by stepwise pressure elevation in isolated dog lung. *J Appl Physiol* 1984;56:862–867.
45. Mizus I, Michael JR, Summer WR, et al: Acid aspiration induced pulmonary pressure rise is attenuated by hypoxia or cyclo-oxygenase inhibition, abstracted. *Am Rev Respir Dis* 1983;127:316.
46. Farrukh IS, Summer WR, Michael J, et al: Thromboxane induced vasoconstriction, involvement of calcium. *J Appl Physiol* 1985;58:34–44.
47. Grega GJ, Svensjo E: Pharmacology of water and macromolecular permeability in the forelimb of the dog, in Staub NC, Taylor AE (eds): *Edema*. New York, Raven Press, 1984, pp 405–424.

18 Pulmonary Vascular Responses to Leukotriene D_4 Are Species-Dependent

Philip J. Kadowitz
Dennis B. McNamara
Jon M. Grazer
Albert L. Hyman

The leukotrienes are a family of biologically active hormones formed from arachidonic acid by way of the 5-lipoxygenase pathway.[1] In the lipoxygenase pathway, which is alternative to the cyclo-oxygenase pathway, the substrate is converted to 5-hydroperoxyeicosatetraenoic acid which is oxygenated to a labile epoxide intermediate named leukotriene (LT) A_4.[2-4] This labile epoxide intermediate which is analogous to the pivotal prostaglandin (PG) endoperoxide intermediate, PGH_2, in the cyclo-oxygenase pathway, can be transformed enzymatically to LTB_4 which has potent chemotactic activity.[2,3,5] Leukotriene A_4 can also be converted to LTC_4 by the addition of glutathione and this leukotriene can be further metabolized to LTD_4 by a γ-glutamyl transpeptidase[1,6,7] and subsequently to LTE_4.

It has been recently reported that LTC_4, LTD_4, and LTE_4 are the main components of the slow reacting substance of anaphylaxis (SRSA).[6,8,9] Since SRSA is a contractile substance which is released by immunologic challenge from the lung, it has been hypothesized that SRSA is an important mediator of symptoms in bronchial asthma and other immediate-type hypersensitivity reactions.[10-12] The effects of the leukotrienes on the lung are of considerable interest because of their postulated role as mediators in asthma.[12] Leukotrienes C_4 and D_4 have potent contractile activity on preparations of airway and vascular smooth muscle from the lung.[12-16] These substances have significant bronchoconstrictor activity in a variety of species.[17-19] However, little has been written about the effects of the leukotrienes on the pulmonary vascular bed. In the monkey the predominant response to injection of LTC_4 is a fall in pulmonary arterial pressure (PAP); whereas aerosol administration of LTC_4 caused a marked rise in PAP.[19] In the rat, injections of LTC_4

caused a dose-related fall in PAP.[20] However, other studies have indicated that LTC_4 may mediate hypoxic pulmonary vasoconstriction in the rat.[21] In contrast to studies with LTC_4 in the rat and monkey, LTD_4 caused a marked increase in pulmonary vascular resistance in the newborn lamb when injected into the pulmonary artery.[22] However, less is known about responses to LTD_4 on the pulmonary vascular bed of the mature animal.[23] The purpose of this report is to describe and compare responses to LTD_4 in the pulmonary vascular bed of cat and sheep under conditions of controlled blood flow using recently described methods.[24-26] The effects of LTD_4 and of the primary prostaglandins are also compared in the pulmonary vascular bed of the cat.

RESULTS

LTD_4 Responses in the Sheep

Pulmonary lobar vascular responses to LTD_4 in the intact-chest sheep were studied in 11 animals and these data are presented in Table 18-1. Under constant flow conditions, intralobar injections of LTD_4 in doses of 0.1 to 1.0 μg caused significant dose-related increases in lobar arterial and small vein pressures without changing left atrial pressure. In the range of dose employed in the present study in the sheep, LTD_4 had no significant effect on systemic arterial pressure. The increases in lobar arterial and small vein pressures were rapid in onset and mean vascular pressures returned to base-line value over a 0.5- to 4.0-minute period depending on the dose of the leukotriene. The lobar arterial to small vein pressure gradient and the gradient from small vein to left atrial pressure increased significantly at all doses of LTD_4 studied (Table 18-2).

Table 18-1
Influence of Intralobar Injections of Leukotriene D_4 (LTD_4)
on Mean Vascular Pressures in the Sheep (n = 11)

	Pressure (mmHg)			
	Lobar Artery	Small Vein	Left Atrium	Aorta
Control	15 ± 1	11 ± 1	5 ± 0	102 ± 4
LTD_4, 0.1 μg	26 ± 2*	15 ± 1*	5 ± 0	103 ± 4
Control	17 ± 1	12 ± 1	5 ± 1	100 ± 5
LTD_4, 0.3 μg	34 ± 2*	20 ± 2*	5 ± 1	100 ± 5
Control	15 ± 1	11 ± 1	5 ± 1	97 ± 5
LTD_4, 1 μg	39 ± 2*	22 ± 3*	5 ± 1	101 ± 4

*$P < .05$ when compared to corresponding control, paired comparison.

Table 18-2
Influence of Intralobar Injections of Leukotriene D_4 (LTD$_4$) on
Mean Vascular Pressure Gradients in the Sheep Lung (n = 10–11)

	Pressure gradient (mmHg)		
	Lobar Artery- *Left Atrium*	*Lobar Artery-* *Small Vein*	*Small Vein-* *Left Atrium*
Control	10 ± 1	4 ± 1	6 ± 3
LTD$_4$, 0.1 μg	21 ± 4*	11 ± 2*	10 ± 2*
Control	12 ± 1	5 ± 1	7 ± 2
LTD$_4$, 0.3 μg	29 ± 4*	14 ± 3*	15 ± 4*
Control	10 ± 2	4 ± 1	6 ± 3
LTD$_4$, 1 μg	34 ± 5*	17 ± 4*	17 ± 5*

*$P < .05$ when compared to corresponding control, paired comparison.

Influence of Cyclo-oxygenase and
Thromboxane Synthesis Inhibitors
in the Sheep

In order to determine if pulmonary vascular responses to LTD$_4$ in the sheep were dependent on formation of products in the cyclo-oxygenase pathway, the effects of sodium meclofenamate, a cyclo-oxygenase inhibitor, and of OKY-1581, a thromboxane synthesis inhibitor, were investigated. After administration of sodium meclofenamate in a dose of 2.5 mg/kg intravenously (IV), the increases in lobar arterial pressure in response to LTD$_4$ were reduced markedly at each dose of the leukotriene studied. The thromboxane synthesis inhibitor, OKY-1581, in doses of 5 to 10 mg/kg IV, also significantly reduced the increases in lobar arterial pressure in response to the three doses of LTD$_4$. However, the inhibitory effects of the cyclo-oxygenase inhibitor on responses to LTD$_4$ were greater than were the inhibitory effects of the thromboxane synthesis inhibitor. Neither OKY-1581 nor sodium meclofenamate had significant effect on pulmonary vascular or systemic arterial pressure in the sheep. The effects of sodium meclofenamate and OKY-1581 on pulmonary vascular responses to an agent whose actions mimic those of thromboxane A_2 (TxA$_2$) were also investigated. U-46619, an agent whose actions are similar to those of TxA$_2$ on smooth muscle, caused dose-dependent increases in lobar arterial and small vein pressures without affecting left atrial or systemic arterial pressure. The increases in lobar arterial pressure in response to U-46619 were not altered after administration of sodium meclofenamate, 2.5 mg/kg IV, or OKY-1581, 5 to 10 mg/kg IV.

In biochemical studies, the effects of OKY-1581 on the metabolism of arachidonic acid and of the prostaglandin endoperoxide, PGH$_2$, by microsomal fractions from sheep lung were investigated. The addition of

1-carbon $14(^{14}C)$-arachidonic acid (20 μmol/L) to the microsomal fraction (200 μg protein) resulted in the formation of 6-keto-prostaglandin $PGF_{2\alpha}$, the stable breakdown product of prostacyclin (PGI_2), 255 ± 21 pmol and TxB_2, the stable breakdown product of TxA_2, 230 ± 19 pmol/h in the absence of the inhibitor. Prostaglandins $F_{2\alpha}$, E_2, and D_2 were also formed. However, when OKY-1581 was added to the incubation medium in concentrations of 10^{-9} mol/L or greater, the formation of TxB_2 was reduced to 37% of control at 10^{-7} mol/L and 31% of control at 10^{-6} mol/L. Moreover, the synthesis of 6-keto-$PGF_{1\alpha}$ was not decreased at concentrations of OKY-1581 up to 10^{-6} mol/L. The formation of $PGF_{2\alpha}$, PGE_2, and PGD_2 was not decreased by OKY-1581 in concentrations up to 10^{-6} mol/L. The effects of OKY-1581 on thromboxane synthesis were also studied in two sheep. In these animals the lungs were removed after the animals were treated with OKY-1581, 10 mg/kg IV. When thromboxane synthesis activity was compared in homogenates from the treated animals, it was found to be markedly depressed when compared to control animals.

The influence of OKY-1581 on endoperoxide metabolism by sheep lung microsomal fraction was also investigated. In the absence of inhibitor, 166 ± 15 pmol of 6-keto-$PGF_{1\alpha}$ and 161 ± 17 pmol of TxB_2 were formed per two-minute period when 10 μmol/L PGH_2 was added to 200-μg microsomal protein. Prostaglandins $F_{2\alpha}$, E_2, and D_2 were also formed from PGH_2. However, addition of OKY-1581 in concentrations of 10^{-9} mol/L or higher reduced the formation of TxB_2, by more than 80% at the higher concentrations of the inhibitor. The formation of $PGF_{2\alpha}$, PGE_2, 6-keto–$PGF_{1\alpha}$, or PGD_2 was not reduced by OKY-1581.

The effects of the cyclo-oxygenase and thromboxane synthesis inhibitors on lobar vascular responses to arachidonic acid were also investigated in the sheep. Intralobar injections of arachidonic acid in doses of 30 and 100 μg caused a significant dose-dependent increase in lobar arterial pressure without affecting left atrial pressure. The increases in lobar arterial pressure in response to arachidonic acid were also decreased significantly after administration of OKY-1581, 5 to 10 mg/kg IV.

Effect of Ventilation on Responses to LTD_4 in the Sheep

The relationship between the effects of LTD_4 on ventilation and on the pulmonary vascular bed was studied in four sheep. In these experiments, responses to LTD_4 were obtained when the left lower lobe was ventilated and when lobar ventilation was arrested at end-expiration by inflating a balloon catheter in the left lower lobe bronchus. In these experiments, the left lower lobe was perfused with arterial blood to lessen the effects of hypoxia on the lung and 1 to 3 mL of a 2% lidocaine viscous solution was instilled into the lobar bronchus to prevent coughing. The correlation between the increases in lobar arterial pressure in response to intralobar injections of LTD_4, 0.1 to 1.0 μg, when the lobe was ventilated and when lobar ventilation was arrested was very good. The correlation coefficient of the regression line was 0.90 ($P < .05$) with a slope of (0.83) that was not significantly different from the line of identity. These data indicate that responses to LTD_4 are similar when the lobe is ventilated and when ventilation is arrested. These results suggest that the effects of LTD_4 on vascular and airway smooth muscle in the lung occur immediately.

Species and Responses to LTD_4 in the Pulmonary Vascular Bed

In order to determine if responses to LTD_4 varied with species, the effects of LTD_4 on the pulmonary vascular bed were investigated in the intact-chest cat and these data are summarized in Table 18-3. Intralobar injections of LTD_4 in doses of 0.3, 1.0, and 3.0 μg caused small but significant dose-related increases in lobar arterial pressure without affecting left atrial pressure. Systemic arterial pressure was increased significantly in response to intralobar injections of the 1.0- and 3.0-μg doses of LTD_4. Although lobar vascular responses to LTD_4 were modest in the cat, U-46619 had marked vasoconstrictor activity (Table 18-3). As described earlier, both LTD_4 and U-46619 had marked vasoconstrictor activity in the sheep pulmonary vascular bed and the dose-response curves for both substances in this species were superimposable. However, in the cat U-46619 had far greater vasoconstrictor activity than did LTD_4.

Table 18-3
Influence of Intralobar Injections of Leukotriene D_4 (LTD_4) and U-46619 on Mean Vascular Pressures in the Cat (n = 6–9)

	Pressure (mmHg)		
	Lobar Artery	*Left Atrium*	*Aorta*
Control	14 ± 1	3 ± 1	110 ± 5
LTD_4, 0.3 μg	16 ± 1*	3 ± 1	113 ± 5
Control	13 ± 1	2 ± 1	110 ± 8
LTD_4, 1.0 μg	16 ± 1*	2 ± 1	119 ± 6*
Control	13 ± 1	3 ± 1	115 ± 10
LTD_4, 3.0 μg	21 ± 2*	3 ± 1	124 ± 11*
Control	14 ± 2	3 ± 1	130 ± 8
U-46619, 0.003 μg	20 ± 3*	2 ± 1	133 ± 7
Control	12 ± 1	3 ± 1	124 ± 9
U-46619, 0.01 μg	23 ± 3*	3 ± 1	130 ± 7
Control	11 ± 2	3 ± 1	118 ± 6
U-46619, 0.03 μg	28 ± 4*	4 ± 2	124 ± 8

*$P < .05$ when compared to corresponding control, paired comparison.

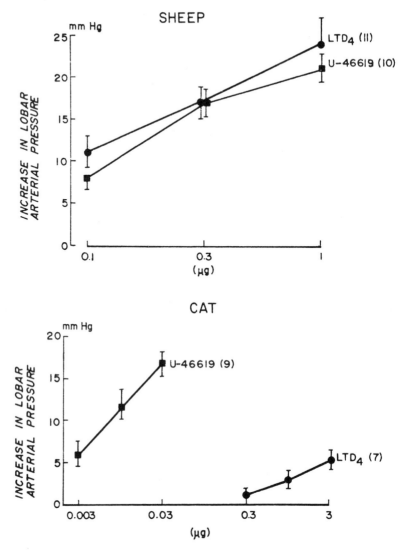

Figure 18-1 Dose-response curves comparing increases in lobar arterial pressure in response to injections of LTD_4 and U-46619 in the sheep (n = 11) and cat (n = 10).

Dose-response curves for LTD_4 and U-46619 are illustrated in Figure 18-1.

In other experiments in the sheep or in the cat, responses to LTD_4 were similar when the lung was perfused with blood or with low molecular weight dextran. The role of the cyclo-oxygenase pathway in the mediation of pulmonary vascular responses to LTD_4 was also investigated in

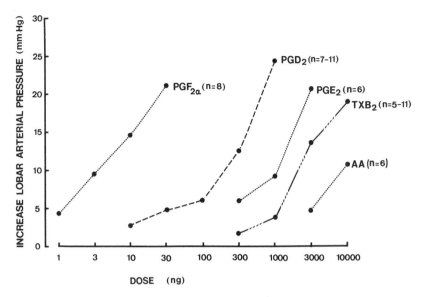

Figure 18-2 Dose-response relationships comparing increases in lobar arterial pressure in response to injections of graded doses of prostaglandins (PG) $F_{2\alpha}$, D_2, E_2, thromboxane (Tx) B_2, and arachidonic acid (AA) in the cat. n = number of cats.

the cat. Administration of indomethacin or sodium meclofenamate, 2.5 mg/kg IV, had no significant effect on pulmonary vasoconstrictor responses to U-46619 or LTD_4 in the cat. The increases in systemic arterial pressure in response to the 1.0- and 3.0-μg doses of LTD_4 were not altered by the cyclo-oxygenase inhibitors. However, the cyclo-oxygenase inhibitors, in the doses employed, significantly reduced the increases in lobar arterial pressure in response to intralobar injections of arachidonic acid. The cyclo-oxygenase inhibitors had no significant effect on pulmonary vascular or systemic arterial pressure in the cat. The effects of the cyclo-oxygenase products of arachidonic acid are shown in Figure 18-2. It can be seen that all products in this pathway had far greater vasoconstrictor activity than did LTD_4 in the feline pulmonary vascular bed.

DISCUSSION

Experiments in the intact-chest sheep demonstrate that intralobar injections of LTD_4 increase pulmonary lobar arterial pressure in a dose-related manner.[23] Since pulmonary blood flow was maintained constant and left atrial pressure was unchanged, the increase in pressure gradient across the lung lobe suggests that pulmonary lobar vascular resistance was increased by LTD_4.[23] The increases in lobar arterial pressure in response to LTD_4 were associated with dose-related increases in small intrapulmonary vein pressure. In addition to increasing lobar arterial and venous pressures, LTD_4 increased the pressure gradient from lobar artery to small vein. These experiments in the sheep suggest that LTD_4 increases pulmonary vascular resistance by constricting intrapulmonary veins and segments upstream to the small vein believed to be small arteries.[23] Results obtained in mature animals are consistent with results in the newborn lamb in which LTD_4 increased pulmonary and systemic vascular resistances and decreased cardiac output.[22,23] It has been reported that LTD_4 has potent coronary vasoconstrictor activity in the sheep that can be associated with left ventricular impairment.[27] However, in the sheep, LTD_4 had no significant effect on systemic arterial or left atrial pressures in the range of doses studied. The effects of LTD_4 on left atrial pressure in the newborn lamb were not measured so that the mechanism of the fall in cardiac output is uncertain.[22] The effects of LTD_4 on the systemic vascular resistance of the newborn lamb appear to be greater than those observed in the mature animal.

In terms of relative pressor activity in the pulmonary vascular bed of the sheep, LTD_4 was very potent with activity paralleling that of U-46619, a stable prostaglandin analog whose actions are thought to mimic those of TxA_2.[28] Moreover, when compared to other vasoactive hormones whose effects have been studied in the sheep, LTD_4 is far more active than other arachidonic acid metabolites, alveolar hypoxia, or histamine, which acts over a similar portion of the pulmonary vascular bed and is released along with the leukotrienes in immediate hypersensitivity reactions.[11,24,26,29]

It has been reported that LTD_4 has potent contractile activity on isolated airway smooth muscle and lung parenchyma and that it increases bronchomotor tone.[13,16-18] However, in the intact-chest sheep, the effects of LTD_4 on the pulmonary vascular bed appear to be independent of alterations in ventilation or those that occur as a consequence of changes in bronchomotor tone or lung volume, since similar responses were obtained when the lobe was ventilated or when lobar ventilation was arrested by obstruction of bronchial airflow. In previous studies, responses to a number of vasoactive substances including cyclo-oxygenase metabolites of arachidonic acid and histamine, were similar when the lobe was ventilated or lobar ventilation was arrested, suggesting that the actions of these vasoactive hormones on pulmonary vascular resistance appear to be independent of alterations in bronchomotor tone.[26,30] In both the cat and in the sheep, pulmonary hypertensive responses to LTD_4 appear similar when the lung was perfused with blood or low molecular weight dextran. Thus, responses to LTD_4 in both species are not dependent on the interaction with formed elements in blood.

In the sheep, pulmonary vasoconstrictor responses to LTD_4 were markedly attenuated after treatment with sodium meclofenamate suggesting that responses to this lipoxygenase product are dependent on the formation of products in the cyclo-oxygenase pathway. In addition, vasoconstrictor responses to LTD_4 were decreased by OKY-1581, a thromboxane synthesis inhibitor. These data suggest that a substantial portion of the pulmonary vasoconstrictor response to LTD_4 is due to the release of TxA_2. The observation that meclofenamate had greater inhibitory effect on responses to LTD_4 than did OKY-1581 suggests that pulmonary vasoconstrictor responses to this lipoxygenase metabolite are dependent on the formation of TxA_2 and other cyclo-oxygenase products such as PGD_2 and $PGF_{2\alpha}$ which have substantial pressor activity in the pulmonary vascular bed.[29,31] It has been shown that injections of SRSA or synthetic LTC_4 and LTD_4 cause the release of prostaglandins and TxA_2 from isolated guinea pig lung.[32,33] The results of the present experiments in the sheep are consistent with data obtained with isolated guinea pig parenchyma and on bronchoconstrictor responses in the guinea pig indicating that responses to LTD_4 are dependent on the release of TxA_2 and prostaglandins.[33,34]

A similar relationship between these inhibitors and responses to arachidonic acid was also observed in that there was a greater reduction in response to LTD_4 after treatment with meclofenamate than after OKY-1581. These data confirm previous studies showing that pulmonary vasoconstrictor responses to arachidonic acid are due to formation of products in the cyclo-oxygenase pathway,[30,35-38] and extend these findings by showing that a portion of the response is due to TxA_2 formation.

Although responses to LTD_4 and arachidonic acid were markedly reduced by meclofenamate, this cyclo-oxygenase inhibitor had no significant effect on pulmonary vasoconstrictor responses to U-46619, an analog whose actions are thought to mimic those of TxA_2.[28] These data indicate that sodium meclofenamate inhibited cyclo-oxygenase activity in the pulmonary vascular bed and that the cyclo-oxygenase inhibitor did not influence vascular responses to the thromboxane mimic. In addition, vasoconstrictor responses to U-46619 were not altered by OKY-1581 in doses that inhibited responses to LTD_4 and arachidonic acid. These results also suggest that the thromboxane synthesis inhibitor did not alter thromboxane receptor–mediated responses and that the effects of the inhibitor were due to inhibition of the formation of TxA_2. These data also suggest that TxA_2 would have marked vasoconstrictor activity in the sheep pulmonary vascular bed if U-46619 actually does mimic responses to this labile hormone. The inhibition of TxA_2 synthesis was also investigated in microsomal fractions from sheep lung. The results of these studies show that OKY-1581 inhibited the formation of TxA_2 as measured by formation of its stable breakdown product, TxB_2. Thromboxane B_2 formation was inhibited over a wide range of concentration of OKY-1581 when either arachidonic acid or the endoperoxide PGH_2 was employed as substrate. Although TxB_2 formation was decreased by OKY-1581, PGI_2 formation, as measured by the production of 6-keto-$PGF_{1\alpha}$, was not inhibited even at very high concentrations of the thromboxane synthesis inhibitor. Prostaglandins E_2, $F_{2\alpha}$, and D_2 were formed when PGH_2 or arachidonic acid was added to the microsomal fractions. It is not known if this prostaglandin synthesis was enzymatic; however, the amount of these substances formed was not decreased by OKY-1581 and in the case of PGE_2 was enhanced by the inhibitor. Since the total amount of product formed from arachidonic acid (6-keto-$PGF_{1\alpha}$, TxB_2, $PGF_{2\alpha}$, PGE_2, and PGD_2) was decreased, although TxB_2 formation was reduced, it is unlikely that OKY-1581 had a significant inhibitory effect on sheep lung cyclo-oxygenase activity. These experiments suggest that effects of OKY-1581 on responses to LTD_4 and arachidonic acid are due to inhibition of thromboxane synthetase activity and not to an effect on cyclo-oxygenase activity or on thromboxane receptor–mediated activity in the pulmonary vascular bed of the sheep. In other experiments in lung homogenates taken from sheep receiving OKY-1581, 5 to 10 mg/kg IV, TxB_2 formation was greatly reduced.

The results of studies in the sheep demonstrate that LTD_4 has very potent vasoconstrictor activity in the pulmonary vascular bed of this species and that this activity is due for the most part to release of products in the cyclo-oxygenase pathway. However, the effects of LTD_4 in the pulmonary vascular bed of the sheep and the cat are different. In the cat, LTD_4 had only modest pressor activity equal to that of arachidonic acid and far less than that of $PGF_{2\alpha}$, PGD_2, or PGE_2 in that species.[31] Furthermore, in this species, cyclo-oxygenase blockers did not modify responses to this lipoxygenase product. Although the relative magnitude of responses to LTD_4 as well as the mechanism of action differ in the sheep and the cat, both species were extremely sensitive to the effects of U-46619. Thus, there appears to be true species variation in the pulmonary vascular response to this lipoxygenase metabolite. This variation was not observed with U-46619 which may operate via TxA_2 receptors in the pulmonary vascular bed. In addition to demonstrating marked species variation in the response to LTD_4, the present data may be interpreted to suggest that LTD_4 itself does not have potent vasoconstrictor activity in the lung when the cyclo-oxygenase system is blocked. Moreover, the remaining pressor activity of LTD_4 in the sheep after cyclo-oxygenase blockade, and the similar pressor activity in the cat, suggest that the activity of this lipoxygenase metabolite is far less than that of products of the cyclo-oxygenase pathway such as TxA_2, $PGF_{2\alpha}$, or PGD_2.[31,39] The data from the present study suggest that it would be difficult to formulate a unified hypothesis on the role of LTD_4, a major component of SRSA, on the pulmonary circulation since species variation is so marked. The present data, however, suggest that LTD$_4$ could have pronounced effects on lobar arterial and small vein pressures in the sheep. These effects on venous pressures could contribute to an increase in capillary pressure and may alter fluid balance in the sheep lung. These hydrostatic effects along with alterations in capillary permeability which could occur as a consequence of lung injury could result in pulmonary edema and marked abnormalities in gas exchange.

SUMMARY

Pulmonary vasoconstrictor responses to leukotriene (LT) D$_4$ were compared in intact-chest sheep and under conditions of controlled lobar blood flow. Intralobar injections of LTD$_4$ in the sheep caused dose-dependent increases in lobar arterial and small vein pressures without altering left atrial or systemic arterial pressure. Leukotriene D$_4$ was very potent in increasing pulmonary vascular resistance in the sheep with activity similar to U-46619, a TxA$_2$ receptor mimic. Pulmonary vascular responses to LTD$_4$ in the sheep were similar when the lung was ventilated and when lobar ventilation was arrested, and when the lobe was perfused with blood or with artificial perfusate. Pulmonary vasoconstrictor responses to LTD$_4$, but not the thromboxane mimic, in the sheep were reduced by inhibitors of thromboxane and cyclo-oxygenase synthesis. In contrast, LTD$_4$ had modest vasoconstrictor activity in the pulmonary vascular bed of the cat whereas U-46619 had marked activity in this species. Responses to LTD$_4$ in the cat were not altered by cyclo-oxygenase inhibitors. It is concluded that LTD$_4$ has marked pulmonary vasoconstrictor activity in the sheep, increasing pulmonary vascular resistance by constricting intrapulmonary veins and upstream segments. In this species, responses to LTD$_4$ were independent of changes in ventilation or the interaction with formed elements but were dependent on the formation of cyclo-oxygenase products including TxA$_2$. However, in the cat LTD$_4$ had very weak pressor activity and this activity was not dependent on the integrity of the cyclo-oxygenase system. In this species, LTD$_4$ had far less vasoconstrictor activity than did prostaglandins E$_2$, F$_{2\alpha}$, or D$_2$. These studies indicate that there is considerable species difference in responses to LTD$_4$, a major component of the slow reacting substance of anaphylaxis, in the pulmonary vascular bed.

ACKNOWLEDGMENTS

Drs Joshua Rokeach and Barry M. Weichman provided the LTD$_4$ used in the study and Ms Alice Landry helped with the biochemical experiments. Ms Janice Ignarro helped in preparing the manuscript. This work was

244

supported by National Heart, Lung, and Blood Institute grants HL11802, HL15580, HL18070, and HL29456.

REFERENCES

1. Hammarstrom S: Leukotrienes. *Ann Rev Biochem* 1983;52:355-377.
2. Borgeat P, Samuelsson B: Arachidonic acid metabolism in polymorphonuclear leukocytes: unstable intermediates in formation of dihydroxy acids. *Proc Natl Acad Sci USA* 1979a;76:3212-3217.
3. Borgeat P, Samuelsson B: Metabolism of arachidonic acid in polymorphonuclear leukocytes: structural analysis of novel hydroxylated compounds. *J Biol Chem* 1979b;254:7865-7869.
4. Borgeat P, Hamberg M, Samuelsson B: Transformation of arachidonic acid and homo-γ-linolenic acid by rabbit polymorphonuclear leukocytes. Monohydroxy acids from novel lipoxygenases. *J Biol Chem* 1976;251: 7816-7820.
5. Ford-Hutchinson AW, Bray MA, Doig MV, et al: Leukotriene B: a potent chemokinetic and aggregating substance released from polymorphonuclear leukocytes. *Nature* 1980;286:264-265.
6. Murphy RC, Hammarstrom S, Samuelsson B: Leukotriene C: a slow reacting substance from murine mastocytoma cells. *Proc Natl Acad Sci USA* 1979;76:4275-4279.
7. Orning L, Hammarstrom S, Samuelsson B: Leukotriene D: a slow reacting substance from rat basophilic leukemic cells. *Proc Natl Acad Sci USA* 1980;77:2014-2017.
8. Morris HR, Taylor GW, Piper PJ, et al: Structure of slow-reacting substance of anaphylaxis from guinea-pig lung. *Nature* 1980;285:104-108.
9. Lewis RA, Austen KF, Drazen JM, et al: Slow reacting substances of anaphylaxis: identification of leukotrienes C and D from human and rat sources. *Proc Natl Acad Sci USA* 1980;77:3710-3714.
10. Kallaway CH, Trethewie DR: The liberation of slow reacting smooth muscle-stimulating substances in anaphylaxis. *Q J Exp Physiol* 1940;30:121-145.
11. Brocklehurst WE: The release of histamine and formation of a slow-reacting substance during anaphylactic shock. *J Physiol* 1960;151:416-435.
12. Dahlen SE, Hansson G, Hedqvist P, et al: Allergic challenge of lung tissue from asthmatics elicits bronchial contraction that correlates with the release of leukotriene C_4, D_4 and E_4. *Proc Natl Acad Sci USA* 1983;80:1712-1716.
13. Dahlen SE, Hedqvist P, Hammarstrom S, et al: Leukotrienes are potent constrictors of human bronchi. *Nature* 1980;288:484-486.
14. Hand JM, Will JA, Buckner CK: Effects of leukotrienes on isolated guinea-pig pulmonary arteries. *Eur J Pharmacol* 1981;76:439-443.
15. Krell RD, Osborn R, Vickery L, et al: Contraction of isolated airway smooth muscle by synthetic leukotrienes C_4 and D_4. *Prostaglandins* 1981;22:387-409.
16. Jones TR, Davis C, Daniel EE: Pharmacological study of the contractile activity of leukotrienes C_4 and D_4 on isolated human airway smooth muscle. *Can J Physiol Pharmacol* 1982;60:638-643.
17. Drazen JM, Austen KF, Lewis RA, et al: Comparative airway and vascular activities of leukotrienes C-1 and D *in vivo* and *in vitro*. *Proc Natl Acad Sci USA* 1980;77:4354-4358.
18. Holroyde MD, Altounyan REC, Cole M, et al: Bronchoconstriction produced in man by leukotrienes C and B. *Lancet* 1981;2:17-18.

19. Smedegard G, Hedqvist P, Dahlen SE, et al: Leukotriene C_4 affects pulmonary and cardiovascular dynamics in monkey. *Nature* 1982;295:327–329.
20. Iacopino VJ, Fitzpatrick TM, Ramwell PW, et al: Cardiovascular responses to leukotriene C_4 in the rat. *J Pharmacol Exp Ther* 1983;227:244–247.
21. Morganroth ML, Reeves JT, Murphy RC, et al: Leukotriene synthesis and receptor blockers block hypoxic pulmonary vasoconstriction. *J Appl Physiol* 1984;56:1340–1346.
22. Yokochi K, Olley PM, Sideris E, et al: Leukotriene D_4: a potent vasoconstrictor of the pulmonary and systemic circulations in the newborn lamb, in Samuelsson B, Paoletti R (eds): *Leukotrienes and Other Lipoxygenase Products.* New York, Raven Press, 1982, pp 211–214.
23. Kadowitz PJ, Hyman AL: Analysis of responses to leukotriene D_4 in the pulmonary vascular bed. *Circ Res* 1984;55:707–717.
24. Hyman AL, Kadowitz PJ: Effect of alveolar and perfusion hypoxia and hypercapnia on pulmonary vascular resistance in the lamb. *Am J Physiol* 1975; 228:397–403.
25. Hyman AL, Kadowitz PJ: Pulmonary vasodilator activity of prostacyclin (PGI_2) in the cat. *Circ Res* 1979;45:404–409.
26. Kadowitz PJ, Hyman AL: Pulmonary vascular responses to histamine in sheep. *Am J Physiol* 1983;244:H423–H428.
27. Michelassi F, Landa L, Hill RD, et al: Leukotriene D_4: a potent coronary artery vasoconstrictor associated with impaired ventricular contraction. *Science* 1982;217:841–843.
28. Coleman RA, Humphrey PPA, Kennedy I, et al: Comparison of the actions of U46619, a prostaglandin H_2-analogue, with those of prostaglandin H_2 and thromboxane A_2 on some isolated smooth muscle preparations. *Br J Pharmacol* 1981;73:773–778.
29. Kadowitz PJ, Joiner PD, Hyman AL: Influence of prostaglandins E_1 and $F_{2\alpha}$ on pulmonary vascular resistance in the sheep. *Proc Soc Exp Biol Med* 1974;145:1258–1261.
30. Hyman AL, Mathe AA, Leslie CA, et al: Modification of pulmonary vascular responses to arachidonic acid by alterations in physiologic state. *J Pharmacol Exp Ther* 1978;207:388–401.
31. Kadowitz PJ, Hyman AL: Comparative effects of thromboxane B_2 on the canine and feline pulmonary vascular bed. *J Pharmacol Exp Ther* 1980; 213:300–305.
32. Engineer DM, Morris HR, Piper PJ, et al: The release of prostaglandins and thromboxanes from guinea-pig lung by slow-reacting substances of anaphylaxis and its inhibition. *Br J Pharmacol* 1978;64:211–218.
33. Piper PJ, Samhoum MN: The mechanism of action of leukotriene C_4 and D_4 in guinea-pig isolated perfused lung and parenchymal strips of guinea pig. *Prostaglandins* 1981;21:793–803.
34. Weichman BM, Muccitelli RM, Osborn RR, et al: *In vitro* and *in vivo* mechanisms of leukotriene-mediated bronchoconstriction in the guinea pig. *J Pharmacol Exp Ther* 1982;222:202–208.
35. Hyman AL, Spannhake EW, Kadowitz PJ: Divergent responses to arachidonic acid in the feline pulmonary vascular bed. *Am J Physiol* 1980;239:H40–H46.
36. Spannhake EW, Hyman AL, Kadowitz PJ: Dependency of the airway and pulmonary vascular effects of arachidonic acid upon route and rate of administration. *J Pharmacol Exp Ther* 1980;212:584–590.
37. She HS, McNamara DB, Spannhake EW, et al: Metabolism of prostaglandin endoperoxide by microsomes from cat lung. *Prostaglandins* 1981;21:531–541.

38. Spannhake EW, Colombo JL, Craigo PA, et al: Evidence for modification of pulmonary cyclooxygenase activity by endotoxin in the dog. *J Appl Physiol* 1983;54:191–198.
39. Kadowitz PJ, Hyman AL: Influence of a prostaglandin endoperoxide analogue on the canine pulmonary vascular bed. *Circ Res* 1977;49:282–287.

19 Relationships Among Endothelium, cGMP, and Relaxation of Pulmonary Vessels

Louis J. Ignarro
Philip J. Kadowitz

The objective of this chapter is to briefly review the critically important role that vascular endothelium plays in modifying pulmonary vascular responses to endogenous vasoactive substances, but not to certain vasodilator drugs, and to review the hypothesis that cGMP is involved in the expression of the vascular smooth muscle relaxant effects elicited by both classes of vasodilator. Substantial experimental evidence has accumulated during the past six years to support the view that cGMP is intimately involved in the expression of the vascular smooth muscle relaxant effects of the nitrogen oxide–containing vasodilator drugs. These include sodium nitroprusside, amyl nitrite, sodium nitrite, and glyceryl trinitrate as well as other organic nitrate esters.[1,2] These vasodilators work by releasing or generating nitric oxide (NO) within the vascular smooth muscle cell, and this reaction may involve the formation of S-nitrosothiols from corresponding endogenous thiols.[3] In either case the liberated NO directly activates the soluble form of guanylate cyclase, resulting in a rapid and marked intracellular accumulation of cGMP which immediately precedes onset of relaxation.[3,4] Unlike the above vasodilator chemicals which are not dependent on vascular endothelium for their effects, various endogenous vasodilators such as acetylcholine are dependent on functioning endothelial cells to elicit their responses.[5-7] These endothelium-dependent vasodilators also appear to involve the actions of intracellular cGMP in mediating vascular smooth muscle relaxation.[8-12] Although vascular endothelium is not required for the cGMP-accumulating response to acetylcholine, the presence of endothelial cells markedly enhances the cGMP responses to acetylcholine.[11]

NITROGEN OXIDE–CONTAINING VASODILATORS

Until recently, the vasodilator effects of sodium nitroprusside, organic nitrites, and organic nitrates had been widely attributed to a "direct" interaction with vascular smooth muscle. The mechanism of action of these vasodilators has now been fairly well established,[1-4] and for this reason we have suggested the use of the more chemically descriptive terminology "nitrogen oxide–containing vasodilators."[3] The latter term is more appropriate than the former and is chemically correct as opposed to the term "nitrovasodilators," which is appearing in the literature. Sodium nitroprusside is actually a nitroso compound (nitrosoferricyanide) and nitroglycerin is a nitrate ester. None of these compounds are *nitro* vasodilators and, therefore, the use of the term nitrovasodilators is chemically incorrect and its use should be discouraged.

NO and Nitrosoguanidines

We first demonstrated that NO gas is a potent vascular smooth muscle relaxant.[13] The objective of this experiment was to ascertain whether chemical agents known to activate soluble guanylate cyclase also relax vascular smooth muscle. The rationale was if sodium nitroprusside, which releases NO, activates guanylate cyclase and if cGMP is involved in eliciting relaxation, then NO, which also stimulates cGMP formation, should cause relaxation. Figure 19-1 illustrates the marked but transient relaxant effect of NO on KCl-precontracted helical strips of bovine coronary artery.

Various hemoproteins inhibited the relaxant effect of NO (Figure 19-1) by sequestering and binding NO gas, thereby preventing the interaction between NO and the smooth muscle.[13] Methylene blue and ferricyanide are oxidants that inhibit soluble guanylate cyclase activity, especially enzyme activation by NO.[14] Methylene blue irreversibly antagonized relaxation caused by NO, although ferricyanide was ineffective (Figure 19-1). The reason for this difference in effects on vascular smooth muscle is that whereas methylene blue (vital biological stain) crosses cell membranes, ferricyanide (highly charged anion) does not. Methylene blue penetrates the smooth muscle cell and enters the cytosolic compartment where it inhibits soluble guanylate cyclase and cGMP formation, and therefore relaxation caused by agents that stimulate cGMP formation.

Several nitrosoamines or nitrosoguanidines were also shown to relax vascular smooth muscle both in vitro and in vivo.[13,15,16] The mechanism of vasodilatation by these agents is attributed to NO, which is readily released in aqueous solution, especially in the presence of free thiols.[17,18] Like NO, nitrosoguanidine-elicited relaxation is abolished by the guanylate cyclase inhibitor methylene blue.

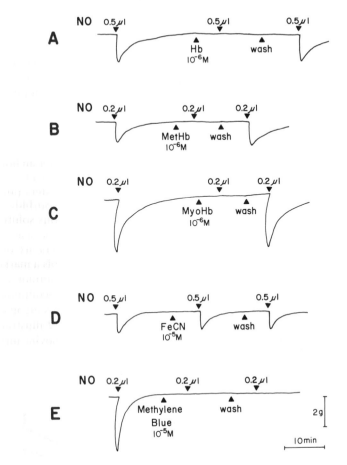

Figure 19-1 Effects of hemoglobin (Hb, panel **A**), methemoglobin (MetHb, panel **B**), myoglobin (MyoHb, panel **C**), potassium ferricyanide (FeCN, panel **D**), and methylene blue (panel **E**) on relaxation of 30 mmol/L KCl-precontracted bovine coronary arterial strips induced by nitric oxide (NO). Volumes of NO bubbled into the baths in these experiments elicited 25% to 50% reduction of induced tone. Note that after exposure to NO, isometric force spontaneously returned to precontracted levels. Rinsing the strips with 30 mmol/L K (wash) reversed the inhibitory effect of the heme proteins but not that of methylene blue. All concentrations are expressed as final bath concentrations. (Reproduced with permission from Gruetter et al.[13])

Vascular smooth muscle relaxation produced by NO is preceded by a rapid and marked accumulation of cGMP, and both smooth muscle responses are inhibited or abolished by methylene blue and hemoproteins.[3,4] Nitrosoguanidines produced similar effects. These observations have been made in bovine coronary artery, mesenteric artery, intrapulmonary artery, and intrapulmonary vein.[1-4,19] An excellent correlation

250

was consistently found between the capacity of these vasodilators to relax vascular smooth muscle, activate soluble guanylate cyclase, and stimulate intracellular cGMP accumulation, all of which were markedly inhibited by methylene blue.

Nitroprusside, Amyl Nitrite, and Nitroglycerin

Aqueous solutions of sodium nitroprusside are unstable after an hour; decomposition results from the discharge of NO gas, which oxidizes to NO_2 and turns the solution a yellow color. Organic nitrite esters (amyl or butyl nitrite) and organic nitrate esters (nitroglycerin, isosorbide dinitrate, pentaerythritol tetranitrate) are more stable in aqueous solution but are readily decomposed to nitrite anion and NO in the presence of thiols at weakly alkaline pH. Organic nitrite and nitrate esters are only weak activators of guanylate cyclase, but in the presence of thiols a marked enzyme activation results from the rapid formation of S-nitrosothiols and NO.[3,18] All of these clinically employed nitrogen oxide–containing vasodilator drugs relax vascular smooth muscle by mechanisms involving S-nitrosothiols, NO, and cGMP accumulation.[1-3] Figure 19-2 illustrates the relaxant effect of nitroglycerin on precontracted strips of bovine intra-

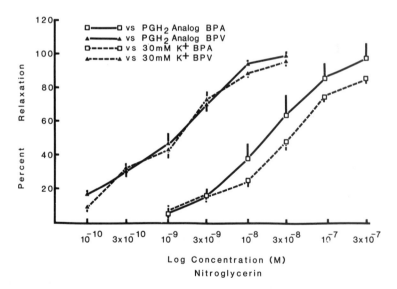

Figure 19-2 Concentration-relaxation curves for nitroglycerin in bovine intrapulmonary artery (BPA) and vein (BPV). Tone was induced with either 30 mmol/L KCl (K$^+$) or 10^{-8} mol/L U-46619 (PGH$_2$ analog) as indicated. Each point represents the mean ± SEM from seven to ten strips. (Reproduced with permission from Edwards et al.[19])

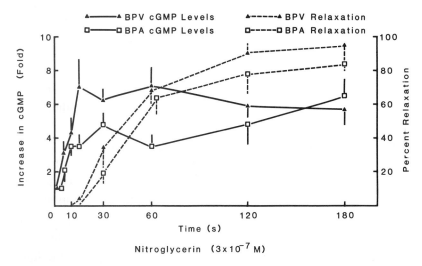

Figure 19-3 Time course relationships for relaxation and cGMP accumulation elicited by nitroglycerin. Tone was induced in strips of bovine intrapulmonary artery (BPA) and bovine intrapulmonary vein (BPV) with 30 mmol/L KCl. Basal cGMP levels were 6.7 ± 0.8 pmol/g of tissue in BPV and 9.4 ± 0.5 pmol/g tissue in BPA. Each point represents the mean $\pm$ SEM from four strips. (Reproduced with permission from Edwards et al.[19])

pulmonary artery and vein. Intrapulmonary veins were more sensitive than arteries to this relaxant effect. Relaxation was preceded by cGMP accumulation, which was more evident in veins than arteries (Figure 19-3). Methylene blue markedly inhibited both cellular responses to nitroglycerin in artery and vein.[19]

Responses very similar to those illustrated in Figures 19-2 and 19-3 were observed with sodium nitroprusside, nitroso compounds, and other organic nitrate esters.[2,19] Although added cGMP itself (8-Br-cGMP) relaxed both arteries and veins, there was no significant difference in the sensitivities between vessel types.[19] These observations suggest that the consistent differences in sensitivities to relaxation caused by the nitrogen oxide–containing vasodilators is attributed to cellular events occurring prior to whatever effect cGMP itself elicits to promote smooth muscle relaxation. We have preliminary evidence that unpurified soluble guanylate cyclase fractions from intrapulmonary vein are more responsive than are those from artery to activation by NO and related agents. Unlike the vasodilators that elevate cGMP levels, those that elevate cAMP levels (isoproterenol) are equipotent in intrapulmonary arteries and veins.[19] Prostacyclin (PGI_2), on the other hand, which also activates adenylate cyclase, is much more potent as a relaxant of intrapulmonary artery than vein.[20]

Bovine intrapulmonary veins may not possess receptors for PGI$_2$,[20] although this tissue is capable of synthesizing the prostaglandin.[21,22]

S-Nitrosothiols

Earlier observations in this laboratory on the enhancement by thiols of activation of vascular soluble guanylate cyclase by nitrogen oxides led to the discovery of the formation of S-nitrosothiols when thiols are allowed to react with the nitrogen oxides.[17,18,23] Several S-nitrosothiols were synthesized and found to relax vascular smooth muscle, cause vasodilatation in vivo, activate soluble guanylate cyclase, and stimulate intracellular cGMP accumulation.[3,19,24-26] S-Nitroso-N-acetylpenicillamine, a stable crystalline material, was found to mimic the relaxant and cGMP-accumulating effects of nitroglycerin in bovine intrapulmonary artery and vein (Figure 19-4). Hemodynamically, systemic injections of S-nitrosothiols elicit responses that cannot be distinguished from those of sodium nitroprusside or nitroglycerin.[3] S-Nitrosothiols are potent systemic vasodilators (Figure 19-5). Moreover, they elicit direct pulmonary vasodilator responses in the intact-chest dog, and these responses are virtually identical in characteristics to those produced by sodium nitroprusside and nitroglycerin.[27] All agents decreased pulmonary arterial pressure and in-

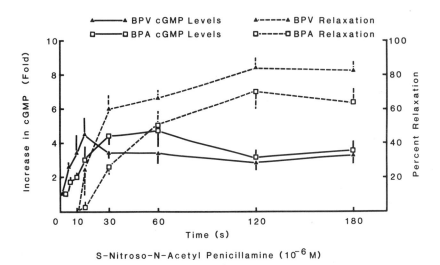

Figure 19-4 Time course relationships for relaxation and cGMP accumulation elicited by S-nitroso-N-acetylpenicillamine. Tone was induced in strips of bovine intrapulmonary artery (BPA) and bovine intrapulmonary vein (BPV) with 30 mmol/L KCl. Basal cyclic GMP levels were 6.7±0.8 pmol/g of tissue in BPV and 9.4±0.5 pmol/g of tissue in BPA. Each point represents the mean±SEM from four strips. (Reproduced with permission from Edwards et al.[19])

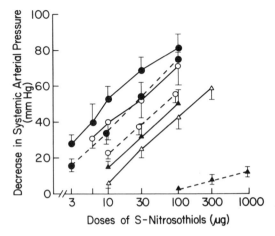

Figure 19-5 Effects of S-nitrosothiols, nitroprusside, nitroglycerin (GTN), and NaNO$_2$ on systemic arterial pressure in the anesthetized cat. Symbols: ●———●, S-nitrosocysteine; ○———○, S-nitroso-N-acetylpenicillamine; ▲———▲, S-nitroso-2-mercaptoethlyamine; △———△, S-nitroso-3-mercaptopropionic acid; ●---●, nitroprusside; ○----○, GTN;▲----▲, NaNO$_2$. Each value represents the mean ±SE for six cats. For experimental details, see Ignarro et al.[3] (Reproduced with permission from Ignarro et al.[3])

creased cardiac output without altering left atrial pressure and these responses were enhanced when pulmonary vascular tone was elevated by infusion of vasoconstrictors that increase pulmonary vascular resistance by constricting intrapulmonary veins and upstream segments. S-Nitrosothiols thereby resemble other nitrogen oxide–containing vasodilators in that they decrease pulmonary vascular resistance by dilating intrapulmonary veins and upstream segments.

Based on our observations and on those made earlier by Needleman and coworkers,[28,29] who suggested that nitroglycerin reacts with thiol receptors to produce its relaxant effect and to inactivate the vasodilator by monodenitration, we offered the view that organic nitrate esters and other nitrogen oxide–containing vasodilators react with thiols to generate S-nitrosothiols, which then elicit vascular smooth muscle relaxation.[3] The generated S-nitrosothiols themselves or more likely NO, which is spontaneously released, activates guanylate cyclase, elevates cGMP levels in smooth muscle cells, and relaxation ensues. Organic nitrate esters probably cause tolerance to vascular smooth muscle relaxation by depletion of critical thiols in the cells.[28,29] Perhaps this results in little or no formation of S-nitrosothiols and therefore NO, and the overall result is little or no cGMP formation or relaxation.[1-3] Tolerance to the relaxant effect of nitroglycerin is associated closely with the development of tolerance to its capacity to stimulate cGMP formation.[30-32] Preliminary observations in this laboratory indicate that S-nitrosothiols do not induce vascular tolerance and that S-nitrosothiols are fully responsive in vessels rendered tolerant to the relaxant effects of nitroglycerin.

All of the above views are strengthened by the recent report by Horowitz et al[33] that patients who had developed severe tolerance to the cardiovascular effects of nitroglycerin were rapidly and dramatically alleviated from this problem after the intravenous (IV) infusion of N-acetylcysteine. This pretreatment also allowed a significant reduction in the doses of nitroglycerin needed to produce responses comparable to those evident prior to the development of tolerance.

METHYLENE BLUE

Until our recent studies with methylene blue, no antagonists of the vascular smooth muscle effects of nitroglycerin or sodium nitroprusside had been known. We reported that methylene blue, an inhibitor of soluble guanylate cyclase,[14] antagonized the vascular smooth muscle relaxant effects of all of the nitrogen oxide–containing vasodilators[13,34] and also the relaxant effects of endothelium-dependent endogenous vasodilators that stimulate cGMP formation.[11,20] Methylene blue is selective for relaxants that work by stimulating soluble guanylate cyclase, either directly or indirectly. Thus, the relaxant effects of isoproterenol, prostacyclin, and calcium antagonists are not affected. Also, methylene blue does not alter resting cAMP levels or the accumulation of cAMP caused by isoproterenol or prostacyclin. More recent experiments in this laboratory[35] indicate that methylene blue and related vital biological stains lower resting levels of cGMP in intrapulmonary artery and thereby enhance contractile responses to potassium, phenylephrine, and other agents. Large concentrations of these stains actually cause slowly developing contractile responses. These actions of methylene blue are more prominent in arteries possessing an intact endothelium as opposed to damaged endothelium. This is explained by the observations that endothelial cells continually generate relaxing factors which activate guanylate cyclase, elevate cGMP levels, and decrease tone. Endothelium-damaged arteries do not behave in this manner. Resting levels of cGMP are about four- to sixfold higher in endothelium-intact than in endothelium-damaged intrapulmonary artery.

Intrapulmonary veins with intact endothelium have lower resting cGMP levels than do arteries and are less sensitive to the contractile effects of methylene blue. Veins appear to have a much lower capacity to generate endothelium-derived relaxing substances both at resting conditions and in the presence of endothelium-dependent arterial relaxants.[2,20,35] In the absence of endothelium, however, the marked relaxant responses to the nitrogen oxide-containing vasodilators are inhibited or abolished by methylene blue.[3,4,19]

Cyanide, a known but weak inhibitor of soluble guanylate cyclase under certain defined conditions,[36-38] was reported to inhibit the relaxant and cGMP accumulating effects of sodium nitroprusside but not that of nitroglycerin.[39] Another group reported that cyanide inhibits relaxation and cGMP accumulation produced by both vasodilators and related agents.[40] Extensive preliminary observations in this laboratory indicate that cyanide inhibits only the responses to sodium nitroprusside and not those elicited by other nitrogen oxide–containing vasodilators or acetylcholine.[35] Moreover, cyanide appears to inhibit sodium nitroprusside by chemically reacting with the nitrosopentacyanoate anion to yield ferricyanide and NO_2. Such a chemical reaction cannot occur with organic nitrites, nitrates, and organic nitroso compounds. Thus, it would appear that cyanide is not nearly as useful as methylene blue as a pharmacologic inhibitor of vascular smooth muscle relaxation caused by vasodilators that stimulate soluble guanylate cyclase.

ENDOTHELIUM-DEPENDENT ENDOGENOUS VASODILATORS

Since the original discovery by Furchgott and Zawadzki[5] that acetylcholine relaxes arterial smooth muscle by endothelium-dependent mechanisms, other endogenous substances have been found to relax arteries by mechanisms necessitating the presence of functioning endothelial cells (see review[12]). These endogenous substances include bradykinin, substance P, certain other peptides, arachidonic acid, histamine, and serotonin in certain arteries, calcium ionophores, and related agents. Most of the published studies have been with systemic arteries, and little work in this regard has been done with pulmonary vessels or with veins.

Acetylcholine

We reported that acetylcholine relaxes precontracted bovine intrapulmonary arterial rings by endothelium mechanisms involving the marked stimulation of cGMP accumulation.[11] Acetylcholine elicits time- and concentration-dependent increases in cGMP levels in intrapulmonary artery with endothelium (Figure 19-6 and 19-7). The endothelial receptors are muscarinic in nature because atropine blocks both relaxation and cGMP accumulation. Soluble guanylate cyclase is involved in the formation of cGMP because methylene blue inhibits both cellular responses. Intrapulmonary veins only contract in response to acetylcholine, an effect that is blocked by atropine and enhanced by methylene blue. Cyclic GMP levels increase slightly but no relaxation is observed. The enhancement of

256

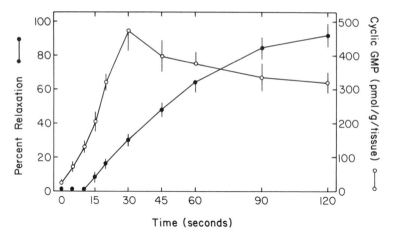

Figure 19-6 Time course of cGMP accumulation and relaxation in bovine intrapulmonary arterial rings elicited by acetylcholine. Arterial rings were isolated with an intact endothelium and were submaximally contracted with 10^{-5} mol/L phenylephrine before exposure to acetylcholine (10^{-6} mol/L). Rings were freeze-clamped at the time indicated. Values represent the mean ± SE using six to 12 arterial rings isolated from three to six separate animals. Relaxation and cGMP levels were determined in the same arterial rings. Relaxation is expressed as the percentage of decrease in phenylephrine-induced tone. (Reproduced with permission from Ignarro et al.[11])

contractile responses by methylene blue is attributed to suppression of formation of cGMP, thereby resulting in enhancement of tone due to removal of the intracellular relaxant cGMP. Similar observations were made with endothelium-damaged arterial rings. The arterial endothelial cells apparently stimulate cGMP formation in smooth muscle even under resting conditions with tension applied. This view is substantiated by the findings that resting levels of cGMP are four- to sixfold higher in endothelium-intact than in endothelium-damaged arteries. The differences in veins are much smaller, and endothelium-intact veins have two- to threefold lower resting cGMP levels than do endothelium-intact arteries.[35]

Arachidonic Acid

Arachidonic acid elicits arterial responses that are more complicated to interpret than those of acetylcholine. Arachidonic acid relaxes bovine intrapulmonary arterial rings by two distinct endothelium-dependent mechanisms involving both cGMP and cAMP.[20] Concentrations of 0.01 to 1 μmol/L arachidonic acid elicit indomethacin-sensitive relaxant responses associated with cAMP accumulation whereas higher concentrations elicit indomethacin-insensitive but methylene blue–sensitive relaxant responses associated with cGMP and cAMP accumulation. Indomethacin

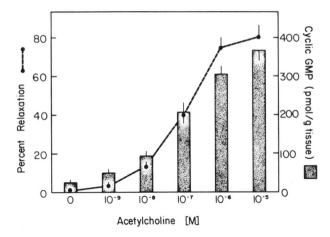

Figure 19-7 Concentration-dependent cGMP accumulation and relaxation in bovine intrapulmonary arterial rings elicited by acetylcholine. Arterial rings were isolated with an intact endothelium and were submaximally contracted with 10^{-5} mol/L phenylephrine before exposure to acetylcholine. All rings were freeze-clamped at exactly 60 seconds after the addition of acetylcholine to bath chambers. Values represent the mean ± SE using six to ten arterial rings isolated from three to five separate animals. Relaxation and cGMP levels were determined in the same arterial rings. Relaxation is expressed as the percentage of decrease in phenylephrine-induced tone. (Reproduced with permission from Ignarro et al.[11])

abolishes cAMP accumulation and also relaxation caused by the lower concentrations of arachidonic acid. In the presence of indomethacin the large relaxant responses and cGMP accumulation caused by 10 μmol/L arachidonic acid are abolished by methylene blue. Therefore, all relaxant responses to arachidonic acid are nearly abolished when the formation of both cGMP and cAMP are markedly inhibited.[20] The indomethacin/cAMP component of the relaxant response is attributed to a vasodilator prostaglandin such as prostacyclin. The methylene blue/cGMP component is attributed to an endothelium-derived relaxing factor that is unrelated to prostaglandins.

Endothelium-Derived Relaxing Factor

The endothelium-derived relaxing factor involved in the relaxant response to arachidonic acid is unknown at this time. Efforts to gain insight into this important problem were unsuccessful in experiments designed to obtain meaningful information with the use of inhibitors such as quinacrine, nordihydroguaiaretic acid, SKF-525A, metyrapone, and iproniazid. All of these agents are nonselective inhibitors of multiple enzymatic pathways and merely confounded the interpretation of our observations.[11,20] The nature of the endothelium-derived relaxing factor(s) is

258

unknown, and appears not to be the same factor as that associated with acetylcholine, or an arachidonic acid metabolite of either the cyclo-oxygenase or lipoxygenase pathway.[11,20,41] Nor does this factor appear to be an oxygen radical,[41,42] as originally proposed.[5,6,12]

Griffith et al[41] have been successful in demonstrating the generation and release of an unknown and highly unstable relaxant substance from arterial endothelium in response to acetylcholine. Through the use of perfusion- and superfusion-cascade experiments, we have been only partially successful in making similar observations. Methods need to be developed to trap and stabilize the endothelium-derived factors in order to study their pharmacologic properties. Recent preliminary experiments in this laboratory indicate that soluble guanylate cyclase purified to homogeneity from bovine lung is partially activated (twofold) when previously depolarized rings of endothelium-intact bovine intrapulmonary artery are submerged in enzyme reaction mixtures fortified with calcium and GSH. Acetylcholine, which does not activate guanylate cyclase, further stimulated enzymatic activity in the presence of arterial rings (four- to six-fold). Neither arterial rings that had been rubbed to remove endothelial cells nor endothelium-intact intrapulmonary veins activated guanylate cyclase in the absence or presence of acetylcholine. Although these observations suggest that arterial endothelial factors directly activate the soluble form of guanylate cyclase, definitive conclusions await the isolation, identification, and testing of the endothelium-derived factor(s).

Endogenous Peptides

Certain peptides appear to relax arterial smooth muscle by endothelium-dependent mechanisms. These include bradykinin, substance P, cholecystokinin, and some others (see review[12]). Preliminary observations in this laboratory indicate that bradykinin relaxes both intrapulmonary artery and vein by endothelium-dependent mechanisms involving cGMP.[43] Bradykinin is the only substance that we have found which relaxes not only artery but also vein by endothelium-dependent mechanisms. A 23-amino acid fragment of atrial natriuretic factor was found to be vasoactive in pulmonary arteries but not veins. This peptide relaxes intrapulmonary artery by endothelium-independent mechanisms involving the accumulation of cGMP but not cAMP.[43] Interestingly, intrapulmonary veins are unaffected by this arterial vasoactive peptide. At first, it appeared that the arterial relaxant response to vasoactive atrial natriuretic factor was similar in mechanism to that of nitroglycerin and sodium nitroprusside because endothelium did not influence relaxant responses. Such is not the case, however, because veins are insensitive to the peptide whereas veins are even more sensitive than arteries to the relaxant responses of nitroglycerin and sodium nitroprusside.[19] Moreover, methylene blue, an inhibitor of soluble guanylate cyclase, abolishes vascular responses to the nitrogen oxides but does not alter the responses to the peptide.[43] Since the cGMP accumulation in response to the peptide is not inhibited by methylene blue and related dyes, soluble guanylate cyclase cannot be involved in the stimulation of cGMP formation. Phosphodiesterase inhibition is an unlikely mechanism because the peptide does not inhibit phosphodiesterase activity in extracts prepared from lung. One possibility is that membrane-bound or particulate guanylate cyclase is stimulated by the peptide, and this view is supported by our findings that methylene blue does not inhibit particulate guanylate cyclase activity. However, we could find no evidence for the activation by the atrial natriuretic peptide of particulate guanylate cyclase prepared from lung, arteries, or liver.

IN VIVO OBSERVATIONS

In intact-chest dogs and cats, intralobar injections of arachidonic acid elevate pulmonary vascular resistance by constricting intrapulmonary veins and upstream segments.[44,45] The conversion of arachidonic acid to cyclo-oxygenase products and the blockade of constrictor responses by cyclo-oxygenase inhibitors indicate that constrictor responses to arachidonic acid are attributed to cyclo-oxygenase products.[45] Injections of small doses of arachidonic acid often cause decreases in pulmonary vascular resistance which are enhanced in the presence of actively elevated pulmonary vascular tone.[44] Prostacyclin elicits similar effects.[44] Cyclo-oxygenase products are likely responsible for both vasoconstrictor and vasodilator responses to arachidonic acid because indomethacin abolishes both responses. These in vivo observations raise some questions regarding the physiologic relevance of the *in vitro* findings that noncyclo-oxygenase metabolites of arachidonic acid markedly relax intrapulmonary artery.[20] More in vivo studies are necessary in order to answer this question.

More recently, responses to acetylcholine and vagal stimulation were investigated in the feline pulmonary vascular bed under conditions of controlled pulmonary blood flow and left atrial pressure.[46] Electrical stimulation of vagal efferent fibers increased lobar arterial pressure but a depressor response was unmasked in the presence of elevated pulmonary vascular tone. Similar responses were produced by injections of acetylcholine.[46] Depressor responses to vagal stimulation and acetylcholine in animals treated with 6-hydroxydopamine were blocked by atropine and enhanced by physostigmine. It is important to note that the lipoxygenase inhibitor, 5,8,11,14-eicosatetraynoic acid, failed to alter vascular responses to injected acetylcholine.[46] The latter observations are consistent with our conclusions from in vitro experiments which suggest that lipoxygenase metabolites of arachidonic acid may not represent the endothelium-derived relaxing factor(s) that mediates vascular smooth muscle relaxation in response to acetylcholine.[2,11,20] Therefore, although it is clear that the feline pulmonary vascular bed is functionally innervated by cholinergic fibers which when stimulated result in pulmonary vasodilatation mediated by vascular muscarinic receptors, the question of whether or not endothelium-derived factors are involved in such physiologic responses remains to be answered.

CONCLUSIONS

The responsiveness of the pulmonary vasculature to vasodilator therapy depends on many factors including the presence and extent of lung injury as well as the type of vasodilator therapy employed. Although many endogenous vasoactive substances relax pulmonary arterial smooth muscle in vitro by endothelium-dependent mechanisms, pulmonary veins generally contract under similar conditions. Thus, endothelium-intact veins behave similarly to endothelium-damaged arteries. One exception is the nonapeptide bradykinin, which relaxes both pulmonary arteries and veins by endothelium-dependent mechanisms. In vitro studies have clearly defined the dramatic influence of vascular endothelial cells on arterial responses to endogenous vasodilators. Questions still remain unanswered, however, as to the role of endothelial cells in vivo in the modulation of local changes in vascular tone in response to acetylcholine and vasoactive autacoids.

Unlike the naturally occurring vasodilators, the nitrogen oxide–containing vasodilator drugs elicit their effects by endothelium-independent mechanisms. Pulmonary vascular responsiveness to the latter vasodilator drugs is very different from responses to agents such as acetylcholine and bradykinin. Nitroglycerin and sodium nitroprusside markedly dilate pulmonary veins and arteries both in vitro and in vivo. Indeed, the veins are generally more sensitive than are the arteries to relaxation elicited by these drugs. Acetylcholine, on the other hand, relaxes endothelium-intact arteries but not veins, at least in vitro. As discussed earlier, an unequivocal statement that endothelium is required for acetylcholine-elicited vasodilation in the intact animal cannot be made at this time.

Despite the clear differences in mechanism of action between the nitrogen oxide vasodilator drugs and endogenous vasodilator substances, the final mechanism of vascular smooth muscle relaxation by both classes of agent appears to be similar, if not identical. All of these vasodilators stimulate the formation of cGMP in a time- and concentration-dependent manner in vascular smooth muscle. Soluble or cytoplasmic guanylate cyclase is the target site for activation because methylene blue, a relatively selective inhibitor of this enzyme, inhibits both relaxation and cGMP accumulation which normally occur in response to nitroglycerin, sodium nitroprusside, acetylcholine, arachidonic acid, or bradykinin. Figure 19-8

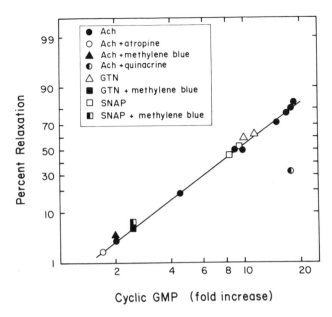

Figure 19-8 Correlation between bovine intrapulmonary arterial relaxation and cGMP accumulation elicited by acetylcholine (Ach), nitroglycerin (GTN), and S-nitroso-N-acetylpenicillamine (SNAP). All values represent those obtained 60 seconds after addition of relaxant agents. Percentage of relaxation is plotted on a probit scale and cGMP levels are expressed as -fold increase on a log scale. Cyclic GMP values were converted to percentage of maximum for calculation of the rank correlation coefficient ($r = .92$). The following concentrations of agents were tested: atropine, 10^{-7} mol/L; methylene blue, 10^{-5} mol/L; quinacrine, 10^{-5} mol/L; GTN, 10^{-7} mol/L; SNAP, 10^{-6} mol/L; and Ach, 10^{-9} to 10^{-5} mol/L. (Data points were taken with permission from Ignarro et al.[11])

illustrates the excellent correlation obtained between arterial relaxation and cGMP accumulation in response to various vasodilators that stimulate guanylate cyclase either directly or indirectly. There is now good experimental evidence that vasodilators, which stimulate cGMP formation in aorta, also stimulate protein phosphorylation.[47,48] Cyclic GMP may cause vascular smooth muscle relaxation by stimulating the protein kinase–mediated phosphorylation of a protein capable of rapidly binding intracellular free calcium.[49]

ACKNOWLEDGMENTS

The authors acknowledge the technical assistance given by Keith S. Wood, Richard G. Harbison, and Theresa Burke, and the assistance of Jan Ignarro in the preparation and editing of the manuscript.

REFERENCES

1. Ignarro LJ, Gruetter CA, Hyman AL, et al: Molecular mechanisms of vasodilatation, in Poste G, Crooke ST (eds): *Dopamine Receptor Agonists.* New York, Plenum Press, 1984, pp 259-288.
2. Ignarro LJ, Kadowitz PJ: Pharmacological and physiological role of cyclic GMP in vascular smooth muscle relaxation. *Ann Rev Pharmacol* 1985; 25:171-191.
3. Ignarro LJ, Lippton H, Edwards JC, et al: Mechanism of vascular smooth muscle relaxation by organic nitrates, nitrites, nitroprusside and nitric oxide: evidence for the involvement of S-nitrosothiols as active intermediates. *J Pharmacol Exp Ther* 1981;218:739-749.
4. Gruetter CA, Gruetter DY, Lyon JE, et al: Relationship between cyclic GMP formation and relaxation of coronary arterial smooth muscle by glyceryl trinitrate, nitroprusside, nitrite and nitric oxide: effects of methylene blue and methemoglobin. *J Pharmacol Exp Ther* 1981;219:181-186.
5. Furchgott RF, Zawadzki JV: The obligatory role of endothelial cells in the relaxation of arterial smooth muscle by acetylcholine. *Nature* 1980;288: 373-376.
6. Furchgott RF: Role of endothelium in responses of vascular smooth muscle. *Circ Res* 1983;53:557-573.
7. Furchgott RF, Cherry PD, Zawadzki JV, et al: Endothelial cells as mediators of vasodilation of arteries. *J Cardiovasc Pharmacol* 1984;6:S336-S343.
8. Holzmann S: Endothelium-induced relaxation by acetylcholine associated with larger rises in cyclic GMP in coronary arterial strips. *J Cyclic Nucleotide Res* 1982;8:409-419.
9. Diamond J, Chu EB: Possible role for cyclic GMP in endothelium-dependent relaxation of rabbit aorta by acetylcholine. Comparison with nitroglycerin. *Res Commun Chem Pathol Pharmacol* 1983;41:369-381.
10. Rapoport RM, Murad F: Agonist-induced endothelium-dependent relaxation in rat thoracic aorta may be mediated through cGMP. *Circ Res* 1983; 52:352-357.
11. Ignarro LJ, Burke TM, Wood KS, et al: Association between cyclic GMP accumulation and acetylcholine-elicited relaxation of bovine intrapulmonary artery. *J Pharmacol Exp Ther* 1984;228:682-690.
12. Furchgott RF: The role of endothelium in the responses of vascular smooth muscle to drugs. *Ann Rev Pharmacol* 1984;24:175-197.
13. Gruetter CA, Barry BK, McNamara DB, et al: Relaxation of bovine coronary artery and activation of coronary arterial guanylate cyclase by nitric oxide, nitroprusside and a carcinogenic nitrosoamine. *J Cyclic Nucleotide Res* 1979; 5:211-224.
14. Murad F, Mittal CK, Arnold WP, et al: Guanylate cyclase activation by azide, nitro compounds, nitric oxide, and hydroxyl radical and inhibition by hemoglobin and myoglobin. *Adv Cyclic Nucleotide Res* 1978;9:145-158.
15. Gruetter CA, Barry BK, McNamara DB, et al: Coronary arterial relaxation and guanylate cyclase activation by cigarette smoke, N'-nitrosonornicotine and nitric oxide. *J Pharmacol Exp Ther* 1980;214:9-15.
16. Lippton HL, Gruetter CA, Ignarro LJ, et al: Vasodilator actions of several N-nitroso compounds. *Can J Physiol Pharmacol* 1982;60:68-75.
17. Ignarro LJ, Edwards JC, Gruetter DY, et al: Possible involvement of S-nitrosothiols in the activation of guanylate cyclase by nitroso compounds. *FEBS Lett* 1980;110:275-278.

18. Ignarro LJ, Gruetter CA: Requirement of thiols for activation of coronary arterial guanylate cyclase by glyceryl trinitrate and sodium nitrite: possible involvement of S-nitrosothiols. *Biochim Biophys Acta* 1980;631:221–231.
19. Edwards JC, Ignarro LJ, Hyman AL, et al: Relaxation of intrapulmonary artery and vein by nitrogen oxide-containing vasodilators and cyclic GMP. *J Pharmacol Exp Ther* 1984;228:33–42.
20. Ignarro LJ, Harbison RG, Wood KS, et al: Mechanism of intrapulmonary arterial relaxation by arachidonic acid: evidence for the involvement of cyclic GMP and cyclic AMP. *J Pharmacol Exp Ther* 1985;233:560–569.
21. McMullen-Laird M, McNamara DB, Kerstein MD, et al: Human lung metabolism of prostaglandin endoperoxide. *Circulation* 1982;66:166.
22. Kerstein MD, Saroyan M, McMullen-Laird M, et al: Metabolism of prostaglandins in human saphenous vein. *J Surg Res* 1983;35:91–100.
23. Ignarro LJ, Barry BK, Gruetter DY, et al: Guanylate cyclase activation by nitroprusside and nitrosoguanidine is related to formation of S-nitrosothiol intermediates. *Biochem Biophys Res Commun* 1980;94:93–100.
24. Wolin MS, Wood KS, Ignarro LJ: Guanylate cyclase from bovine lung: a kinetic analysis of the regulation of the purified soluble enzyme by protoporphyrin IX, heme and nitrosyl-heme. *J Biol Chem* 1982;257:13312–13320.
25. Ignarro LJ, Wood KS, Ballot B, et al: Guanylate cyclase from bovine lung: evidence that enzyme activation by phenylhydrazine is mediated by iron-phenyl hemoprotein complexes. *J Biol Chem* 1984;259:5923–5931.
26. Ignarro LJ, Wood KS, Wolin MS: Regulation of purified soluble guanylate cyclase by porphyrins and metalloporphyrins: a unifying concept. *Adv Cyclic Nucleotide Res* 1984;17:267–274.
27. Kadowitz PJ, Nandiwada P, Gruetter CA, et al: Pulmonary vasodilator responses to nitroprusside and nitroglycerin in the dog. *J Clin Invest* 1981;67:893–902.
28. Needleman P, Johnson EM: Mechanism of tolerance development to organic nitrates. *J Pharmacol Exp Ther* 1973;184:709–715.
29. Needleman P, Jakschik B, Johnson EM: Sulfhydryl requirement for relaxation of vascular smooth muscle. *J Pharmacol Exp Ther* 1973; 187:324–331.
30. Keith RA, Burkman AM, Sokoloski TD, et al: Vascular tolerance to nitroglycerin and cyclic GMP generation in rat aortic smooth muscle. *J Pharmacol Exp Ther* 1982;221:525–531.
31. Axelsson KL, Andersson RGG, Wikberg JES: Vascular smooth muscle relaxation by nitro compounds: reduced relaxation and cyclic GMP elevation in tolerant vessels and reversal of tolerance by dithiothreitol. *Acta Pharmacol Toxicol* 1982;50:350–357.
32. Axelsson KL, Andersson RGG: Tolerance towards nitroglycerin, induced in vivo, is correlated to a reduced cGMP response and an alteration in cGMP turnover. *Eur J Pharmacol* 1983;88:71–79.
33. Horowitz JD, Antman EM, Lorell BH, et al: Potentiation of cardiovascular effects of nitroglycerin by N-acetylcysteine. *Circulation* 1983;68:1247–1253.
34. Gruetter CA, Kadowitz PJ, Ignarro LJ: Methylene blue inhibits coronary arterial relaxation and guanylate cyclase activation by nitroglycerin, sodium nitrite and amyl nitrite. *Can J Physiol Pharmacol* 1981;59:150–156.
35. Ignarro LJ, Harbison RG, Wood KS, et al: Role of endothelium-derived relaxant factor (EDRF) in regulation of vascular smooth muscle cGMP levels and tone: properties of methylene blue. *Fed Proc* 1985;44:1235.
36. Kimura J, Mittal CK, Murad F: Activation of guanylate cyclase from rat liver and other tissues by sodium azide. *J Biol Chem* 1975;250:8016–8022.

37. Gerzer R, Böhme E, Hofmann F, et al: Soluble guanylate cyclase purified from bovine lung contains heme and copper. *FEBS Lett* 1981;132:71-74.
38. Ohlstein EH, Wood KS, Ignarro LJ: Purification and properties of heme-deficient hepatic soluble guanylate cyclase: effects of heme and other factors on enzyme activation by NO, NO-heme, and protoporphyrin IX. *Arch Biochem Biophys* 1982;218:187-198.
39. Kruszyna H, Kruszyna R, Smith RP: Nitroprusside increases cyclic GMP concentrations during relaxation of rabbit aortic strips and both effects are antagonized by cyanide. *Anesthesiology* 1982;57:303-308.
40. Rapoport RM, Murad F: Effect of cyanide on nitrovasodilator-induced relaxation, cyclic GMP accumulation and guanylate cyclase activation in rat aorta. *Eur J Pharmacol* 1984;104:61-70.
41. Griffith TM, Edwards DH, Lewis MJ, et al: The nature of endothelium-derived vascular relaxant factor. *Nature* 1984;308:645-647.
42. Kontos HA, Wei EP, Povlishock JT, et al: Oxygen radicals mediate the cerebral arteriolar dilation from arachidonate and bradykinin in cats. *Circ Res* 1984; 55:295-303.
43. Harbison RG, Wood KS, Hyman AL, et al: Endothelium-dependent and independent regulation of cyclic GMP formation and relaxation of intrapulmonary artery by peptides. *Fed Proc* 1985;44:1235.
44. Hyman AL, Mathe AA, Leslie CA, et al: Modification of pulmonary vascular responses to arachidonic acid by alterations in physiologic state. *J Pharmacol Exp Ther* 1978;207:388-401.
45. Hyman AL, Spannhake EW, Kadowitz PJ: Divergent responses to arachidonic acid in the feline pulmonary vascular bed. *Am J Physiol* 1980;239:H40-H46.
46. Nandiwada PA, Hyman AL, Kadowitz PJ: Pulmonary vasodilator responses to vagal stimulation and acetylcholine in the cat. *Circ Res* 1983;53:86-95.
47. Rapoport RM, Draznin MB, Murad F: Sodium nitroprusside-induced protein phosphorylation in intact rat aorta is mimicked by 8-bromo cyclic GMP. *Proc Natl Acad Sci USA* 1982;79:6470-6474.
48. Rapoport RM, Draznin MB, Murad F: Endothelium-dependent relaxation in rat aorta may be mediated through cyclic GMP-dependent protein phosphorylation. *Nature* 1983;306:174-176.
49. Lincoln TM, Corbin JD: Characterization and biological role of the cGMP-dependent protein kinase. *Adv Cyclic Nucleotide Res* 1983;15:139-192.

Index